Prepared to Care

Contents

Acknowledgements

I am indebted to a considerable number of people who have helped me to identify, access and integrate diverse and extensive sources of information about nurses and nursing in Alberta. Dr. Pauline Paul contributed a chapter on the history of diploma schools of nursing and through her doctoral work on the history of the Edmonton General Hospital and the work of the Grey Nuns as well as her assistance on two projects funded by the Alberta Foundation for Nursing Research has been a wonderful colleague and supporter of the project. Alice MacKinnon's interest and tremendous assistance with archival data gathering in the Edmonton area was invaluable in the funded projects and contributed to the availability of historical information on nursing. I am also deeply indebted to Dr. Helen Sabin for her expert data gathering on materials about Alberta nurses and nursing held at the Glenbow Alberta Archives in Calgary. Doreen Reid, Tracy Shaben, Hafiza Hemani and others also assisted in the collection and assembling of information which was essential to the project.

The Alberta Association of Registered Nurses provided a great deal of encouragement and assistance over the duration of the project. I am grateful to Evelyn Henderson, Information Officer prior to her December, 1995 retirement, for her unfailing commitment to the history of nursing and the publication of this book. Lorraine Mychajlunow assumed responsibility for the AARN from January, 1996 and has been very helpful to me in various ways including the selection of photographs and illustrations from archival collections. I am grateful also to AARN members who served as members of the Provincial Information Committee, the committee responsible for the project for their patience, perseverance and ongoing support. To the Provincial Office Staff of the Association and Provincial Council members throughout the gestation of this book, I express my appreciation for their deep interest and unflagging commitment. From 1859 on, it has been the nurses of Alberta who have worked unfailingly in the public interest who made this history what it is. To all of them, I offer my respect and my gratitude.

I am also most appreciative for assistance given by those who reviewed this book for the University of Alberta Press and provided excellent recommendations for improving the manuscript. Evelyn Henderson and Dr. Helen Sabin also reviewed the manuscript at my request and gave me substantial suggestions and comments. I am particularly grateful to former AARN Executive Director Yvonne Chapman who provided excellent critical commentary as well as suggested revisions of several drafts of particular portions of the manuscript. Mary Mahoney-Robson of the University of Alberta Press has provided ongoing and substantial assistance over several drafts of the manuscript. Her unfailing good humour and editorial expertise has helped to guide and nurture the development of the manuscript in important and helpful ways. The support of Norma Gutteridge initially and after her retirement of Glenn Rollans, Director of the University of Alberta Press, has also been critical to the direction of the project, and to both of them I am deeply grateful.

Finally I would like to express my appreciation to colleagues and students of the Faculty of Nursing, University of Alberta and to AARN members from all of whom I have learned a great deal and whose confidence in me helped me to take on and complete this project. To my family I also express my appreciation for their understanding of the time and effort it has taken to write this book and for their belief and trust in me.

Preface

In writing *Prepared to Care: Nurses and Nursing in Alberta,* my focus is the evolution of nursing as a professional discipline in the context in which it developed in Alberta. In pursuing this objective, the intent is, in part, to attempt to record some important milestones for the profession as well as contributions of nurses in Alberta over 137 years. My purpose is also to present a perspective on the meaning of nurses' work and its relation to the social fabric of the province and to the status of women in society. The approach that has been taken throughout has been to identify and explore social, political and economic forces which were at play in terms of their influence upon the course of nursing history in Alberta. This is important as it assists in understanding the profession in the context of a particular period and in providing reasonable explanations for events and developments in the profession over time.

Prepared to Care is organized around the themes and questions which defined and circumscribed the nursing profession throughout its 137 years in the region now known as Alberta. The challenges that women faced in the early settlement period of Alberta are explored in the first chapter as religious sisters came to the territory to offer their services to native people and an increasing number of settlers. They were joined in their work as time went on by lay nurses. The development of hospitals and the way in which nurses and nursing formed a part of this essentially twentieth century movement are examined at some length in the next two chapters. The public health movement as it played out in Alberta is the focus of the analysis in the following two chapters. As a special case of public health nursing, district nursing involved midwifery services to women in remote and largely unsettled areas of the province and is explored in the second of the two chapters devoted to public health nursing.

Nursing education, a vital element in bringing the profession to its current status as a modern and knowledge-based discipline, is explored in two segments. The first chapter on the subject deals with education at the diploma level, and the second the development of university nursing education in the province. The issues and problems which nurses faced in ensuring accountability to the public in the orderly development of the nursing education system are outlined. Because nursing was seen as women's work, improving the educational status of women who sought to become nurses was difficult and the struggle to ensure that the standards of education were on a par with those in other postsecondary fields was a long one. Alberta nurses served their country with distinction during several periods of international conflict and their work and the challenges they faced in war-ravaged areas of the globe are examined in the chapter "Alberta Nurses in the World Wars."

Finally, issues and directions relevant to the nursing profession with the approach of the twenty-first century are examined in an attempt to identify how these themes, which characterized the struggles of the profession in the previous two centuries, may be important in the next. Remarkable developments in knowledge of health and illness have both shaped and transformed nurses' roles in this century. Since the pace of developments

has accelerated in recent decades, nursing has emerged as a highly specialized professional discipline whose practitioners offer a whole range of front
line health care services in hospital and community health agencies. As it is
likely that there will be many more important scientific advances in health
in this and the next century, nurses' roles will continue to change and
require advanced assessment and decision-making skills. In the modern
Alberta context, health care reform has led to a regionalized health system
where there is new emphasis upon community-based care and individuals
and families are active participants in health decision-making and caregiving. Important issues in the preparation of nurses for advanced practice
roles and in the structure and financing of care are examined in this final
chapter.

Each new generation of nurses must review the history of the profession
from its own perspective. The last time a definitive history of nursing in
Alberta was undertaken was more than three decades ago. Since that time
the profession has undergone a remarkable transformation with the evolution of health knowledge, technological advances in health care and evolv-
ing roles for women in society. The changing context of society of which
nursing forms an integral part mandates that all previous historical work
be reviewed from the standpoint of both historical accuracy and the appropriateness of conclusions when viewed from a contemporary perspective.
Such have been the tasks inherent in this work and they have extended
from one end of the province to the other, inspired new historical nursing
research projects and led to the identification of new information about
the past not available to previous researchers. The Alberta Association of
Registered Nurses has been instrumental over time in encouraging historical studies of the profession and all of the general studies which are currently known have been undertaken with the support of this organization.
The current work is no exception and stands as a tribute to the ongoing
interest and commitment of the members of this organization to valuing
and documenting their history.

Introduction

Nurses have been central to the development of health care and to the growth of its primary focus of activity, the hospital, from an early point in the settlement of Alberta. By the end of the twentieth century, nursing had emerged as a profession with a sophisticated knowledge base and a highly specialized and educated workforce. The increase in knowledge and skills was so great that new health professions were spawned along the way. As nursing has been defined by its knowledge and practice, it has increasingly been recognized as an essential component of the health care system, without which the system could not function. Pioneer nurses, both religious sisters and lay women, set a course of dedicated and high quality service to those in need of care from an early point in the settlement of the territory. At the outset when health knowledge was limited, the Grey Nuns demonstrated that nursing made a difference, and, at that time, nursing was almost the only therapy available for those whose bodies were ravaged by infectious diseases. When knowledge of how to prevent disease appeared, the specialized area of public health nursing developed to offer immunizations, health assessment, health screening and advice and teaching on health and hygiene. The remarkable developments in health knowledge in the latter half of the twentieth century led to tremendous specialization in nursing as hospitals became tertiary care centres with highly sophisticated equipment, services and personnel. Modern nursing has met the challenges and developed a highly sophisticated educational system for preparing nurses for roles in hospitals and community health practice. The emergence of strong nursing organizations to take a leading role in health issues of concern to nurses began in the second decade of the century and the professional association and nursing unions achieved impressive public profiles and their advice was sought when important health issues were at stake.

The measure of a profession's contribution to society is to be found in the value of its service to people. While it is not easy to identify how nursing has been perceived over a long period of time, the task is enhanced by records of the work performed by nurses as described in their own accounts as well as in those of recipients of their care and of others. Nurses have been central to the development of health care and to the growth of its primary focus of activity, the hospital, from an early point in the settlement of Alberta. The arrival of the first nurses in Alberta in 1859 parallels the resurgence of nursing and its recognition as a suitable endeavour for lay women in Britain. The movement to improve standards of care for the sick and wounded was spearheaded by Florence Nightingale. Critical public acclaim for her work in the Crimea in which the lives of thousands of wounded British soldiers were saved through good nursing riveted public attention upon the need for change. The comparability between the types of roles fulfilled by nurses trained by Nightingale in her school and the roles customarily expected of women in nineteenth century Britain was sufficiently evident that nursing achieved respectability and acceptance as a suitable field of work for women outside the home. In making this transition, nursing joined teaching which had been the first area of work to beckon to lay women.[1] As with teaching, altruism and service were key elements in achieving public acknowledgment of nursing as particularly appropriate for women's abilities. Thus, at the outset, nursing became an instrument of women's emancipation. Remarkable advances in health and health care and the rise of the hospital as a centre for care created a need for an increasingly large nursing workforce and the nursing profession became one of the most significant avenues of work for women in this century.

There have been limited attempts to identify the major themes in nurses' work and to integrate existing work into a meaningful and comprehensible portrayal and explanation of developments in nursing. Some important narratives have been written about Alberta nurses' experiences in hospitals, district nursing assignments and public health units that contribute to an understanding of how services provided by nurses developed in the province. There is a need to understand the past in nursing in order to shed light on the present and to point the way to the future. The historic invisibility of women and the lack of recognition given to their work in the home and voluntary work in the community finds a parallel in nursing. Inadequate attention has been given to nurses in the historical record and their contributions have been minimized and undervalued. It is not unusual to find histories of hospitals in which nurses and nursing are hardly mentioned.[2] Many consist of a descriptive record of physicians and surgeons who served the institution as practitioners or as chiefs of services. Although members of the nursing profession have recognized and pointed out the invisibility of nursing as it has been played out in numerous examples, other professionals and the public have been slow to recognize it.

Historians who, like Susan Reverby, have chosen to study the profession, have been startled at the discovery of "nursing's supposed unimportance except to those in the field" and "pervasive sexism."[3] In her review of the various paradigms which have been put forward to explain nursing's difficulty in achieving a status in society comparable to that of certain other professions, Kathryn McPherson[4] refers to "interpretive frameworks" used to explain the transformation of Canadian nursing in the twentieth century. These frameworks include professionalization where the primary emphasis has been the struggle for professional legitimization and status, proletarianization or the application of industrial methods of production to a service field such as nursing, and gender focusing upon the gender-segregated nature of the nursing profession. S.J. Roberts's[5] postulation that nurses constituted an oppressed group in the modern context was startling to members of the profession when her ideas were initially put forward. Nevertheless, it led to considerable analysis of the status of the profession and a search for supporting documentation, both current and historical to explore the thesis. These studies have all been important in helping nurses to see themselves as others have seen them and to determine the legitimacy of the arguments that have been put forward to explain the nature of their work and the directions they have taken as a profession. This represents the background information that illuminates my study of nurses and nursing in Alberta.

In attempting to understand the traditions and values which character-ize a society and underscore its identity, it is important to pay particular attention to the contributions of its citizens through their institutions, organizations and individual efforts. Following the European emigration to North America beginning in the sixteenth century, new communities sprung up all over the continent. Nursing was an early and fundamental part of social organization in the settlements that developed in Canada, including Alberta. At a time when knowledge of disease was in a primitive state, technology was virtually nonexistent and a few herbal remedies were the only medicinal therapies available, the practice of nursing developed as an integral part of the emerging health system serving the population. Nursing care was often the sole weapon in fighting infectious disease and its importance is underscored in accounts of the devastating epidemics of smallpox, typhoid, diphtheria, cholera, typhus, trachoma, scarlet fever and other infectious diseases that ravaged the new settlers and native popula-tion in continuing and successive episodes. Epidemics of infectious dis-eases were commonly brought to various communities by settlers and visi-tors from elsewhere. Following an epidemic, just as the population had regained its health and begun to put the problems of infectious disease in the community to one side, another would strike with a vengeance and emergency conditions would again prevail. The accounts of the Grey Nuns in nineteenth century Alberta provide ample evidence that those who ben-efited from their ministrations were eminently better off than those who, for one reason or another, could not, providing some early evidence that nursing made a difference in the care and treatment of those with infectious diseases.

This account of the development of nursing in Alberta is aside from native healing methods and traditional herbal remedies, which were known at the time of the European migration. Native healing has continued to be important in the native community, and indeed is believed to constitute important alternative and/or complementary methods of care and treatment. A number of those involved in the health care professions have incorporated some of these remedies and methods within the scope of their practice. Although little data that might have shed some light on the status of native healing and herbal remedies in the nineteenth and twentieth centuries is available, it is known that the European immigrants and the native peoples offered assistance to each other in a number of different realms. Health care was no exception to this.

In presenting a perspective on the history of a profession such as nursing, its relationship to other professions and to the health system are of interest, as to a certain extent these relationships define the nature of the service and the structure within which work is performed. Nursing has made remarkable progress towards the achievement of professional status in society if one examines the changes that have occurred relative to criteria that have been proposed as defining the elements of a profession. Abraham Flexner's[6] original criteria for judging whether or not an occupation could be considered to be a profession were put forward in the second decade of the twentieth century. The nursing literature as late as the middle of the twentieth century confirms that nurses had difficulty categorizing theirs as a profession according to these criteria because of the requirement for a knowledge base and the scholarly inquiry needed to support it.[7] Certain elements that characterized practice were considered to hold more import in nursing including altruism, humility, self-sacrifice, and compliance. Economic reward was considered self-serving and inconsistent with the altruistic ideals of the profession. This was undoubtedly a reflection of the expectations of Victorian gentlewomen of the time. Nightingale did not see nursing as an endeavour for which compensation would be an important element. Women of the time were generally expected to do good works but to reject compensation for it. Thus nurses were discouraged from seeking salaries and wages commensurate with their work. Independent thinking and decision-making were thought to be the province of the physician, not the nurse. Medicine was well-established by the latter half of the nineteenth century, while nursing was in its infancy. Even though nurses came to reside in communities to practice their profession prior to physicians in some areas, the fact is that medicine embraced a dominant role in health care and physicians assumed leadership roles in all areas of health care when they arrived to practise in Alberta.[8]

Gradually with increasing complexity of practice, ongoing development of the discipline, and the improved status of women in society, nurses would recognize that questioning, independent thinking and discovery of new knowledge were fundamental to outstanding nursing practice. As consumerism came to the fore, health consumers began to demand that all those who had responsibilities in relation to their health were accountable for their services. This was supported in the courts where nurses along with other health professionals were deemed to be responsible and accountable under the law for their actions. Over time professionalism would acquire a deeper meaning and nursing would move rapidly towards a new definition of its practice and its role in health care. The relevance of gender as an issue in defining roles in the health system with a male-dominated medical profession and a female-dominated nursing profession would come to the fore much later when restricted roles and differential treatment of women in society came under intense scrutiny. Over the decades, considerable advancement has occurred in the profession, and this refinement and development in the professional role can be attributed to public perception that nursing was important to the health and well-being of the community.[9] Although nursing had always been considered to be an art, the view that it was also a science developed more slowly. In the final decades of the twentieth century, it can be said that nursing has become established more firmly as a science through research and scholarship. The scope of knowledge required in nursing is broad and, in view of its scientific and humanitarian aspects, there is a need for scholars in nursing who can ask key questions about health from the perspective of nursing.

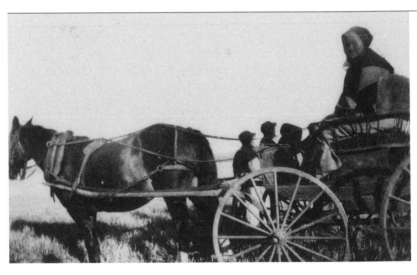

☙ *Grey Nuns using an ox-cart (1928–1930) not unlike*
the ones that carried them to Alberta in 1859.
(ASGME).

The Origins of Nursing

The benefits of settlement on the Canadian prairies had not come to public consciousness at the time the first nurses—the Grey Nuns—headed west from Quebec to what is now Alberta to work with the native peoples. The diminishing size of the buffalo herds as well as a severe winter climate and short growing season were common knowledge. The fur trading posts, including Edmonton House which had been operating since 1795, were the first white settlements in Rupert's Land.

It was not until the 1860s that interest in settlement in the west grew in eastern Canada for economic and political reasons. Exploration and mineral discoveries established the economic potential of the region. The findings of the Palliser Expedition, 1857–1860, identified for the first time immense deposits of coal, vast timber resources and agricultural possibilities on the plains, in addition to exploring and assessing transportation and communication corridors.[1] Just after Palliser's report was released, gold fever hit the Alberta region. The mere suggestion that gold might be in the area was responsible for the doubling of the population within a decade.[2] Although the intensity of the gold rush in Alberta dimmed with the discovery that deposits found near Rocky Mountain House were insignificant compared to those found in the Klondike and later in British Columbia, the new focus upon the economic value of western resources commanded the attention and interest of those in the eastern part of the country.

Political concerns also played a major part in the interest in the western region. There had been increasing tension with the United States from encroaching settlement from the American frontier, but the outbreak of the Civil War in 1861 temporarily relieved the situation. Canadian public opinion was largely hostile to the Union states and sympathetic to the Confederacy. For these reasons the British began to favour confederation of its colonies in order to foster an effective defence against the possibility of an American invasion.[3] Confederation of the four British colonies, Nova Scotia, New Brunswick, Quebec and Ontario occurred on 1 July 1867.

With the transfer of the ownership of the powerful Hudson's Bay Company in 1863, wheels were set in motion for assumption of responsibility for the territory by a federal government. Following Confederation, Prime Minister John A. Macdonald immediately made an agreement with the Hudson's Bay Company to transfer to Canada jurisdiction over most of the land west of the Rockies and north of the 49th parallel, creating the North-West Territories and the Province of Manitoba in 1870.

The findings of the Palliser Expedition, the results of subsequent surveys and the gold rush in the west and north led to widespread acceptance of the need for a railroad linking east and west. The inherent usefulness of the availability of such transportation in moving people and trade goods vast distances with a minimum of disruption was appealing. Thus the idea of a transcontinental railway had political, social as well as military value and was critical to the extension of Confederation, retention of national jurisdiction over the western territories and ultimately to the settlement of western Canada. The transcontinental railway became an instrument of change in the settlement of western Canada. Although the French-Canadian nuns had expected to work mainly with native people, and indeed this was the case for a number of years, the completion of rail lines meant an influx of large numbers of settlers. The growing need for health care for this new population dramatically shifted the focus of the established nurses in the area.

In French Canada, a legacy of strong women's roles emerged from the patterns established in New France since there was "reason to believe the women's social/political position, both in marriage and outside it, as well as their economic position, was stronger in New France than elsewhere in the seventeenth and eighteenth centuries."[4] This legacy provided an important context for women's activities and for the heritage of nursing in Canada. Nurses who were recognized as nurses established and maintained the first system of health services in early Canada, physicians and professional medicine coming later. In Alberta, the Grey Nuns brought with them their traditions of competence, independence, self-sufficiency, and determination. In that these women were the first nonnative women to come to settle in the area, the example they set for the community in terms of what women could do was a powerful one. Their independence and determination to control those areas which were rightfully theirs was not lost with the passage of time as these characteristics were applied in their day-to-day operations.

They Came By Ox-Cart — The Pioneering Grey Nuns

The story of nursing in Alberta begins with the arrival of three Grey Nuns, Sisters Alphonse, Emery and Lamy, by ox-cart at Lac Ste-Anne in 1859.[5] They had come to the Catholic mission northwest of Edmonton House at the request of Father Albert Lacombe primarily to serve the native and Métis peoples in the area by offering health care, education and shelter to those in need. Their mission was an integral part of their religious commitment and from the outset they made their services available to anyone who requested help regardless of their ability to pay for the service. Settlement at nearby Edmonton House was centred around the fur trade, and as James MacGregor noted, "In 1858 the prairies, which were merely a part of Rupert's Land, which in turn was only that part of British North America

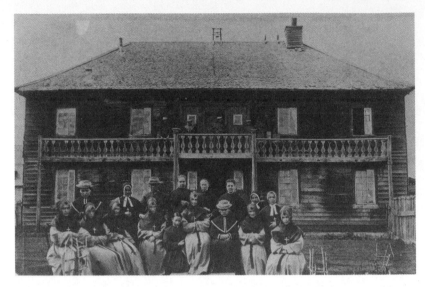

↬ *Grey Nuns hospital-school-orphanage in St-Albert built in 1863. Sister Emery, one of the first three Grey Nuns to come to Alberta is seated fourth from the left. (ASGME 5129–22(2))*

belonging to the Hudson's Bay Company, were an empty land still controlled by a few fur traders."[6] The Catholic mission to which the sisters came had been established in 1843 at Lac Ste-Anne by the pioneering Oblate missionary priest Reverend Father Jean-Baptiste Thibault long before settlement was to reach the area.

Their long journey began at the motherhouse in Montreal and the sisters travelled by rail through the northern United States, disembarking south of the area which is now Manitoba. From there they made their way to the Grey Nuns' mission at St-Boniface where they spent the next ten months learning about native culture and studying the Cree language. They set out on 4 August 1859 walking beside their ox-carts on the journey to Lac Ste-Anne, a journey which would end some 50 days later on 24 September. An account of their experiences written by Sister Alphonse describes the hardships of traveling over the rough prairie trails in their ox-carts, sleeping in a tent with the benefit of only one blanket all the time battling clouds of mosquitoes.[7] The last few miles between Fort Edmonton and Lac Ste-Anne were done on horseback which Sister Emery particularly enjoyed as she had been raised on a farm. The sisters took up their activities immediately after their arrival, which included nursing, teaching and farming to provide food for the mission.

A move to St. Albert four years later by the Catholic mission occurred for several reasons. The nuns had found that potatoes and barley were the only crops that did well at Lac Ste-Anne; the more fertile soil[8] at St. Albert was necessary to grow enough food. A significant number of independent fur traders resided in the Lac Ste-Anne area and were operating in competition with the Hudson's Bay Company, clearly in violation of its charter. They offered more favourable prices for goods as well as alcohol to the Métis population willing to trade their furs. Since it was essential for the Oblate missionaries and the Grey Nuns to maintain very good relationships with Company officials, they undoubtedly had to take some action to distance themselves from the free traders.[9] After all, the Company had clear and undisputed authority over the region, and this was frontier territory where one neighbour depended upon another. From an ethical standpoint, it was evident that consumption of alcohol was devastating to the native and Métis peoples. For the missionaries to stay at Lac Ste-Anne would have represented tacit endorsement of the practice of selling alcohol to this vulnerable population. These reasons were sufficiently powerful to justify relocation to an area where conditions were more favourable for the pursuit of their activities.

THE FIRST HEALTH CARE AGENCY IN ALBERTA IS ESTABLISHED BY NURSES

From their arrival in 1859, the Grey Nuns cared for the sick and the poor in their living quarters. Their ministrations on behalf of their patients were well-received by the native peoples and settlers, and demands for their care increased dramatically as their reputation grew, the number of settlers rose and the population was hit by a succession of epidemics of infectious diseases. The sisters recognized that they would soon need a separate area to care for the increasing number of people who sought their help. In 1870 they built an in-patient hospital ward in their convent in St. Albert for those who required constant care. This proved over time to be inadequate for the still-rising number of settlers seeking aid, and in 1881, they constructed a separate hospital building at the St. Albert mission to receive patients. The sisters are credited with developing the first hospital in

Alberta as early as 1870. Since from the beginning they took in patients who needed special nursing care to their convent, they perhaps should more properly be credited with providing hospital services and operating a health centre or hospital from the time of their arrival in 1859.

However, home visiting was clearly the principal nursing activity of the Grey Nuns prior to the establishment of facilities with space for all who came. The sisters reported that between August and December 1864, 48 home visits had been carried out with 100 patients receiving treatment.[10] Sister Emery reported that staffing was an issue, for they had limited time to attend to home visiting and thus were not able to respond to all requests for help. When a devastating smallpox epidemic hit the area in 1870, the sisters soon filled their new patient ward built at the Mission. It is reported that of the population of 900 in St. Albert, some 600 contracted the disease and 320 succumbed to it.[11] Sister Emery noted that the nuns assisted 692 families that year, providing 351 vaccinations and 392 meals. Sister Alphonse commented on the impact of the epidemic on children, the need for precautions to prevent nurses from contracting smallpox during an epidemic and the benefit of nursing care for those who could be accommodated in the hospital:

> The disease ravaged the people, and we already have lost four of our children, with a fifth close to death. There is nothing so sad, it is a real shame! All the time that we care for them, it is necessary to cover the nose tightly. Those outside the hospital are dying quickly because they lack care.[12]

The nuns worked tirelessly for some six months until the worst of the epidemic was over. Of some interest is Sister Charlebois's account that Bishop Vital-Justin Grandin was so worried about the sisters' health that he assigned priests to take on night duty to help out during these emergency conditions.[13] Their small hospital was filled to capacity during succeeding epidemics of typhoid in 1881 and 1884, and measles in 1886.[14]

The expansion of the work of the mission to other parts of present-day Alberta and the Northwest Territories began soon after the arrival of the sisters in the mid 1800s. The first was the settlement at Lac la Biche where there was a group of Métis and Cree families to whom the priests had been ministering on a traveling basis for a number of years. At the request of

Bishop Taché, three Grey Nuns were sent there in 1862 in order to expand the services which could be offered to the population. It was to remain on a permanent basis until 1898 during which time it served as a point of departure for missions to the north. Undoubtedly the much smaller population in the area made it less viable in a long-term sense as a mission field. Writing from the Hôpital Général de la Providence à la Rivière MacKenzie, Sister Ward raised a different and deeply unsettling problem the sisters had encountered during a period when the caribou had disappeared from the area, that of cannibalism on the part of a man who had eaten his wife and children in the face of the general conditions of famine. From the account, this event was clearly very horrifying to the sisters, and such a practice would appear to be as controversial then as it is today.[15]

Other missions of the Grey Nuns involved the establishment of schools exclusively, and there were numerous modifications made in the nature and extent of services in different areas as needs changed. Several missions to provide health care were established in the latter part of the century in the southern part of the province including a major commitment in Calgary with the founding of the Holy Cross Hospital in 1892. In the next year, the hospital and school on the Blood Reserve at Standoff near Cardston were established. In the north, the Grey Nuns moved their centre of operations once more in 1895, this time from St. Albert to Edmonton in response to a request from Edmonton physicians to provide leadership in establishing hospital services. These were badly needed as a result of the exponential population increase due to the initiation of rail services and the settlement that followed.

The heritage that the Grey Nuns brought with them to Alberta was one founded upon the exemplary health service developed at Quebec in the seventeenth century. The contrast between nursing in Quebec and nursing in Britain at the time is significant. Following Henry VIII's renunciation of the Catholic church in 1534, the nursing orders of nuns staffing the large London hospitals were ejected from these institutions.[16] With them went a high quality of nursing offered by knowledgeable and caring individuals. They were replaced by women of low character and morals of the Sairey Gamp ilk in the character popularized by Dickens. In Canada, nursing never fell to the level seen in Britain at the time because the first settlement at Quebec was established as a colony of France. Since the Protestant Reformation had failed to take hold in France, the nursing orders of the

Roman Catholic Church remained in control of nursing and as a result, nursing did not regress as in Britain. Young women of suitable character and who came from good families were recruited to the church in France and pursued nursing as an integral part of their religious commitment.

Even after the British conquest, the French hospital and nursing system survived largely intact because it was so effective in providing a needed and highly regarded service to the population. The larger French than English population for a long period of time after the conquest, the inability of the colony to access supply ships and difficult communication with Britain for a substantial part of the year because of winter freeze-up of the St. Lawrence River undoubtedly were factors that maintained the French influence in health care following Confederation. As John Gibbon and Mary Mathewson explain:

> If the settlements along the St. Lawrence River had been colonized in the seventeenth century by the English instead of by the French, the history of nursing in Canada might have been very different. Fate, however, decided in favour of the French, and that was fortunate both for the Huron and Algonquin Indians and for the white pioneers, since in the wake of the fur traders and coureurs de bois, came the Augustinian Hospitallers or Nursing Sisters of Dieppe to Quebec and the St. Joseph Hospitallers of La Flèche to Montreal on their missions of healing and of mercy—missions which had no counterpart in the colonizing efforts of the Protestant English in North America.[17]

A Canadian nursing heritage is both unique in comparison to other countries and strong by virtue of its traditions of quality and excellence established initially by the nursing orders of the Roman Catholic Church. In western Canada in general and Alberta in particular, the foundations laid by the Grey Nuns provided a standard of service that other hospitals and health agencies have had to work diligently to meet.

THE EXPANDING DOMAIN OF NURSING

With the establishment of schools of nursing in Britain on the Nightingale model from 1860 on and the spread of this pattern of nursing education to North America, increasing numbers of nurses who had been prepared for practice began to arrive in Alberta as it opened up to settlement. The first North American school of nursing to be established was at Bellevue Hospital in New York in 1873, and a Canadian school was founded the next year in association with the St. Catharines General and Marine Hospital through the efforts of Dr. Theophilus Mack.[18] It was a model that would be widely emulated throughout Canada including the west in the years to follow. Lay nurses figured prominently in the mission work of Protestant churches. Like the Catholic missions "Increasingly the Church served homesteads and agricultural communities, rather than Indian Missions."[19] In the work of the Church of England in Canada, the establishment of the Diocese of Athabasca in 1873 led to the establishment of churches, residential schools as well as hospitals, and "women workers" as they were called, served in missionary roles as teachers, nurses and matrons of schools. According to Meredith Hill, *Synod Journals* listed women as part of the diocesan staff of lay workers as early as 1907, this being much earlier than in other dioceses. Hill notes that the lay women who worked in the Athabasca diocese had outstanding attributes and capabilities and many came from the Deaconess and Missionary Training House in Toronto. There are many fundamental similarities between the expectations for the work of these lay women and the Catholic sisters, for in society generally it was expected that "In hospital and school missions, women's work was seen as the expression of women's nature—nurturant, rescuing, protecting."[20]

The first lay nurse who is reported to have come to present-day Alberta was Miss Mary Newton, sister of Canon Newton of the Anglican mission at the Hermitage, eight miles downstream from Edmonton. A graduate of Queen Charlotte's Maternity Hospital in London and a teacher there until she became ill, she took up residence at the Hermitage.[21] A report in the *Edmonton Bulletin* announced her arrival and indicated that she planned to offer nursing services to the community, health permitting.[22] Subsequently, she began to practise her profession at the mission and in 1891 "she advertised that she was prepared to do nursing and midwifery in homes—fee ten dollars per week."[23] Her work carried out in a missionary enclave of the Church of England was consistent with what the church aimed to provide as a service to people, particularly in sparsely populated areas where the needs were great.

The Canadian Methodist and Presbyterian churches, later to join as the United Church of Canada, approached home missions in frontier western areas in similar fashion to the other Christian missions. Beginning with the establishment of small mission hospitals in British Columbia in 1898, small hospitals were established in Alberta by 1906 at Smoky Lake and Lamont in 1912. This would expand to 22 hospitals by 1937, all of which depended upon lay nurses "with not only good academic qualifications but also a high sense of civic responsibility."[24] Many of the nurses who were recruited for duty in these hospitals were also graduates of the United Church Training School in Toronto. As many of these hospitals were built in very remote areas where health care was desperately needed, the work carried on by these lay nurses was a tremendous challenge, requiring both courage and commitment. As time went on the number of those prepared to undertake nursing increased and some of these nurses were available for private duty in the homes of those who were ill since that was the dominant mode of practice in the late nineteenth and early twentieth centuries.

HEALTH CARE EXPANSION AND NURSING SERVICES

After the turn of the century, health care organizations were founded in many of the new settlements around the province. These initiatives were universally assisted and supported by nurses. In many cases, nurses initiated and directed efforts leading to the establishment of hospitals. The hospitals that were founded in small centres across the province in the first and second decades of the twentieth century were, for the most part, small operations and could perhaps be better described as health centres or nursing stations. Nevertheless they offered front-line health services and provided essential health care to the settlers who had come west to homestead and carve out new lives for themselves.

The fundamental importance and meaning of religion in the nineteenth century explains the deep interest of a number of Christian religions in converting the native peoples to their beliefs. With the establishment of fur trading posts, Christian groups established missions in Alberta to minister to the native and Métis peoples. These included a number of Roman Catholic organizations. Bishop Grandin requested the Sisters of the Misericorde to establish another hospital in Edmonton devoted to maternity care because the Grey Nuns had believed that a separate building and personnel were required. They were involved in general hospital care for those with communicable diseases and did not want to spread disease between the patients. Also a number of other groups of nuns from various congregations came to Alberta to provide nursing services.[25] The Sisters of Providence went to Daysland in 1907, Athabasca in 1913, McLennan in 1929 and High Prairie in 1937.[26,27] The Sisters, Servants of Mary Immaculate, who were from Poland, went to Beaver Lake (Mundare) in 1903 and Willingdon in 1935.[28] In 1909 the Sisters of Charity de Notre Dame d'Evron established their work at Trochu and in 1910 at Vegreville and 1919 at Bonnyville.[29] Most of these religious congregations limited their work to a small number of facilities that they could manage with the expertise and resources available in their orders. The Sisters of Service took over the Edson hospital that had been established in 1928 and founded another institution in Vilna in 1929.[30] The Daughters of Jesus operated hospitals at Lac la Biche from 1939 and took over the operation of the hospital in Pincher Creek in 1924.[31] In 1940, the Hospitalières de St. Joseph of the Hôtel Dieu in Montreal founded and began to operate a hospital in Barrhead.[32] The Sisters of Charity of St. Vincent de Paul of Halifax operated three hospitals: Westlock from 1927, Hardisty from 1929 and Jasper from 1930.[33] The Sisters of Charity of the Immaculate Conception of St. John began a hospital at Radway in 1926 and in 1911 the Daughters of Wisdom established one in Castor. The Sisters of St. Martha operated St. Michael's Hospital in Lethbridge from 1929 and the Seton Hospital in Banff beginning in 1930.[34]

Missions under the auspices of Protestant churches were also founded in a number of other Alberta communities. The Methodists were the first of the Christian organizations to arrive in Alberta and the Reverend Robert Rundle took up residence in the area in 1840. The Methodist church sent missionary nurses and physicians to Star and Pakan in 1901 and Morley in 1906. The initiative at Star moved to Lamont in 1903 and became a larger endeavour in later years culminating in the construction of the Lamont Public Hospital in 1912. The Presbyterian Church initiated projects at Vegreville in 1906, Grande Prairie in 1910 and Bonnyville in 1917. At Grande Prairie, efforts of missionary physicians led to a gradually expanding enterprise. Upon the departure of one of the first nurses to be sent to the area, Miss Agnes Baird, the *Grande Prairie Herald* noted that: "The value of her experience and knowledge of medicine and the handling of patients at a time when it was impossible to obtain the services of a medical practitioner, was inestimable, and she in no case spared herself when called upon in an emergency."[35] The Anglican Missionary Society was active in initiating a cottage hospital at Onoway in 1913. Other hospitals established through community efforts included Lacombe (1907), Camrose (1910) and Lloydminster (1914). Local physicians sometimes set up hospitals close to their practices in small communities, and hospitals in Wetaskiwin (1906), Bawlf (1906), Olds (1912), Consort (1912), Bassano (1915) and Drumheller (1915) were initiated in this way. Individual nurses also were responsible for establishing small hospitals in a number of communities. The Van Haarlem hospital in Lethbridge was a highly successful enterprise that began under the direction of Elizabeth Van Haarlem in 1910. The institution was eventually taken over by the Sisters of St. Martha as St. Michael's Hospital in 1929.[36] Nurses were also primarily responsible for opening hospitals in Lacombe[37] and Rimbey[38] in 1907, Vermilion in 1913,[39] Vulcan in 1917,[40] Rocky Mountain House in 1922,[41] Fairview in 1924,[42] and undoubtedly many others as well.

Voluntary organizations such as the Victorian Order of Nurses (VON) were influential in providing initial and continuing support for the building and operation of a number of hospitals in Alberta. The VON's objective was to identify areas of need, to initiate the needed nursing services and to maintain them until such time as community organization developed and a permanent agency could take over their operation. VON financial support for small hospitals initially came from "a special fund to provide suitable buildings for Cottage Hospitals, to accommodate either six or ten patients, two nurses and a maid."[43] The first initiative of the VON in Alberta opened as the Lady Minto Cottage Hospital in Red Deer in 1903. Later, the VON sustained a commitment to assisting to develop needed services in Alberta and assumed responsibility for managing hospitals in High River (1909) and Athabasca (1917) and for operating Lady Minto Cottage Hospitals in Islay (1912) and Edson (1914).[44] The small hospitals begun by the VON across the country had largely been transferred to other groups such as local municipalities and lay corporations by 1924.[45] However, the thrust of VON efforts moved more to community nursing initiatives after this time.

The burgeoning settlement brought with it the need for health services, and concerned citizens worked very hard to ensure that care was available to them when it was required. In a local history of the area around Hanna, Freda Viste observed that "Of all the tribulations faced by the early settlers, the lack of hospitals and doctors was one of the greatest."[46] When wives and families began to join their pioneer husbands on the frontier, "the

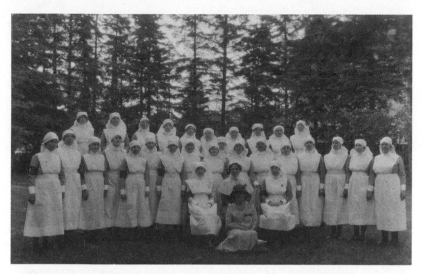

↜ *A class of lay women who had taken the home nursing course taught by registered nurses employed by the St. John Ambulance; inspection by Mrs. Lancelot Dent, June 9, 1926; pictured center front is Mrs. Ida H.I. Bannister, RN, Lady Divisional superintendent. (St. John Ambulance Provincial Archives 97–E–17, received on loan from Alice MacKinnon, chairperson.)*

need for hospitals became more evident."[47] Viste went on to say that "Occasionally there was a nurse among the pioneers' wives. They were a godsend to any community, often being called upon to administer aid in the absence of a doctor. They ran into situations where they had to set broken bones, or sew up and dress wounds without anesthetic."[48] However, on the frontier, neighbour helped neighbour to the best of their abilities. It was usually women who were asked to care for others or to assist in the delivery of babies where no physicians or nurses were available. Many of these pioneer women became skilled in providing health care to their friends and neighbours and gave of their time and energies to help those in need.

Nurses with formal training became more numerous from the second decade of the twentieth century on, but there continued to be many women who did not have formal training who offered their services to the public. The goal of professional nursing legislation fuelled the formation of the International Council of Nurses in 1899 and several North American nursing organizations. However it was recognized that in Canada, professional legislation was a provincial issue since jurisdiction for health rested with the provinces. The Calgary Association of Graduate Nurses was one of the first in the province in 1904, and by 1912 had joined forces with the Edmonton Association of Graduate Nurses to work for legislation to ensure registration of nurses. By 1914 they had formed the Graduate Nurses Association of Alberta and made a strong case for the development of legislation. The passage of the Registered Nurses' Act in 1916 protected the title of "registered nurse," so that from that time on, no one could purport to be a registered nurse if not duly registered by the Alberta Association of Registered Nurses (AARN). Nurses had worked very hard to achieve this legislative standard as it provided a measure of public protection and gave status and credibility to the work that they performed competently and diligently across the vast area of the province. Social organization in the province had now reached the point where there were many facilities in operation to deliver health care. Also, the number of health professionals who had been duly prepared in educational programs and had taken up residence in both urban and rural areas in order to provide care to the populace had grown exponentially after the widespread development of schools of nursing and after the passage of the Registered Nurses Act.

———————

Health care services became firmly established in Alberta through the efforts of a religious order of Catholic nuns beginning in 1859. Their work expanded to Calgary, Edmonton and many points in the north prior to the dawn of the twentieth century. The nuns were joined by other religious orders who settled in many areas of the province and offered health services. These women and their successors would provide solid leadership in nursing service, administration and education. The quality of nursing they offered would serve as a model for other institutions in the province. Lay nurses who had received their training elsewhere also began to arrive in Alberta prior to the twentieth century and made many important contributions to health in this largely unsettled area of the country. With the increasing acceptance of single women in the workforce and with the burgeoning service needs of frontier communities, positions for nurses were created in increasing numbers with the establishment and growth of hospitals. As the twentieth century began, the birth of the province was drawing near. Status as a province in 1905 would make Alberta a full partner in Confederation, and with the passage of time it would become an important player in matters of national scope, including those in the area of health. As settlers arrived by the trainload, the movement to develop hospitals gathered momentum in response to the tremendous population explosion and the resulting health needs of the burgeoning society. In an era where knowledge of health and disease was in its incipient stages, illness was ever-present in the form of infectious disease and there were few known cures for common health problems. Despite the fact that health was considered to be the responsibility of the individual and the family rather than of the society, the community gradually recognized that it was to the benefit of all to develop systematic provisions for the care of those who were afflicted by diseases. Hospitals became an early form of community action to support the health and well-being of early settlements in frontier areas in the province of Alberta, and nurses were instrumental in their establishment as well as in their operations from the outset.

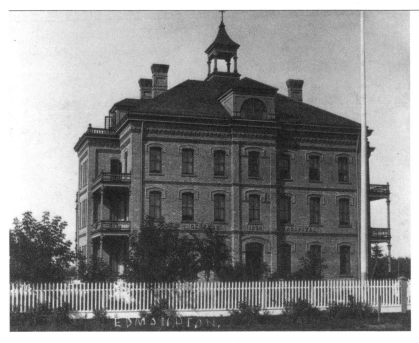

↬ *Edmonton General Hospital, 1895. (*PAA*, received on loan from* AARN P93*)*

2

Nurses and the Establishment
of Early Hospitals

The hospital of the nineteenth century was defined as much by need and exigency as by illness and contagion. At the outset North American hospitals represented alternative centres for care that could also be provided within the confines of the home. Since hospital care offered no particular benefit to citizens who could afford to hire nurses privately to provide care in the home, hospitals tended to be frequented by those of less fortunate circumstances. These people lacked financial and/or family resources to help them endure an illness and were in need of someone to care for their needs. That these patients did not have the means to employ nurses to provide care in their homes gave the early hospital its image as a charity institution or almshouse. It became increasingly recognized however that hospitals were institutions where medicine and nursing could be provided both more effectively and efficiently on a continuous basis to a larger number of patients than was the case if they were scattered throughout the community. On the frontier, the establishment of hospitals was prompted by the need for an organized approach to immediate and urgent requirements for health care for an increasing population of settlers, large numbers of whom found themselves afflicted at regularly recurring intervals by epidemic disease.

Even though hospitals founded by religious groups had originated as a mission of care of both a spiritual and physical nature for native peoples, the need for hospitals became all the more urgent because the natives were hit hard by infectious diseases brought to the west by the Europeans. They were highly susceptible to these very foreign diseases since they had had no previous exposure to them. Natives were decimated by outbreak after outbreak of diseases of epidemic proportions. In frontier areas as well, social institutions and services were in an embryonic state and arrangements to provide health care for both settlers and native peoples had to be made according to the needs as well as the resources of particular settlements. In areas where there were religious groups with a mission to care for the native peoples, the quality of the care tended to be considerably higher since these missionaries were committed to doing everything in their power to promote healing among those who were sick.

As settlements became larger and more sophisticated, physicians increasingly began to see hospitals as laboratories where they could practise their profession more productively because they could see their acutely ill patients easily, as frequently as necessary and with relative ease. There were also nurses who remained in the setting to provide continuous nursing to these very sick patients when physicians were not present. Thus, changing modes of practice led to visits by physicians to the patient's home being replaced by hospital and emergency or visits by the patient. This saved professional time and expense for physicians while, at the same time, requiring the patient to leave home and enter the institution for the required length of time. Despite the efficiencies and economies of scale for physicians, it was nevertheless science and technology that provided the primary impetus for the widespread development and pro-

liferation of hospitals after the turn of the century. Increasing professionalization and bureaucratization of hospitals parallelled the introduction
of scientific and technical innovations and coincided with the rise in the
status of the hospital as the paramount centre for the treatment and care
of a multitude of diseases and health problems.[1] The transformation of
the hospital over the course of the twentieth century was a revolutionary
development made possible by persuading the public that the hospital was
the only place where scientifically based care could be given. Because of
the need for technology and expertise centred in the hospital, the highest
quality of care could no longer be provided in the home. Even though
hospitals had existed since the seventeenth century in Canada, the professionalization of hospitals was essentially a movement which occurred in
the twentieth century.[2]

Developments in Southern Alberta

As traders and miners settled in southern Alberta, hospitals soon were
established. The pattern that developed was quite different from northern
Alberta where the Hudson's Bay Company was able to maintain tighter
control over trading and settlement from its trading post at Fort
Edmonton. When the Company gave up its jurisdiction over Rupert's
Land, it was relieved of the increasingly difficult task of maintaining its
authority over the expansive territory, especially in the south. The free
traders, private traders or whisky traders as they were variously called, were
in almost all cases Americans lured north by the prospect of profiting from
the fur trade. These traders had no scruples about how they plied their
trade; liquor was the principal item traded for furs. The number of independent traders operating in the territory had increased considerably by
the mid-1860s and by 1873 there were more than a dozen whisky posts
operating in the southern prairie region including Fort Whoop-Up. After
the transfer of Hudson's Bay Company authority over Rupert's Land, "a
lawless hiatus which allowed the Americans to operate north of the forty-
ninth parallel" developed in southern Alberta and Saskatchewan.[3] As C.M.
MacInnes observed, the free traders "interpreted the end of the Company's
rule to mean the beginning of a period of anarchy in which might was right
and justice the will of the strong."[4] It was clear that something had to be

done if order was to be maintained, and the North-West Mounted Police (NWMP) force was established in response to this need in 1873. Following recruitment and training of a force, a party set out for the west in the summer of 1874 under the command of George French with James F. Macleod second in command. Doug Owram commented that "the police brought that security and justice to the North West and in so doing transplanted some of the most important characteristics of civilization."[5]

The intent of the establishment of a small hospital at the NWMP post at Fort MacLeod in 1874 was to serve the 150 member NWMP force initially sent to bring law and order to the southern Alberta area. The establishment of the hospital at Fort MacLeod was a unique development and one that occurred early in the history of health care in Alberta. The health needs of members of the Force, Indians of the Northwest plains, Hudson's Bay Company employees and white independent traders all came within the mandate of the operation of this hospital,[6] which was initially run by NWMP surgeons assisted by orderlies. However, by 1896 women who were nurses were employed by the Force to manage the hospital and provide nursing care.[7] The broad mandate of those who could be cared for shows that the Force intended to provide assistance to virtually all who requested their assistance. Not unexpectedly, this hospital took on characteristics of other small hospitals and employed lay nurses as staff members to provide care. Later the Force established a similar post hospital at Fort Calgary. Many members of the Force married nurses and these women were often called upon to provide care to people who required it in a variety of locations across the prairies. In *Red Serge Wives*, Joy Duncan describes the experiences of a number of these women called upon to provide nursing in remote western and northern locations.[8] However, the scope of operations of the NWMP hospital at Fort MacLeod was relatively small and would remain small compared to those that developed in areas where the population base was much larger.

In Calgary, the population had expanded to over 500 when it was incorporated as a town in 1884. Two physicians had arrived to take up residence and practise medicine in 1883, but there were no health care facilities for the care of those afflicted with the inevitable epidemics of infectious diseases. As the railway brought trainload after trainload of settlers from the east to southern Alberta, the population of Calgary grew very quickly. The problems associated with a burgeoning population where prospective settlers arrived before adequate housing was available meant that there was substantial overcrowding of housing that was adequate for the climate. This situation led to the widespread use of inadequate tents and shacks. Community indignation ran high in several cases where Calgary citizens succumbed to illnesses alone and untended. Hattie Price died of heart disease alone in a tent, George Shaw succumbed to typhoid fever untended in a shack near the Elbow River and finally Jimmy Smith died of tuberculosis in a room in the Royal Hotel.[9]

Jimmy Smith's deathbed bequest of $600 towards the construction of a public hospital may also have been a catalyst to action. Public concern bordered on outrage as it was recognized that citizens were dying who might have been saved had they received appropriate care in a hospital. A public meeting was convened on 16 November 1886 of a group called the Hospital Committee chaired by the incumbent mayor, Mr. G.C. King, a former member of the NWMP who had been a member of the troop that founded Fort Calgary in 1875.[10] The group met for several years and was successful in 1889 perhaps due to the efforts of the mayor of the day, a physician, Dr. Lafferty in obtaining from the territorial government a grant of a parcel of land 4 1/2 acres in size to the north of the Bow River. Finally a hospital charter was adopted and letters of incorporation for the Calgary General Hospital drawn up and temporary quarters for the hospital found at 7th Street and 7th Avenue. The official opening of the hospital took place on 24 November 1890 and health care services were offered under the direction of the first Matron, Elizabeth Hoade, a nurse from Winnipeg whose husband, Nelson Hoade was employed as night nurse and general handyman. Even though married women were not generally hired as nurses in these early days of hospitals and nursing, there were exceptions on the frontier where suitably qualified staff were not always available. In that the Matron and her husband were somewhat unconventional employees of the hospital, it is likely that it was an arrangement that was not entirely satisfactory, as it lasted only a short time.

By 1887 the population of Calgary was close to 3,500 and the only hospital beds were offered by the rather primitive NWMP post that had been established at Fort Calgary. The Bishop of St. Albert, Vital-Justin Grandin approached several religious communities in the East for one that would be

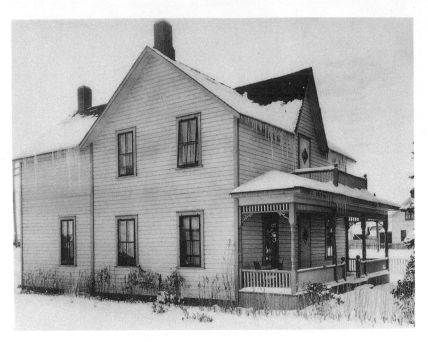

 ✧ *Calgary General Hospital in 1895.* (GAA NA–8–281/AARN P239)

willing to establish a hospital that was desperately needed. Only the Grey Nuns responded, deciding in 1889 to take on the challenge in Calgary.[11] After two years of preparations and fund raising, four sisters led by their superior, Sister Agnes Carroll, arrived by rail in the bitter cold at 2:00 a.m. on the 21st of January 1891. Finding no transportation available, they trudged the quarter of a mile to the Sacred Heart Convent where they sought shelter for the night. They were accompanied by Father Hippolyte Leduc who had been in charge of the construction of their hospital prior to their arrival and who had gone to St. Boniface to meet them.[12] The first hospital building of the Holy Cross Hospital was small beginning with four, then eight beds, and plans were made early the next year to construct a large building and fundraising began in earnest for this much more substantial building. The number of beds was still small in comparison to the need and Sister Carroll "taught the women of Calgary to care for the sick at home; with so few hospital beds available, good home nursing was essential."[13] Once again the Grey Nuns had put their resources together and pooled their efforts in order to establish needed health care services to serve the health needs, this time of the population in this growing metropolis where the Calgary General Hospital had been established just a few months prior to the Holy Cross Hospital.

In 1894, the Calgary General Hospital engaged the services of Miss Mary Ellen Birtles, a graduate of the Winnipeg General Hospital as Superintendent of Nurses. Miss Birtles remained until 1903 and was responsible for the development of the School of Nursing. Correspondence from Miss Birtles to Marion Moodie, the first graduate of the school indicated the varied career that Birtles enjoyed and the many places where she worked and traveled. The nine years of her appointment in Calgary was comparatively long as judged by the tenure of the majority of her successors as superintendents of nurses. Undoubtedly the services of nurses with excellent credentials were in great demand in these years, and this may have explained in part the fact that superintendents tended not to remain in their positions for lengthy periods of time. Decorated by the Governor General of Canada in an investiture held in 1935 at his Ottawa Rideau Hall residence, Miss Birtles was recognized as one of the pioneers of early nursing in Alberta.

The construction of the transcontinental railroad brought settlers in large numbers to the southern area since the Canadian Pacific Railway, the first of the transcontinental lines, traversed the southern prairies. The initial wave of settlers consisted mostly of men involved in coal mining and railway construction including the private entrepreneurs who were responsible for the development of these industries. These businessmen were confronted soon after their arrival with the needs of their workers and those of their families for health care services. They sent for physicians who were promised suitable remuneration in return for caring for mine and railway employees. These company physicians were given full authority to open hospitals and the institutions they initiated were modeled after those they were familiar with in Britain and in which lay nurses, also trained in Britain, were hired. The hospitals were administered at the outset by a matron who had authority over the day-to-day operation of the institution subject to the jurisdiction of all-male boards of directors that exercised ultimate control.

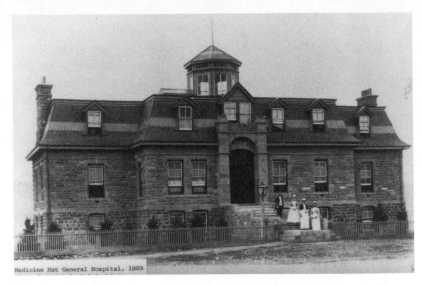

Medicine Hat General Hospital, 1889

✣ *Medicine Hat General Hospital, 1889. (PAA, received on loan from AARN P278)*

NURSING AS A WOMANLY VIRTUE

The establishment of the Medicine Hat General Hospital in 1890 with Miss Grace Reynolds as Matron and Miss Mary Ellen Birtles as her assistant was an important development in southern Alberta since it was one of the first to be established in the area and occurred just prior to the founding of the Calgary General Hospital. Since the idea of establishing a training school for nurses had all but become synonymous with sustaining hospital operations, a school of nursing was established four years later. The annual report of the medical superintendent two years prior to the establishment of the school states:

> The time has also come when a training school for nurses should be started. We are constantly receiving applications from young ladies who are anxious to acquire a nurse's training. This could be done with very little additional outlay. There are few ways in which the hospital can benefit the public more than by being able to supply a nurse's training to those who are anxious and willing to acquire one and who are often willing to give their time and work gratuitously for the sake of the information they receive.[14]

The time and talents of women were sought to provide the nursing care essential to the operation of the hospital. However, the nurses were also subject to an array of rules and regulations governing their conduct as well as the way in which they pursued their lives:

> The nurses are enjoined to observe carefully at all times, the ethics of nursing, and to cultivate the professional spirit which includes a cheerful, willing obedience to authority. Dignity, decorum, and quietness of manner must be observed and the entire time of duty devoted to the welfare of the patients. When off duty nurses should participate in only wholesome recreation, and at all times must guard against anything that would bring dishonour to their school or their profession.[15]

Nurses were expected to work for little remuneration—in other words to subsidize the operation of the hospital almost as volunteers. It is unlikely that this situation was unique in western Canada or in North America, as the new schools were established based on the service of women. Some two years later, it was noted that:

> The commencement of a training school for nurses has filled a long felt want in connection with this Institution. Since August 1st lectures have been given weekly to the nurses. A number of ladies of Medicine Hat having expressed a desire to attend these lectures, it was decided to allow all interested ladies [of Medicine Hat] to attend.[16]

The widely-held view that nursing was often viewed as useful preparation for marriage and motherhood in terms of the knowledge that might be gained about caring for the health of others is reflected. Even though married women of the time did not generally seek employment outside the home, the provision that the married women of Medicine Hat could attend the classes in order to gain skills they would presumably apply in the home underscores the fact that the knowledge gained from studying nursing was seen as valuable, and that women were seen as being capable of mastering it. It is also clear from the open invitation to lay women that nursing was seen as a natural activity for women for which they would have innate abilities. This would allow them to take advantage of that knowledge and skills that would be taught in the program of study.

Company hospitals were originally created to serve the needs of their workers primarily in the coal mining and railway industries, workers who were prone to injury and accident. As the population increased these hospitals began to expand their operations to treat immigrants and settlers as well. The Galt Hospital of Lethbridge established in 1892 as a mine hospital was operated and maintained by the Alberta Coal and Railway Company. In the words of Nelle Chapman Higinbotham:

> For the first year that I was in the Hospital, our patients were mostly men, accidents in the mines, and stabbing affrays . . . filling up the wards. The miners made very good patients and except for coal dust, were very clean; we never found "live-stock" on them, such as we found on dock workers at the MGH [Montreal General Hospital, her alma mater]. The work in the hospital varied a great deal. For some weeks all beds would be occupied with additional camp beds placed wherever possible. Time off duty was almost impossible except when we were able to get outside help, which we could occasionally, there being a very capable practical nurse in Lethbridge, a Miss Barnes, whom we used to get in for extra night duty, but as she was always nearly dated up for maternity cases, she was only occasionally available.[17]

These words are echoed and corroborated by nurses who were contemporaries of Mrs. Higinbotham in both the north and the south of the province. They also indicate the incredibly adverse conditions under which nurses worked as judged by today's standards. It was clear that they truly were expected to sacrifice almost all of their personal time and lives for their work. The question of the inequity between what was expected of women and men in terms of their work arises, for even the coal miners were granted leisure hours. It may be that the value placed upon the work that women did in nursing was simply not considered in the same realm as work done by men to earn a living to support their families.

The suggestion that Miss Barnes was constantly dated up for maternity cases is consistent with the writings of others. In 1910, Marion Dudley Cran published *A Woman in Canada*. Her book included the results of her observations on the life of women in western Canada, and she paid particular attention to the issues for women relative to childbirth. Cran (born in

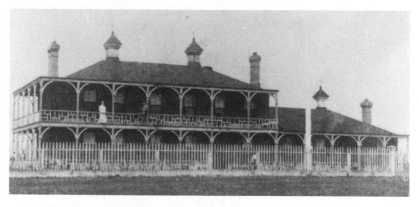

↩ *Galt Hospital, Lethbridge, 1891.* (PAA, *received on loan from* AARN *P96*)

South Africa and raised in Britain) had trained as a nurse and later taken up journalism.[18] Her understanding of the nursing profession made her observations quite powerful. The absence of government-organized maternal-child care was disturbing to her, as were the poor working conditions experienced by most nurses. She met with various government authorities who listened, but were unresponsive to her requests for change. She wrote: "This was a game of battledore and shuttlecock, the need of the women being the shuttlecock between the greater and lesser governments."[19] From the continued inaction in response to her requests, it is apparent that women's needs were not a matter of government priority. Without the devoted work of the few lay midwives available such as Miss Barnes, and Van Haarlem in Lethbridge, of nursing orders of various religious denominations, women would have been almost entirely without maternity services in this area.

Building Hospitals in Northern Alberta

As it became increasingly easy for prospective settlers to travel to Edmonton with the completion in 1891 of the spur line to Strathcona from the transcontinental line of the Canadian Pacific Railway in Calgary[20] and with the arrival of the Canadian Northern Railroad in Edmonton in 1905,[21] the rapidly expanding population in Edmonton was in desperate need of health services. Although many physicians were practising in Edmonton by

1895, the only hospital was that operated by the Grey Nuns at the St. Albert mission. The nine-mile trek over the rough road from Edmonton to the St. Albert hospital was an inconvenience for the increasing number of settlers requiring hospital care as well as for the physicians who were charged with their care. The size of the population and the need for hospital care for those who contracted epidemic diseases provided the rationale for a hospital in Edmonton by 1895. The decision by the Grey Nuns to construct and operate Edmonton's first hospital, the Edmonton General Hospital, in that year following an invitation to do so by six Edmonton physicians was a significant step taken by the sisters and represented a milestone for health services in the growing town of Edmonton as well as for their religious congregation. The account of the development of this hospital just prior to the turn of the century sheds light on the relationship between nurses and physicians, on the status of nurses and physicians in society, on the relative importance of the association between religion and health care and finally on the degree to which religious tolerance existed among the various denominations.

With the increase in population, more physicians moved to the area and began to use the services of the hospital run by the nuns in St. Albert. However, following completion of railway lines terminating in Edmonton, the town became the centre of population growth in the area. A request from physicians practising in Edmonton to build a general hospital in Edmonton was put forward to remedy the lack of a facility in Edmonton for the care of the sick.[22] The physicians' request was not made directly to the nuns but to "his Lordship Bishop Grandin":

> We the undersigned medical practitioners of the Town of Edmonton do hereby agree that we will do all that is in our power to support a general hospital to be built by the Grey Nuns in the Town of Edmonton; and that we will agree to support it to the exclusion of any other Hospital, provided that it be built this year with accommodation in proportion to the size of the town and that it be run as a general hospital under the management of the sisters without a resident doctor.
>
> Signed by H.C. Wilson, H.L. McInnis, P.S. Royal, James H. Tofield, J.D. Harrison and E.A. Braithwaite.[23]

The reply from Bishop Grandin came promptly only three days later. Such a timely reply to such a formal request seems rather startling, but it may be that the suggestion was one that had been discussed within the Mission:

> Although I don't have any direct authority over the administration of the Reverend Sisters of Charity, I considered it my duty to talk to them about your letter. Consequently I am writing today to their superior general to entreat her to undertake the establishment of a general hospital at Edmonton, and to provide qualified sisters for this work. N.B. This hospital will have to be close to the Catholic church.[24]

In advising Mère Deschamps of this development on the same day, Bishop Grandin indicated:

> You will remember that I told you before, the last time we met on the 18th of last March, that I was not in favour of a hospital in Edmonton.[25]

Apparently, the matter had been discussed previously and Bishop Grandin had taken the negative point of view. His reply to the physicians indicates that he had changed his stance on the matter whatever the reason. He went on to say:

> However you will tell me that it is necessary to have the funds to do this. Undoubtedly it is necessary my dear Mother, and knowing how much your daughters will know how to economize and manage their affairs wisely, I would not be afraid to borrow the necessary sum, convinced that the sisters would be able to pay reasonable interest and pay down the capital within a few years. Sister Carroll is far from being in such an advantageous position as in Edmonton, and although she is complaining about this, she is paying interest on the debt and reduction of the capital.[26]

The sisters decided to respond positively to the request to move the base of their operations to Edmonton and proceeded to make plans to construct the new hospital. Their decision may have been facilitated by the successful developments in Calgary where the order had established the Holy Cross Hospital some five years previously. Community support for building the hospital appeared high as noted in the following petition from citizens to the Town Council for financial assistance to support the effort: "On August 22, 1894, 850 persons sent a letter to the Mayor and Councillors of Edmonton. . . . "[27] The group of citizens had requested $10,000 to assist the Grey Nuns' building fund. When Mr. Beck, a lawyer acting on behalf of the citizens, presented the petition to Council " . . . it was moved by J.H. Picard and seconded by C.F. Strang" that in answer to "the prayer of the Petitioners, that a grant of $1,000 be given towards the erection of a General Hospital in Edmonton."[28] The land for the site was purchased from the Hudson's Bay Company and these negotiations had to go through Company headquarters in London. In a letter to C.C. Chipman, Commissioner of the Hudson's Bay Company, Sister Brassard, Supérieure of the St-Albert mission stated: "I was waiting to receive the money from Montreal and as it has not come to date, I have written ordering a cheque for the sum of $2,300 to be sent directly to you as payment for the lots 21/66 block 11. Please have the transfer made in favour of the Corporation of 'The Sisters of Charity of the North-West Territories'."[29] It seems that such matters then as today could founder in the bureaucracy, as it was necessary for Sister Xavier who had been appointed to direct operations at the hospital to write as follows to the Mayor and Council of Edmonton on 22 October 1895:

> Some time ago, as you are aware, your Council promised one thousand dollars ($1,000) to help in the construction of a General Hospital. This building being now very nearly completed, and being myself the principal manager at the present of the Institutions, I take the respectful liberty of asking your Corporation to give us this sum now if possible to help in the settling of bills.[30]

A letter of thanks written on November 6 of that same year indicates that the promised $1,000 had been received.

At the outset of hospital operations, patients were charged 50 cents per day for a bed in a general ward if the person was able to pay. The declaration in that "Be it well understood that the hospital has nothing to do with paying the medical men; all patients who have not the means of paying a

Doctor, will be under the care of the Physician of the month; . . . all who pay, can have any Doctor they may choose" supported the nuns' firm contention that they would care for all, regardless of ability to pay.[31] This document also included a paragraph stating that clergy of all faiths could visit patients and the reminder that "never a pauper patient has been refused admittance." It was evident from a review of the records that the Grey Nuns cared for a large number of indigent patients and that despite the funds raised by the Hospital Ladies' Aid Society, there were continuing difficulties in financing this care. Funds were received from both the federal Department of the Interior and from the city to assist with caring for this large group of patients. The problem in financing this care would continue to be a thorny one as time went on.

However, the mortar had barely set in the new building when a more troublesome issue arose relative to the professional relationship between the nuns and the physicians who cared for patients in the Hospital. According to the *Edmonton Bulletin* "The medical board of the Hospital here consisting of Doctors Wilson, Harrison, Braithwaite and McInnis has resigned."[32] Although the basis of the conflict was ostensibly professional decision-making, the question took the form of a power struggle between the nuns and the physicians, the physicians maintaining that they should exercise complete control over admissions of nonpaying patients to the hospital and that they should not have to serve as the physician of the month for these people. The nuns refused to back down from what they viewed as their rightful authority even though the physicians argued that the nuns might unknowingly admit an infectious case to a public ward of the hospital where the individual might be in contact with those who could be vulnerable to the infection. The argument was labelled as a weak pretense at controlling admissions when Father Leduc refuted it in his letter of reply published in the newspaper in which he supported the nuns right to determine who would be admitted to the hospital as follows:

the right to admit patients to the hospital was given under a secondary pretext used by the physicians. The real reason they have difficulty with this is found in the last clause of their article [to the newspaper] in which they say that they have no authority in the hospital. But was it not these same physicians who asked that the General Hospital be built? Did they not think that the sisters would not run the hospital according to the rules of their order? Did the doctors have complaints to make against the administration of the hospital by the nuns or against the care given to the sick? . . . The Sisters of Charity who, have for a number of years helped the doctors, filled their prescriptions, cared for all kinds of their sick patients, and studied medical care, have surely enough knowledge of medicine to be able to detect a case of infectious disease such as erysipelas, scarlet fever, blood poisoning etc. If there is the least suspicion of this, the person with the disease is immediately isolated until the physician can make his diagnosis.[33]

In this rather public disagreement between the physicians and the nuns, the issue was put forward as one dealing with medical judgement. The more covert and important issue was control over admissions to the Hospital. The physicians chose to resign from the staff of the hospital and to fight their battle publicly in the newspaper. Considerable discussion may have taken place behind the scenes to no avail, and they thought their options were such that they could take the risk of public disclosure. Father Leduc's rebuttal, also published in the newspaper, puts forward the sisters' side of the story and attempts to put the fundamental issues of disagreement before the public. He pointed out that it was the same physicians who had beseeched the Grey Nuns to undertake the construction of a general hospital in Edmonton who now wanted to exercise control over all patient admissions on a pretext of the need for a physician to first make a diagnosis prior to admission of indigent patients. A document that describes the physicians' point of view in the dispute asserts:

> The disagreement which has taken place between the Doctors of the Medical Board, . . . was over the right of admission of patients.
>
> We claim that all patients must have a card of admission from a Dr.
>
> That card, in case of private or paying patient [is] to be signed by a Dr.; as long as he is a duly qualified physician, only that private patients must have such care and the Dr. who signed such card shall be the one to look after such patient.
>
> In pauper cases the card must be from one of the Drs. of the Hospital Board. Emergency pauper cases need not have a card but can be admitted and the Dr. for the month must be sent for.

Now, the answer given by Father LeDuc for the Hospital is that the building belonging as it does to the Grey Nuns. They, through the Mother Superior here, have the right to admit who they please and need not in any case refer to any Doctor. Nor need they have those admitted placed under the care of any Dr.

Next the physicians attempted to provide a rationale for their conclusion that they must exercise control over all hospital admissions:

One reason why we wanted to have control of the pauper cases is Mother Superior admits a patient who may have some infectious disease as Erysipelas, Scarlet Fever, Diphtheria or Blood Poison and such may be placed in the public wards. Such diseases certainly would spread and one or perhaps more deaths would occur. Especially would this be so if a case of Erysipelas were placed in a ward where there were patients suffering from wounds, or an accident, or recovering from an operation.

Again, who is the one but the Drs. to say whether a person is a fit and proper subject for Hospital treatment? No one! Not even the Mother Superior. But cases are admitted and we are called upon to treat as paupers those who have been able and are willing to pay for their treatment. As a matter of fact there have been quite a few such cases and they have paid us from $10. to $40. still at the same time the sisters told us they were paupers and as far as we know were down on the books as such.

Because while having to assume the responsibility of the cases and attention of the so-called patients, no matter how admitted, we had no authority or say in the admission, management, nursing or discharge or general work of the Hospital. We agreed to attend the present Institution as a General Hospital. We did so, furnishing our own instruments, giving our time, etc. but we did not agree to attend to a private Hospital or an Institution as Father LeDuc told us 'was more than a Hospital'. In fact it is a mixed Institution, part Hospital, part Almshouse and part a Boarding house.[34]

There can be little doubt that this conflict represented a deep impasse between the sisters and the physicians. Such a familiar power struggle between the male physicians and the female nursing sisters is intriguing given that the situation occurred almost a century ago, prior to suffragist and feminist movements, before nursing was legitimately constituted as a profession, and prior to the declaration by the Privy Council of Great Britain that according to the British North America Act women were "persons." Argumentation was indirect in defence of the nuns' position and was addressed to the physicians by another man, rather than by the nuns directly. Although somewhat circuitous and rather oblique from a contemporary point of view, this undoubtedly enhanced their position and communicated to the physicians that they would not be given free rein to determine the operation of the General Hospital. Another facet of the dispute was that the original appeal by the Edmonton physicians to the Grey Nuns to build a hospital contained the names of five English-speaking physicians and one French-speaking physician. With the publication of the details of the dispute including the resignation of the members of the medical board, it was clear that only four English-speaking physicians had resigned. The French-speaking physician and one other physician had refused to join the revolt and thus the decision to abandon the hospital was by no means unanimous. Another French-Canadian physician arrived to take up a practice in Edmonton just as the hospital was being built, and over the next decade several more would come, so that soon there would be six French-Canadian physicians practising medicine at the Edmonton General Hospital.

As in so many other disagreements, there were no clear winners and losers. The nuns held fast in their contention that they would continue to admit patients to the Hospital, and the physicians did not retract their resignations from the Medical Board of the Hospital. How the physicians received the news that the nuns were not willing to capitulate to them in terms of the admission of patients is not known. However, it is clear from Father Leduc's statements in the newspaper that the nuns strongly disputed the physicians' argument that the nuns could not be expected to organize patient placements so that those suffering from infectious disease would not be placed adjacent to those who were potentially susceptible to the disease. The resolution of the dispute appears to have led directly to the establishment of the another hospital in Edmonton. The development of another hospital may have seemed to those involved with the Edmonton General to be unnecessary at the time. However with the rapid population growth further to completion of the spur line from the main line of the CPR in from Calgary to Strathcona on the south bank of the North Saskatchewan River in 1891, and the Canadian Northern Railway to Edmonton in 1905, it was clear that these as well as other new facilities would be badly needed in the immediate future.

It may be that the decision had already been made by a group of citizens to press for another hospital in Edmonton and that the physicians who disagreed with their lack of complete control over admissions at the Edmonton General considered this as their "third option." Even though the development of another hospital was a very difficult issue for the nuns, their institution was well-established and was in no danger of losing its medical staff. Their major achievement was that they had held fast in the dispute with the physicians relative to their assertion that they possessed the professional judgement and therefore had the right to admit individuals to their hospital. Nevertheless, the plans to construct another hospital in Edmonton soon unfolded as fund-raising began in earnest to support this effort.

A Women's Aid Society to raise money for the hospital had gone to work a year prior to this, and it was somewhat startling to reflect on the information that:

> At the October meeting, 1901, Rev. Mr. Gray and Mr. Alex Taylor were present as a committee from the Board of Directors to ask the ladies to assume the responsibility of the debt on the Hospital, while they would keep up the maintenance and pay the interest on the principal. They reported that the debt amounted to the modest sum of eight thousand dollars or eight thousand two hundred dollars. The ladies (always agreeable, and never flinching at the call of duty, large or small), agreed to undertake the work, and since that date have applied all monies towards paying off the indebtedness, and are proud to report that the liabilities have been reduced by three thousand six hundred and seventy-one dollars and seventy cents.[35]

The first location of the little frame house with 25 beds that served as the hospital was on Boyle Street, at 97th Street and 103A Avenue, and the institution was often referred to as the Boyle Street Hospital. According to Christina Dorward and Olive Tookey, "Miss Jessie Turnbull was chosen from amongst several applicants and became the first matron at a salary of

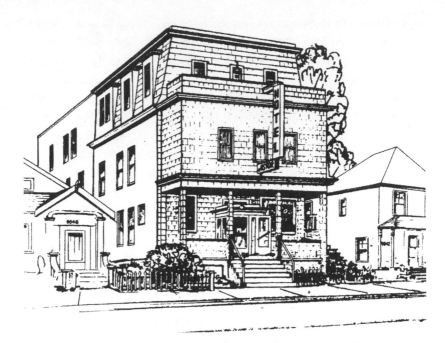

↬ *A drawing of the original Boyle Street Hospital (later Royal Alexandra Hospital); building was demolished in 1976. (Illustration by George Weber, provided by Murray W. Ross)*

$35.00 per month. She was assisted by an undergraduate nurse at a salary of $25.00 per month."[36]

The construction of larger facilities was necessary because of rapid population growth, although it did not proceed without difficulty. There was public controversy over the passage of a hospital bylaw enabling a grant of $175,000 for construction of a new hospital, and a 20 June 1910 article in the *Edmonton Bulletin* reported a demonstration in favour of such a bylaw. At this demonstration, Alderman J.D. Hyndman is quoted as saying: "he thought people should be compelled to contribute to hospitals as they are . . . necessities of a modern city. Under the system which had prevailed the burden has fallen on the few." In the same article, the work of nurses was referred to as follows:

"We have in the present hospital," said Mr. Fraser, "as good a staff of nurses as is to be found anywhere. It is only because we have such an excellent staff that we have been able to do even passable work, with the inadequate facilities of the existing building."

In addition, references to the work of the nuns at the Edmonton General Hospital some years after the dispute were complimentary:

Mr. Fraser, continuing, stated that in expressing the wish for a new hospital he did not wish in any way to cast reflections on the work done in the institutions managed by the sisters of the Roman Church. He was proud of the work they had done, and were doing, but he believed that the establishment of a thoroughly modern citizens' hospital would help all the existing institutions.[37]

The ordinance of the North-West Territories to incorporate the Edmonton Public Hospital was put forward and assented to by the Lieutenant Governor and the Legislative Assembly of the Territories on 4 May 1900, although the hospital did not open its doors until the 1st of December of that year. It thus became the third hospital in Edmonton, as the operations of the Misericordia Hospital had begun just a few months earlier.

Operated under the auspices of the Roman Catholic Church and the sisters of the Misericorde, the Misericordia Hospital opened just a short time prior to the Public Hospital (also called the Boyle Street institution and later the Royal Alexandra Hospital). Although it was Bishop Grandin who was given formal recognition for requesting the formation of a mission in Edmonton by the Sisters of the Misericorde, a reference was found in the archives of the Grey Nuns to the effect that they had asked the Bishop to find an order of nuns willing to take on the construction of another hospital that would be devoted entirely to maternity care. Because they were involved in general hospital care and admitted many patients with communicable diseases to their institution, they felt a separate building and different personnel were necessary to prevent the spread of infection. There may have also been some relationship between the founding of the Misericordia Hospital and the dispute between the physicians and the sisters as there was a measure of competition between the Edmonton General and the Public Hospital that was at least partly sectarian in nature. In direct response to Bishop Grandin's request, four Misericordia Sisters from Montreal and one lay nurse from their Ottawa establishment arrived in Edmonton to open "a

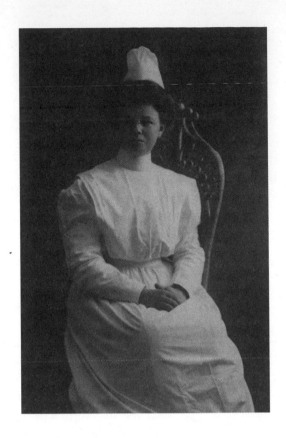

↝ Nurse M.J. Kennedy came to Edmonton with the Misericordia Sisters in May of 1900 from their Ottawa Mission where she had nursed as well. (Archives of the Misericordia Hospital, Montreal)

small maternity hospital in a converted warehouse in the Oliver district."[38] Their first residence had four rooms on the first floor and a type of loft arrangement on the second, all heated by a stove-pipe that extended through the two floors.[39] The first Mother Superior was Sister St. Francois d'Assise and the nuns were accompanied by a lay nurse, Miss Mary Jane Kennedy who came to Edmonton as an integral part of the group. As far as is known, Miss Kennedy was the first lay nurse in a Catholic institution in Edmonton, a unique situation at the time. The sisters came imbued with the need for a cost recovery approach because their Motherhouse had indicated that the order was not in a position to subsidize the work.[40] The diocese of St. Albert, for its part agreed to provide for:

the housing and maintenance of the Sisters until they were self-sufficient. . . . The stipulation in the contract meant that the diocese

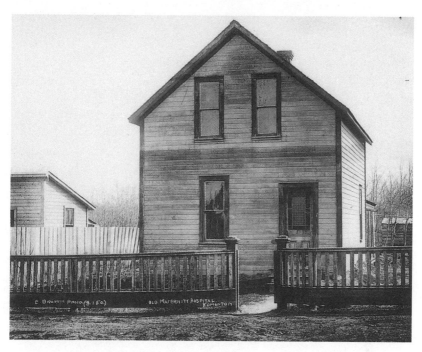

➣ *First residence used by the Misericordia Sisters in Edmonton upon their arrival in Edmonton in 1900. This building was located at 9937–110 Street, across from St. Joachim's church.* (PAA B.3782)

agreed to pay in whole or in part the rent on the interim accommodation to be used by the Sisters pending the completion of the hospital. The St. Albert Diocese also agreed to give them a complete block, surrounded by four streets, in Strathcona. This land was to be provided only if the two parties, after a certain unspecified trial period, decided that the mission was to be permanent. Under the contract, the St. Albert Diocese was to be responsible for the loans which the Community would have to arrange in order to construct the new hospital on the site provided by the diocese.[41]

Although their intent was to provide an institution to care for unwed mothers and their babies, and in fact the chronicles for 1 September 1900, reported that the first patient who arrived was not an unwed mother-to-be, but a young woman who arrived with her husband who wanted to stay

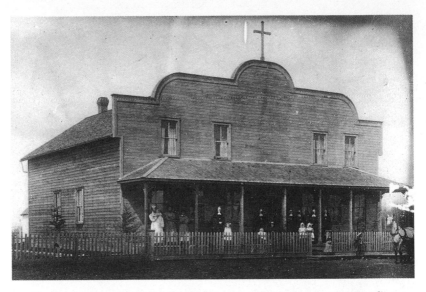

⇾ *The first building of the Misericordia Hospital established by the Misericordia sisters in 1900. The building had been a warehouse used by the Norris and Carey firm as a general store until purchased by the St. Albert Diocese and remodelled for use by the sisters. A utility pole carried the telephone line between St. Albert and Edmonton. (Archives of the Misericordia Hospital, Montreal)*

with his wife during her confinement.[42] As time went on, it was clear that the major thrust of the hospital became general maternity care for the population. Soon after it opened, the hospital became an institution which offered general medical care of all kinds. The sisters also took in boarders and tended a large garden and livestock in the lot south of the hospital that the sisters purchased in 1902 for $50.[43] Private citizens played substantial roles in the ongoing support of the hospital through donations of food, and the Town Council provided tax remissions, presumably in recognition for the service rendered to the citizens of Edmonton. Although a Strathcona location for the hospital the Misericordia Sisters would build had been considered from the outset, and although the Strathcona Municipal Council offered a yearly grant to assist with operating expenses, the sisters decided upon a location to the north of the Edmonton General Hospital in St. Joachim's Parish.[44] The offer by the Strathcona Council had been substantial—$50,000, but the attached condition was one that they could not accept—that the institution be managed by a public board. Again the issue was one of control, and again the sisters refused to allow any incursions on their authority. Although they experienced great financial difficulty in establishing themselves and staying on a firm financial footing in order to be able to secure loans for the construction of new and expanded facilities, this all came to fruition in the winter of 1906 when their new hospital was ready for occupancy.

It was reported in the 18 February 1901 edition of the *Edmonton Bulletin* that the municipal councils of Strathcona and Edmonton met and agreed that a quarantine hospital was needed and agreed to share the costs of furnishing and renting a building in which the hospital would be housed.[45] Later it was decided that this institution would be located "in the rear of the [Public] Hospital grounds" and "under the control of the Board of Directors of the Public Hospital and that the city would give a grant of one thousand dollars a year toward its maintenance."[46] An isolation hospital was established in 1905 to enable health officials to respond to the increase in communicable disease in the city with the sizable and continuing growth in the city's population in this era.

Some years later, public concern arose over conditions at the isolation hospital, which was under the jurisdiction of the Medical Officer of Health. An altercation between the physician who was the Medical Officer of Health and the nurses who staffed the hospital led in 1913 to a "fierce verbal contest with nurses . . . over the issue of job descriptions and wage settlements."[47] The nurses courageously marched to city hall where they demanded a meeting with the mayor. In the aftermath of the march, the superintendent of nurses was fired, but she sued the Board for wages owed according to her contract. The ensuing court case resulted in questioning of the powers and authority of the Medical Officer of Health over the isolation hospital by the presiding judge and eventually to the transfer of its operation to the authority of a municipal hospital board.[48]

The fifth major hospital facility in the Edmonton area was established in 1906 as the Strathcona Hospital on the south bank of the river. A hospital in Strathcona had been talked about for some years and in 1901 the "health officer of the Northwest Territories said a 'pest house' was needed in the district for epidemics"[49] resulting in the establishment of the isolation hos-

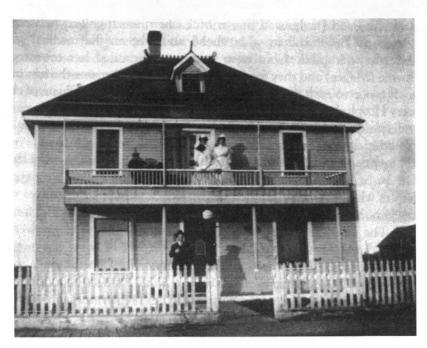

An early photo of the Strathcona Hospital, 105th Street and Whyte Avenue, circa 1909 or 1910. (From More Than a Hospital*)*

pital on the north side of the river to which the municipal council of Strathcona contributed annual sums of money. However, in 1903 the subject of a hospital in Strathcona came up again when physicians presented a petition signed by 96 citizens stating: "We the undersigned ratepayers of the town of Strathcona request that you may be pleased to submit a bylaw to raise the sum of $10,000 for the purpose of purchasing land and erection of a hospital . . ."[50] Although no action took place right away, the idea must have germinated, and it was recognized that funds for the construction of the hospital were small by comparison with what would be needed to operate it.

After the province was established in 1905 and the first premier installed, the CPR was to become involved in the provision of operating funds for the hospital in return for care of their employees. On 6 April 1906 the hospital commenced operation with Florence Tofield as matron and another nurse for assistance in a building on the northwest corner of 78th Avenue and

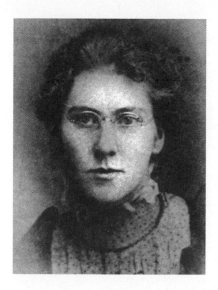

*Jessie Dickson, lady superinten-
dent of Strathcona Hospital,
July, 1906 -April, 1911. (From
More than a Hospital)*

105th Street. The first matron was quickly succeeded by Miss Jessie
Dickson, who remained until 1911, and a scroll expressing the appreciation
of the citizens of Strathcona for her service is preserved in the archives of
the institution.

After the University of Alberta was founded in 1908, Dr. Henry Marshall
Tory recognized that a hospital was important for achievement of his goal
of establishing a medical school at the University. Many sites and much
wrangling later, it was decided that the new hospital would be built on the
campus. It is noted that the hospital board "relied heavily on Miss Baird"
during this period of time[51] and that "Older, larger hospitals of the east
were run by gentleman medical superintendents with M.D.'s, but on the
local scene the lady superintendent was still chief executive officer."[52] She
was able to perform all administrative functions except the signing of
cheques, a task reserved for the board.[53]

THE VALUE OF NURSES' WORK IN HOSPITALS

In the decade just before and after the turn of the century, hospitals had
been established in the major cities of the province in Calgary, Edmonton,
Lethbridge and Medicine Hat. Nurses played prominent roles in both the
administration and care services from the outset. The status of women was
vastly different in the early part of the twentieth century. Alberta repre-

sented the Western frontier in the late 1800s and early 1900s and this afforded women the opportunity to play more significant and substantial roles than might otherwise have been the case in an established community. Nurses were pioneers arriving to provide nursing services in some regions before resident physicians came to the area. Their daily lives in the early years were very difficult as subsistence for themselves and for those to whom they gave care was dependent on their own resources. Thus they became gardeners, farmers, and ranchers to carry on their operations. They were also steadfast of purpose when their intent was challenged. Their services were critical in the implementation of care in the institutions that were created as a result of their efforts. The work of these nurses would serve as a model for the development and expansion of health services in the years which followed.

Both lay nurses and nurses belonging to religious orders functioned in similar roles. For both groups the availability of outside assistance when it was badly needed presented difficulties. The conditions under which nurses worked were related to cultural views about women's work common throughout the western world where women were expected to satisfy the needs of others even if this meant personal sacrifices in terms of their own needs. The same values also explain, at least in part, why specific health services designed to meet women's health needs were the last to emerge. However, some of the struggles of these early nurses were also related to specific cultural differences in the degree of responsibility that was given to nurses for administrative decision-making in British and French-Canadian hospitals.

The establishment of hospitals in major population centres in the northern and southern regions of the province began in the last decade of the nineteenth century continued and gained its major thrust in the early part of the twentieth century. The image of the hospital as almshouse serving the sick-poor of mid-nineteenth century Britain underwent a significant transformation as new developments in health care necessitated situating patients regardless of financial means in a location where they could be observed and given treatment and care as needed. Also as Rosenberg has observed, by the end of the nineteenth century the hospital was becoming "far more central, both in the provision of medical care and in the careers of ambitious physicians."[54] The institutions that were established in this period of time expanded their facilities and personnel and offered a full range of health care services of high quality to the population. With the advances in medicine and in health technology, hospitals would undergo significant changes in order to adapt to advances in practice, the economics of health care and the ever-changing health policy context.

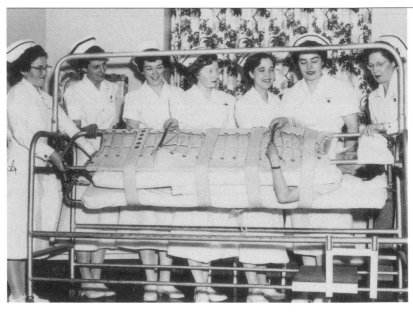

⤷ Nurses at the Calgary General Hospital turning a patient on a Stryker frame, circa 1955. (GAA NA–2600–49/AARN P344)

3

Diligence, Dedication
and Distinguished Service

Nurses in the Modern Hospital Era

Throughout the establishment of the early hospitals around the turn of the century, nurses' work was viewed as being uniquely suited to women since they were deemed to have natural abilities to nurture and care for others. As hospital nursing grew more sophisticated and public health nursing flourished over the remainder of the century, nurses' roles were scrutinized closely in the context of the women's movement, which came to the fore and gained momentum from the 1960s and 1970s onward. Changing societal views on the disparate capabilities of men and women would lead to the opportunity for members of both sexes to enter nontraditional fields of study and work. However, an analysis of the rate at which traditionally male fields of work beckoned to women as compared to the rate at which traditionally female fields of work beckoned to men from the 1930s onwards revealed some stark contrasts, particularly in the latter decades of the twentieth century. The much slower progress in the entry of men to nursing compared to the entry of women to medicine may have reflected a lingering stigma attached to fields of endeavour occupied primarily by women.[1] Clearly this phenomenon is true of other fields where women continued to predominate such as dental hygiene and home economics. The social pressure for men to enter fields such as science and technology, business and management remained strong, albeit somewhat mediated by more open attitudes in society generally about career paths for men. While the number and proportion of men entering nursing continued to be relatively low in the final decade of the twentieth century, there had been a steady increase. Societal attitudes change very slowly and the rate of entry of women to fields of work that have traditionally been dominated by men and are viewed as valuable by the public has been much higher than the rate of entry of men to fields traditionally viewed as women's work and therefore less valuable to society.

Attitudes to nursing have gradually shifted from a view of nursing as solely or primarily nurturing or caring for the needs of another person at an emotional level to a view that places value on the complex knowledge base that is necessary to practise nursing competently. Such an attitude shift did not appear to denigrate the caring or nurturing aspects of nursing as these continued to be seen as an essential component of nursing. As it became recognized that both men and women possessed the ability to nurture and care for others, the issue in learning to become an excellent practitioner of nursing was mastery of the knowledge necessary for practice as well as the willingness and ability to reach out to others who had important health needs. In the future, men will enter the nursing profession for many of the same reasons as women. The attractiveness of a profession or field of work to potential practitioners has been related to such factors as whether or not the field offers meaningful work, good working conditions, reasonable compensation and attractive career potential. With the enhancement of nursing roles in the workforce through educational advancement, higher salaries and more complex responsibilities for client care, there have been radical changes in the health care system over time and in the associated professional scope of practice in nursing.

Pervasive questions of gender have been at work since the emergence of the profession. These have been underscored more recently by the prominence of the women's movement. As a consequence of the relative degree of value accorded the work of the profession with its predominantly female workforce, visibility of nurses and recognition of their achievements have always been somewhat less than desirable or reasonable under the circumstances. Nurses have been in the forefront both of the settlement of the community in Alberta and have established and sustained major health care organizations. As has been amply demonstrated in the years since nurses decided to argue vigorously and indeed do battle for better wages, benefits, and working conditions, the profession has been a primary force in health care institutions and few, if any, hospitals have been able to stay in business without the expert services offered by registered professional nurses.[2] There can be little doubt that the latter is as true in the present as it has been in the past.

Because of the apprenticeship system of hospital training, the majority of the nursing care provided in hospitals was rendered by students for most of the first four decades of the twentieth century. This was a system in which operations of the hospital were heavily subsidized by nursing students who received little or no recompense for the work they performed. If comparable work had been done by graduate nurses, the cost would have been substantially higher. Because of the financial incentive for the hospital, this was a system that was very difficult to dislodge and that persisted long after it had been widely discredited as being both exploitive and detrimental to students in both a personal and educational sense.[3] As Sister Marie Bonin aptly put it: "So deeply time-honoured became this system of nursing education ... that it became difficult to imagine nursing, like other professions, as belonging to a university setting for the education of its practitioners."[4] Because an apprenticeship system was in place where the apprentices provided the majority of the nursing service, there was little or no opportunity for graduate nurses to be employed to provide expert care in hospitals. Since a great deal of care was provided in homes until hospitals offered more complex and specialized care, graduate nurses were able to find work as independent practitioners engaged primarily in private duty nursing in patients' homes and paid directly by patients and their families. However, with the onset of the Depression in the 1930s, nurses lost their clients because potential patients no longer had sufficient funds to engage them to provide nursing services in the home.

Widespread unemployment among nurses during the 1930s produced great hardship for nurses, because remuneration from private duty was essential to the well-being of most. Unemployment was the subject of discussion at many Council meetings of the Alberta Association of Registered Nurses and in an address to the 1932 Annual Convention, Miss Gilbert summed it up as follows:

> The Year of our Lord, 1931, will go down in our memory as one of the blackest. We hear the words "depression and unemployment" every day until we are weary of the sound of them. Probably none is unaffected by their reality. In our profession, the private duty nurses felt it the most, as (our) ranks are swelled by nurses who formerly had regular employment.[5]

Since hospitals were rapidly undergoing technological advancement with the advent of new knowledge and techniques in health care, nursing administrators began to call for the creation of permanent positions for graduate nurses on their rosters: "Instead of adding to the output of graduate nurses during these difficult years by increasing the enrolment of our school of Nursing, we have created employment for those who otherwise would have been obliged to enter an overcrowded and highly competitive field".[6] It was inevitable that the move to employment of nurses by hospitals was associated with loss of some of the independence practitioners had enjoyed. Although individual nurses had often formed partnerships with physicians, caring for the patients of particular general practitioners in private homes,[7] they nevertheless had certain prerogatives which they had to give up when they became employees of the hospital and were duty-bound to conform to its rules and regulations relative to their contract to provide service. At the time nurses were grateful for the opportunity to move into hospital employment, for there was no work otherwise when the cloud of the Depression settled firmly over the country.[8] Although all Canadians felt its harsh effects, it is reported that the impact on the west was particularly vehement[9] for the worldwide economic recession was compounded by a series of droughts and crop failures in western Canada.

Changing Definitions of Professional Work

Tremendous change took place in the nursing profession following the widespread establishment of hospitals in the province, a development which was due, at least in part, to the discovery of new knowledge and associated progress in the availability of treatment for particular illnesses. Deborah Gorham observes that the rise of medicine and its development into a modern and scientific profession was accompanied by "a parallel process . . . in nursing—the most important of the modern health care occupations dominated by women."[10] She states:

> Modern nursing in Canada, like modern medicine, aspired to professional status and to connecting both its training and its practice to science. But . . . the professionalization of women's work as healers did not take place without struggles with the medical profession. From the late nineteenth century, Canadian medical men proved willing to absorb women healers into the modern institutions they created, but only if the women would do so on the physicians' terms.[11]

Many authors have provided some evidence of the struggles nurses have had in establishing their practice as a legitimate area of activity requiring a broad base of knowledge and a wide range of skills. From the outset, nursing was recognized as an art. However, recognition as a science was not generally acknowledged until much later.

There has been relatively little study of how nursing measured as a science in a historical sense. One of the few historians to give careful study to a number of important questions concerning scientific aspects of nursing over time, Kathryn McPherson suggests that on hospital wards, "science played a larger role in everyday life of nurses than the scholarly literature suggests."[12] The elaborate procedures and techniques that nurses were required to master were "based on the theoretical understanding and practical application of the germ theory of disease."[13] McPherson suggests that feminist historians, "committed to critiquing gender asymmetry, have been hesitant to seriously examine nurses' relationship to science in this era [the 1930s and 1940s]."[14] Another relevant issue in the elaborate detail with which procedures were outlined was the application of principles of scientific management to the work in order to allow hospital administrators and physicians to retain control of nurses' work.[15] Her example of the seventeen step process for giving a subcutaneous injection, while serving as a summary of actions required, also helped managers identify the relative amount of nursing time required to perform the procedure and to allow them to institute procedures to improve efficiency.[16] McPherson underscores the need to identify the scientific aspects of the tasks undertaken by nurses to treat and care for patients, for example those relating to assuring asepsis. These were often "interpreted by historians as evidence of nurses' subordinate domestic status" when in fact they took on "new importance when seen as part of a larger system of asepsis for which nurses were responsible."[17] Nurses accepted the need for precision and detail in defining their work, but McPherson argued that rather than submissiveness, such acceptance "empowered nurses to define for themselves what constituted good nursing, . . . Domestic and therapeutic functions were embedded in even the simplest of tasks, such as making a bed"[18]—a task that could be construed as domestic work, but which was vital to patients' comfort and to prevention of pressure sores. McPherson's research suggests an important basis for deeper understanding of nursing practice over time and the context of knowledge and theory that were essential to safe and effective care.

With increasing technology and diversification in nursing roles from the 1950s on, nurses were required to become highly skilled technically in order to perform complex procedures required by their patients in hospitals. Transfer of functions from physicians to nurses has been a continuous process over time. For example, the procedure of taking a temperature rested originally with the physician and was transferred to the nurse around the turn of the century.[19] Many nurses in practice today can remember when initiating intravenous fluids and administering intravenous medications were procedures carried out exclusively by physicians. Today most such procedures are performed by nurses. Where highly complex procedures were needed on an around-the-clock basis, their transfer to nurses became almost inevitable because nurses were in a position to provide such care to hospitalized patients on a regular basis. However, the new and complex procedures were increasingly more difficult to perform and held greater risk in terms of their potential for patient complications. Thus, nurses were increasingly placed in a more vulnerable position in terms of the increased frequency of adverse patient responses to such procedures and also to the possibility of lawsuits. Along with the transfer of functions from physician to nurse, there was a corresponding transfer of functions from the nurse to the licensed practical nurse, formerly called the registered nursing assistant and before that certified nursing aide. The practical nurse emerged as a new category of health worker as a result of the acute shortages of nurses that occurred throughout World War II. The increasing complexity of the role of the registered nurse led to more and

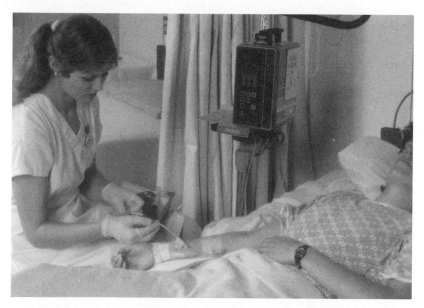

↣ *Monitoring intravenous administration of fluids.* (AARN P321)

more duties being given to the practical nurse to perform under the supervision of the registered nurse.

Although, it is tempting to define professions in terms of tasks performed by their members, the change that has occurred over time in the tasks normally performed by various health disciplines due to advances in knowledge points out the difficulties and problems associated with defining professions in this way.[20] One author has described nursing's functions as instrumental or task-oriented and expressive or people-oriented, where nurse and physician are compared in that the nurse is to "expressive" as the physician is to "instrumental."[21] A task-oriented definition tends to accommodate attempts by hospital managers to associate the task with a specific amount of time, and to fail to allow for broader patient needs. The components of nursing practice put forward by the American Nurses Association in its position paper on nursing education[22] identified three areas which distinguish nursing and the other health disciplines, principally medicine, namely care, cure and coordination. Although these have provided an interesting basis for considering and comparing the work of nurses and physicians, it is somewhat doubtful if any one of these areas is unique to nursing or medicine. Another frame of reference treats nursing functions as either dependent, independent or collaborative; that is, dependent functions are performed under the jurisdiction of the physician, independent functions are performed independently by the nurse and collaborative functions are those which are performed together.[23] Martha Rogers[24] however, categorically denied the existence of dependent functions, asserting that "As a learned profession, nursing has no dependent functions but, like all other professions, has many collaborative functions that are indispensable to providing society with a higher order of service than any one profession can offer." These descriptions of nursing functions relate primarily to physician-direction and physician-interaction. Simplistic approaches to the constructing organizational frames of reference to explain the work of nurses ultimately may fail both the health care consumer and the individual nurse expected to provide care of high quality, but they are useful in that they provoke analysis of the various dimensions of professional work. Nursing along with medicine and the other health professions will continue to undergo sweeping evolutionary alterations and a broader approach to conceptualizing the work of the various professions including nursing is warranted.

Nursing During the Expansionary Era, 1948 to 1980

Both the size of the profession and the scope of nursing practice grew exponentially from 1948 to 1980. The passage of the National Health Grants Act in 1948 was inspired by the similar Hospital Survey and Construction (Hill-Burton) Act in the United States in 1946. In Canada, as in the U.S., such incentives for the development of hospitals heralded an unprecedented era of hospital construction. New hospitals were built and existing hospitals were enlarged and modernized over this period of time. Although national health insurance had been the subject of discussion amongst federal legislators since the 1930s and a series of provincial plans had been enacted, the passage of The Hospital Insurance and Diagnostic Services Act in 1957 was the cornerstone for medicare in Canada, for it was the Act that provided for national hospitalization insurance. On 1 April 1958, the Alberta Hospitalization Benefits plan went into effect and,

Within a year of the commencement of the hospitalization plan, the Alberta government undertook to pay the capital cost of building and equipping hospitals as well as the operating costs. Outstanding capital funded debt on existing hospitals, whether publicly or privately owned, was taken over by the province and future construction was undertaken only with provincial approval and was funded through government-guaranteed debentures.[25]

The Medical Care Act of 1968 provided for national insurance for medical costs and completed the initial series of federal legislative acts establishing a national system of health insurance. This act allowed for federal funds to be transferred to the provinces in reimbursement for physicians' services. Although nursing services were not identified specifically for reimbursement they were covered under the costs of hospitalization. Since the new and expanded hospitals required greater numbers of nurses in order to provide services to the public, expanded career opportunities for nurses arose as a result of the financial impetus for the development of hospitals provided by the federal legislation.

As an example of the tremendous expansion in the number of nurses employed in hospitals, at the University of Alberta Hospital in Edmonton, the number of registered nurses employed in 1952 was 143, while in 1961 it was 342, an increase of approximately 240 percent.[26] In the same period of time, the total number of nursing students went from 286 to 385, an increase of about 135 percent.[27] Nursing students were still being used to provide a considerable amount of service to the hospital in 1962, but the percentage increase in students was less than half of that of registered nurses, undoubtedly evidence of changing times. Criticism of the continued use by hospitals of an inexpensive pool of student labour had begun with the Weir Report of 1932[28] and had become stronger over time. By 1962, there was increasing consensus among nurses across the country about the need for nursing education programs to be an integral part of the general education system. It was believed that students required broader learning opportunities than was possible in single purpose educational agencies operating in association with hospitals. Further it was believed that nursing students who were primarily female should have the same educational options as men and women students in the universities and colleges of Canada. The magnitude of this expansion in nursing staff at the University Hospital was seen again and again in hospitals around the province, institutions that were large and small, urban and rural.

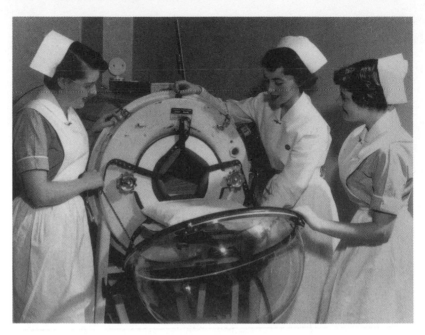

↝ *M. McKay Sproule teaching nursing students to care for patients in an iron lung, circa 1955. (UAA 74–154–53, received on loan from AARN P372)*

With the availability of antibiotics after 1940 and the discovery of vaccines that prevented the occurrence of certain infectious diseases such as polio, the nature of patient populations in hospitals changed radically. Those with infectious diseases and infections were remarkably fewer in number since diseases could now be prevented or treated and the need for hospitalization avoided. Polio was common in Alberta from the 1920s and 1930s and epidemics raged throughout the 1940s and 1950s culminating in the "last terrible outbreak of polio in 1953–54."[29] Nurses played important roles in the care of patients in special wards in hospitals. The development of the iron lung to provide mechanical stimulation for respiratory systems impaired by the disease process offered a way of saving the lives of those who were temporarily or permanently incapacitated by the disease. Nurses volunteered in great numbers for the polio work even though it meant exposing themselves to the causative agent of the disease. Many contracted the disease and for some it was fatal. The altruism of those who offered to care for others who were ill with this disease of unknown origin is evident. The work was physically demanding because it involved heavy and challenging care of patients who had limited ability to carry out personal hygiene activities. There was constant anxiety about electrical power. If there was a power failure, the machines had to be operated manually by the nurses and other attendants in order to maintain the breathing of the patients: "The rule in the University Hospital was that if the power went off, all free staff members ran for the polio wards. One summer evening the power went out three times."[30] The class of 1944 at the Galt Hospital in Lethbridge wrote that: "The hiss and chug of the iron lung still rings in the ears of those who worked with it. Some of the class went through the experience of having to man the lung when there was a power failure."[31] The development of the Salk and Sabin vaccines for polio would make a dramatic difference in the number of people who would contract the disease in the future. At the Red Cross Children's Hospital in Calgary, there were 161 cases in 1952, its first year of operation, 292 in 1953 and 162 in 1954. The figure for 1964 after widespread use of polio vaccines dropped dramatically to 44.[32] Such remarkable changes occurred in many areas of health care and had a dramatic impact upon the work of nurses as a result of new scientific approaches to preventing illness and facilitating recovery from illness.

Development of new surgical techniques occurred in tandem with greater understanding of disease causation and effective treatment. Even though fewer patients were admitted for infectious diseases that could now be prevented and for infections that could be controlled through antibiotic administration, horizons began to widen for patients with health problems for which there would have been no treatment only a few years earlier. This occurred as a result of basic and applied research in a number of fields including anatomy, physiology, pharmacology and pharmaceuticals, microbiology, biochemistry, immunology, medicine and surgery. Large areas of hospital in-patient facilities began to be devoted to the care of surgical patients and new surgical treatments became possible in rapid succession. This was a process that would continue and accelerate with the discovery of new knowledge, and it had a dramatic impact upon the practice of nursing. A great number of nursing positions were required to operate many surgical units in the large hospitals. While surgery had been thought to be feasible in the home on kitchen tables in the first few decades of the century, increasing knowledge of asepsis and the need for specialized equipment to carry out complex procedures meant that major surgery was concentrated mainly in urban areas in large hospitals, with rural hospitals limiting their work to minor procedures. Because surgical methods required rigid adherence to aseptic technique before, during and following surgery, nurses' knowledge and skills were needed to provide wound care applying the principles of asepsis to prevent infections of operative sites. Changing surgical dressings required significant amounts of nursing time, and these were tasks for which nurses were uniquely prepared. As time went on, the number of beds devoted to surgical patients in the large hospitals increased and surgical specialties developed rapidly. Thus, patients were assigned to nursing units on the basis of the nature of their surgery. Developments in surgery spawned a whole host of other specialized areas in hospital in the 1960s including operating room suites, recovery rooms, and intensive care units. Since low nurse-patient ratios were required in these specialized units, considerable numbers of registered nurses with the appropriate skills were needed to staff them.

A chronic shortage of registered nurses that began with the onset of hostilities during World War II when registered nurses signed up in large numbers for active service continued until the 1970s. Although the shortages lasted for a considerable period of time, they were most acute in the 1940s and 1950s and were still considered serious in the 1960s. The minutes of the 1946 Annual Meeting of the Alberta Association of Registered Nurses contains a number of references to the nursing shortage: "the shortage of nurses in Alberta remains acute without any immediate prospect of a rapid return to a normal adequate supply of nurses."[33] Two years later in 1948, Rae Chittick, President of the Canadian Nurses Association and a Past President of the Alberta Association of Registered Nurses, commented to members at the Annual Meeting of the Canadian Nurses Association that:

> When we met in Toronto two years ago, our greatest concern was the insufficient number of nurses in Canada to meet the increasing demands for their services. . . . In spite of the fact that hospital schools are graduating the biggest classes in their history, the actual shortage of nurses in institutions and in the public health fields remains about the same. In fact, a survey made by the Canadian Nurses' Association in 1947 showed that about 28 per cent more nurses were needed to staff existing services. . . . Canada needs about seven thousand more nurses to carry our existing services. It would seem that in the past two years we have accomplished nothing to alleviate the shortage of nursing personnel.[34]

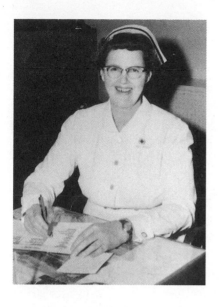

⭐ *Eileen Jameson, Director of Nursing Education, Calgary General Hospital School of Nursing from 1961 until the closing of the school a little over a decade later. (GAA NA–3195–2)*

The striking expansion of hospitals further to the development of national health insurance meant that the size of the nursing workforce needed became much larger. Chittick went on to say "Nurses across Canada continue to view the situation with growing apprehension. Hospital authorities are becoming more and more anxious and the public is both demanding and uneasy. One hears the question asked on all sides, 'What is being done to give us more nurses?'"[35] The minutes of the Annual Convention of the Alberta Association of Registered Nurses of 21 May 1952 indicate that Miss Eileen Jameson reported on problems at the Calgary General Hospital and the concern of the Calgary General Graduate Nurses Association about such issues as shortage of graduate staff, the use of students as staff, the inability of nursing students to attend classes, and the lack of a response to letters of complaint sent to the Medical Superintendent. The Council expressed its support of the position taken by the staff association.[36]

So desperate were nursing and hospital administrators for staff that they hired from categories of nurses who would not have been hired under normal circumstances. These categories included male nurses, those from ethnically diverse backgrounds and also married nurses.[37] Significant social pressure had prevented upper and middle class married women from working prior to World War II. A reference in the Minutes of the Annual Meeting of the Alberta Association of Registered Nurses of 1939 included a discussion of whether or not married nurses should be included in the District Associations. It was suggested that married nurses be allowed to vote on local matters only where it would not interfere with provincial or national policies. Another recommendation made in the same discussion was that married nurses be considered associate members of the Association. They would thus be permitted to vote on matters of local interest, but not on matters of policy.[38] Although married women were enticed into the workforce during the war years to fill the shortages caused by men who had left their civilian posts when they entered the armed forces, upon the cessation of hostilities there was a well-orchestrated campaign to encourage women to leave the workforce and return to their homes. This included the cancellation of national day-care programs in 1945, programs which had been implemented in 1942 to entice women into the workforce.[39] Since nursing was a field of work that was not considered to be suitable for men, the profession was perhaps affected in a less direct way by the bias against women in positions thought to belong more properly to men. Although a dramatic expansion in the hospital nursing workforce occurred in the postwar years, and although the participation rate of married women in the workforce remained generally low, married nurses were actively sought for nursing employment in hospitals in order to alleviate the acute shortages of nurses in the late 1950s and 1960s. Despite the fact that some nursing and hospital administrators were either sufficiently enlightened or thoroughly realistic about the shortage in hiring married women who were registered nurses to staff hospitals, continuing suspicion of married nurses even in the nursing workforce by nurses themselves remained. The minutes of the Annual Meeting of the Alberta Association of Registered Nurses of 1950 contained a reference to a question raised during discussion about private duty nursing "Should private duty *married* nurses whose husbands have an adequate income be placed on a separate call list?"[40] Further, there is some indication that married nurses may have required the permission of the Association to practise, since there is a reference in the minutes of the Annual Meeting of 1947 to a request to the Council by Mrs. Florence Powers who wished to obtain a temporary permit to nurse in Alberta as a married nurse. The need to make such a request was likely related to her graduation from a school outside Alberta, the New York City Hospital from which she graduated in 1913, following which she had done private duty in Calgary and Golden, British Columbia. It was also

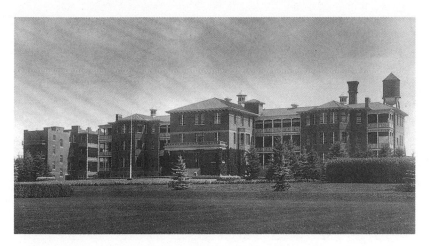

⊷ Provincial Mental Hospital, circa 1928, Ponoka. (PAA A.11, 837)

reported that she had operated a private hospital in Calgary from 1944 to 1946. Although there was gradual acceptance of married women in the workforce over time, it can be seen that even in a profession where married women were encouraged to enter the workforce to alleviate nursing shortages, there was reluctant acceptance of the legitimacy of their full participation in it.

Staffing questions were important ones for many hospitals over time and these became particularly acute during expansionary eras. In the mental health area, staffing shortages were key administrative issues and can perhaps be attributed to the location of facilities at a distance from population centres as well as to reluctant public acceptance of mental health as a legitimate and viable area of health care. The opening of the Provincial Mental Hospital at Ponoka in 1911 underscored a new era in the care and treatment of Albertans with mental health problems. This was an area that would continue to expand over time and Alberta Hospital, Edmonton was opened in 1923 on a site in a remote northeastern section of the city. When the Michener Centre opened in 1923 in Red Deer, originally as the Provincial Training School for Mental Defectives, there would be three institutions accepting mental health patients in the province. The transition in the care offered to patients from the outset of these institutions until the early 1950s was considerable. It was a complete change in approach and therapy from custodial care to active treatment attributed primarily to the introduction of the tranquilizing group of drugs.[41] The use of individual and group counseling for patients was an adjunct to medication, and soon the patients who had been kept in psychiatric institutions on a long-term basis began to be discharged from them following recovery. Records indicated that of those who were hospitalized for less than three months in a psychiatric facility in Alberta, 58 percent were discharged in 1956, while that figure had risen to 79 percent by 1967.[42]

Although staffing of the mental health hospitals would continue to be a problem, recognition of the field of mental health/psychiatric nursing was an important step forward in legitimizing this field of work for nurses. When nursing registration examinations were first instituted, psychiatric or mental health nursing was not considered a separate field of nursing. This is confirmed in the 1918 minutes of the Annual Meeting of the Alberta Association of Registered Nurses that refer to establishing a Board of Examiners under the Registered Nurses Act to test three areas of nursing practice: medical nursing, surgical nursing and obstetrical nursing.[43] It was not until 1933 that the question of whether mental health nursing should be considered to be a separate area was raised.[44] As the number of patients in these facilities and in the psychiatric units of general hospitals grew, mental health/psychiatric nursing became a legitimate area of practice. Because a broad range of knowledge was required to practise in this field competently and because mental health/psychiatric nursing was considered to be fundamental knowledge essential to all other areas of nursing, a separate examination was developed to ensure that nursing graduates were competent to practise in this area.

As it was recognized that there was much to be learned through theory and application of knowledge in clinical areas, affiliation programs in psychiatric/mental health nursing began to develop throughout the province. Schools of nursing sent their students for a period of concentrated practice primarily to the large facilities at Oliver in Edmonton and at Ponoka. Such a program began in the spring of 1956 for four Edmonton schools of nursing, the Edmonton General Hospital School of Nursing, the Misericordia Hospital School of Nursing, the Royal Alexandra Hospital School of Nursing and the University of Alberta School of Nursing.[45] In 1958, students from the Holy Cross Hospital and the Lethbridge Municipal Hospital began their affiliation at the Provincial Mental Institute at Ponoka, and in 1960 St. Joseph's Hospital in Vegreville and the Archer Memorial Hospital in Lamont joined the affiliation program.[46] Chronic shortages of staff members plagued these institutions, particularly Ponoka over the years, but there would be marked improvements in care and in nursing practice in mental health from the time when these institutions opened through the time when advances in drug therapy and in knowledge of mental illness occurred. By the 1980s, decreases in the patient census in the large facilities occurred due to changing approaches to treatment emphasizing community-based care and temporary care in units in active treatment hospitals near the patient's home when short-term hospitalization was required.

Winnifred Stewart was a pioneer in the care of mentally handicapped children. She was a registered nurse who had a son needing special care and a program designed for his needs. As no such programs were available, Stewart began doing "experimental teaching . . . and also medical experimental work"[47] as early as 1934 and formed the Edmonton Association for Retarded Children in 1953. Community-based programs were uncommon even in the 1960s for mentally handicapped children, and many children were institutionalized in such facilities as the Michener Centre in Red Deer for a number of years after that. The school Stewart established was designed to promote the health and social development of these children. It became a model that would be emulated around the province, and the country as community-based care and programming for mentally handicapped children became the dominant model. Stewart's nursing background and courageous determination led her from the role of citizen with broad understanding of the needs of the mentally handicapped to activist persistently presenting the needs and struggling to ensure appropriate educational and care facilities for mentally handicapped people.

CURRENT TRENDS IN HOSPITAL NURSING AND HEALTH CARE REFORM

The rapid expansion of the postwar years with its central focus upon the acute care hospital continued unabated through the 1980s, but came crashing to a halt in the 1990s. Costs had risen dramatically as new treatments and diagnostic tests had become available and under the existing health insurance arrangements, there were no limits to care and to treatment. Governments became increasingly concerned about rising costs and attempted to limit the operating grants given annually to hospitals from provincial and federal coffers. Although in Alberta, there was widespread renewal of hospital facilities and construction of new hospitals in the 1970s and 1980s, this policy was reviewed and reversed when the government of Premier Ralph Klein decided to downsize spending for health care by 25 percent following the provincial election in 1992. The cuts took place over a three-year period and were accompanied by regionalization whereby responsibilities of the provincial Department of Health were transferred to the 19 health regions. The regions became accountable for administering the health system in each of these jurisdictions. Major changes resulted and in the cities large hospitals were closed. In Edmonton, the Edmonton General and Charles Camsell Hospitals were closed, and the Misericordia and newly-constructed Grey Nuns Hospitals were dramatically reduced in size and designated community health centres. In Calgary the Grace Hospital, the Colonel Belcher Hospital and the Holy Cross Hospital were closed and a decision was made to close the Bow Valley Centre, the site of the first hospital in Calgary, the Calgary General Hospital. In Medicine Hat, Lethbridge, Grande Prairie and Fort McMurray, downsizing was very much in evidence with the closing of beds in existing institutions. By 1997, public outrage over problems in accessing hospital care had reached a peak, and along with a corresponding upturn in the economy led to decisions to open some of the beds that had previously been closed.

Nurses were dramatically affected by the cuts in health care. The health system in which nurses formed the largest professional group of employees was questioned not only in terms of its efficiency and effectiveness, but also in terms of whether health care needs justified its size. Decisions were made to close beds and reduce the number of nursing positions required for staffing. Thus, large numbers of nurses found that their positions had been declared redundant and that the opportunity for employment in a field that they had thought was secure had disappeared overnight. Approximately 8,275 employed registered nurses lost their jobs between 1992 and 1995; this figure represented 43 percent of active and employed registered nurses in the province.[48] Short of the Depression when large numbers of nurses were involuntarily put out of work across the country, seldom has the country or indeed any single Canadian province witnessed layoffs of professional nurses on such a large scale and with such speed. Loss of income and opportunity for employment in Alberta led to personal agony, family disruption and loss of morale amongst nurses, one of the largest as well as most highly educated groups of women in the workforce.

There was an associated move to carry on a great deal of what had gone on in hospitals previously in the community. The home became the centre for care to clients and day surgery became the modus operandi for those requiring surgical procedures ranging from cataract implants to those with masectomies. Those hospitalized for major surgery or serious illnesses were no longer allowed to stay for extended periods of time. Even those requiring heart bypass operations found themselves going from an intubated state to home within a few days. Public health nursing and home care nursing became central services as the focus of health care moved from the hospital to the community. Nurses who had previously been employed in the acute care sector now required community nursing knowledge and skills in order to move into the community where there were new opportunities. Although nurses had been recommending a shift in focus from hospital to community care for at least two decades, they were shocked to find that it was carried out with little or no planning and with lightning speed. Although the public and professionals alike have questioned the rationale for the cuts, Kevin Taft criticized the fundamental basis of Premier Klein's rationale for health spending cutbacks beginning in 1993 as being a deliberate attempt to delude the public into believing that health spending was out of control and responsible for the annual deficit and increasingly large public debt. He provided evidence to support his contention that the cuts were not necessary in the first place and that "it wasn't overspending on public programs that caused Alberta's debt to grow. Ordinary Albertans were blamed and punished for something they did not do."[49] One might add that Alberta's highly skilled nursing workforce was also punished for something it did not do.

Despite the difficult employment situation from 1993 onwards, nurses have been highly enterprising and versatile and have developed new skills in order to move to the community as opportunities arose in practice in that setting. It is likely that these trends will persist in the health care system of the future and that the skills of nurses will be essential to ensure that the chaos and confusion of the implementation of change will not be repeated. It is also likely that nurses will continue to be important colleagues and partners on the professional health care team in both hospital and community settings. The hospital of the future will be quite different from that of the past with the acuity level of patients being much higher than previously. As in the past, nurses will be a central health discipline providing care in hospitals, albeit the nature of their care will be much more specialized and intense.

First public health nurses in Alberta, 1918. Back row, left to right: Maude Davidson, Christine Smith (Director), Lillian Sargent. Front row, left to right: Elizabeth Clark, Gladys Thurston. (Royal Alexandra Hospital School of Nursing Archives, received on loan from AARN HN–15)

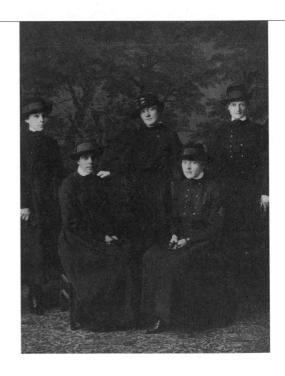

4

The Public Health Movement
and the Emergence
of Public Health Nursing

The emergence of health consciousness as a public good involved a gradual shift in thinking from health as a personal or private responsibility to health as a collective or community responsibility. At the outset, hospitals were a part of this shift in thinking because health was inherently associated with treatment or cure for disease, concepts that were not considered to be different from prevention at a time when the causes and transmission of infectious disease were not well understood J.J. Heagerty points out that the phrase "public health" had not been coined at the time of Confederation.[1] Public thinking had not made the transition to the need for measures of control and care at the community level.

Health care focused upon individual responsibility rather than the idea that it was a public responsibility. The British North America Act of 1867 did not place responsibility for health in the hands of the federal government, and this meant that authority for health was left to the provinces. Health was not thought to be a public responsibility or sufficiently important to be retained as a federal area of responsibility. Social consciousness about public versus private responsibility for health care and for promotion of health and prevention of disease developed over the period since Confederation and the public-private debate relative to health care continues to be controversial.

Changing public attitudes about responsibility for health were a product of fundamental changes in lifestyle occasioned by the move from agrarian to industrial economies in western society. Industrialization in eastern Canada led to overcrowding and high rates of disease, similar to what occurred earlier in Britain. As disease began to decimate the ranks of those living in ghetto conditions, the threat to the health and ultimately the productivity of society began to galvanize public opinion in favour of taking action to protect the health of the population. At issue were hygiene, nutrition, sanitation and the treatment and prevention of infectious disease. Governments were pressured at all levels to take action to support and promote the health of people and to prevent disease and conditions that would lead to the outbreak of disease.

Gradually the public accepted the idea that the devastating epidemics, which had ravaged society throughout the ages, were caused by infectious diseases whose spread could be controlled by proper hygiene and other preventive measures. A succession of scientific discoveries led to new knowledge of the causes and modes of transmission of devastating infectious diseases. Although Edward Jenner had discovered a vaccine that could prevent the development of smallpox in exposed individuals in 1796, the significance of his discovery in terms of universal vaccination did not occur quickly. It took over a century for smallpox vaccination to become widespread practice and it was not until the 1970s that the World Health Organization declared that the disease had been eradicated worldwide.[2] Since strategies for prevention were now possible, the new knowledge raised awareness of the need for public health measures to prevent and control infectious diseases in the community.

The home continued to be the primary setting for the care of the sick for many years beyond the turn of the century. At a time when little could be done for a patient in a hospital that could not be done in the home, the person who could afford care at home was loathe to seek care in hospital. Since hospitals had earlier been associated with poverty and poor quality of care, the shift from home to hospital was a transition that took place slowly and from the public standpoint, reluctantly. Gradually a separation occurred between "illness care" in the hospital and "health care" in the community. As advances occurred in knowledge and technology, hospitals assumed more importance and public acceptance of hospital care was matched by incremental increases in the level of public resources allocated to their support. Public health became increasingly defined as promotion of health and prevention of illness and was a domain in which nurses were front line professionals. Thus, nurses developed and extended knowledge of health promotion and became knowledgeable about the nature of health behaviour and facilitating changes in lifestyle to benefit health.

COMMUNITY ORGANIZATION TO PROMOTE HEALTH

The gradual recognition that the devastating impact of epidemic diseases could be reduced if not eliminated by preventive measures involving the individual as well as the community led to key measures involving changes in social organization and the passage of public health legislation. Because individuals who failed to meet their responsibilities could have a negative and devastating impact on the whole community, the case for authority vested in the community in certain aspects of health promotion and care was strengthened. Nevertheless, the progression to social responsibility for health was hesitant and extended over a considerable period of time. C.A Dawson and E.R. Younge noted that "The establishment of health and hospital services was essentially a twentieth century development. Until the late nineteenth century, illness was everywhere considered an individual or family responsibility,"[3] and in such matters government intervention was seen as intrusive. In society, the health and lives of individuals and families could be put at risk through the inadvertent or careless actions of other members of that society. Eventually the emerging population in Alberta had to come to terms with the need to institute regulations to ensure good health practices and sanitation to which all citizens were obliged to conform.

The first public boards of health in Canada were formed in 1832 "as a reaction to the advance of cholera creeping across the Atlantic."[4] Such boards were later formed on an ad hoc basis when a threat of an epidemic was imminent, and typically were disbanded after the emergency passed. By the early 1870s, the focus of ad hoc boards of health and governments turned to specific strategies to prevent spread of infectious diseases. Quarantine was the first of the defensive strategies to combat the spread of infectious disease and this was applied both to people and to objects with which they had been in contact. Quarantine stations were established on islands in the St. Lawrence where those coming to Canada were required to stay for two weeks to demonstrate they were not carrying an infectious disease.[5] The pitfalls of such an approach soon became apparent as the impossibility of ensuring that all arrivals passed through the quarantine stations became clear. Local isolation of infected persons and quarantine in their homes was also a strategy that was used widely into the 1940s to stop the spread of disease, again with limited success. Disinfection of trade goods that might carry infection was practised in local areas to prevent the transfer of organisms. Such a strategy also had inherent flaws as regulations were easy to ignore and it was impossible to monitor regulations involving such matters.

Sanitation was an ongoing hazard for the population as water supplies in most cities were unsafe because of contaminants dumped in bodies of water that were sources of drinking water. Garbage disposal presented hazards as rotting contaminants from material of human and animal origin were placed in sites too close to human habitation and without proper attention to safe disposal. Thus, there was a need to establish safe water supplies and ensure that sanitation was maintained as urban populations grew rapidly with the arrival of thousands of immigrants to settle in Alberta and elsewhere in the west. Towns and cities gradually developed regulations for safer disposal of wastes in order to keep the potential hazards to the population at a minimum. Evidence of organized community action to prevent the spread of infectious disease "began in western Canada with the appointment of a Territorial Board of Health in 1870. . . . as a public response to do something to counter a raging smallpox epidemic amongst the Indian tribes."[6] The incorporation of the town of Edmonton in 1892 was in part motivated by the desire to develop an organized community response to threats of epidemic disease and the need for regulations pertaining to health and sanitation.[7]

As the larger Alberta towns made the transition from a fur trading and agricultural economy in the decades prior to incorporation, the population multiplied many times over and there was a pressing need for health and sanitation standards to reduce hazards of disease from overcrowding and squalid living conditions. The threat of disease to citizens in the middle of the summer of 1892 when an outbreak of a virulent strain of smallpox in British Columbia appeared first in Calgary, then in Edmonton, caused the citizens of Edmonton to mobilize their resources to attempt to prevent an epidemic. This situation provided the impetus for the development of a by-law permitting the establishment of a permanent Board of Health, the first in what is now Alberta. The terms of the by-law permitted members of the Board of Health to inspect private premises and to order a cleanup if necessary by the occupant or owner.[8] The assistance of local constables could be enlisted to ensure that recalcitrant individuals followed the directives of the Board, and a Medical Officer of Health was empowered to order persons who were deemed to be a danger to others to be taken to hospital or elsewhere as long as such movement would not be hazardous to the person's life. A quarantine order could be placed upon homes where there were infectious diseases and disinfection of articles within could be required. Those who died of infectious diseases had to be buried immediately and outside city limits.[9]

After the establishment of Alberta as a province in 1905, a provincial officer of health was appointed the next year. This development was followed in 1907 by the passage of the first Public Health Act in the province and the formation of a provincial Board of Health, signaling new interest provincially in setting standards of health and sanitation for the mutual benefit of all citizens.[10] The Act also saw the province divided into health districts under local health boards. The provincial board was responsible for the operation of the local boards, the inspection of hospitals, jails and orphanages, as well as collecting vital statistics and any other matters relating to health that arose.[11] A new Public Health Act was passed in 1910 that extended the scope of operations of the Board of Health considerably and reduced the size of the board to three members. However, public health services were not extensive at this point in time so that there was considerable dependence upon other health agencies for assistance. Primary matters of concern to the Board were ensuring safe milk and water supplies because of the crucial nature of these in preventing disease. The Alberta Provincial Laboratory, established in 1907, offered a means of testing water and milk supplies to ensure these were safe, and they also engaged in the development of vaccines.[12]

Some smallpox vaccine began to become available in Alberta as early as 1870. However, use of the vaccine was evidently not widespread as outbreaks of smallpox of epidemic proportions were seen well into the second decade of the twentieth century. A mandatory smallpox vaccination program for children was passed by the Edmonton Board in 1908 and most children were vaccinated. Predictably, there was some opposition to this by a few who perceived the effects of vaccination to be potentially negative: "Rather than realizing this as a blessing many parents were openly hostile. They claimed that an injection of this dreadful germ would cause horrible illness and even death. The newspaper was swamped with stormy letters of protest."[13] In 1915 smallpox vaccination became a compulsory program for all school children in the province as it was clear that such a program was essential in reducing the morbidity and mortality toll in an area.[14] Successive epidemics of other infectious diseases including diphtheria, scarlet fever, tuberculosis and typhoid fever in the period between 1910 and 1914 led the Board of Health to recognize that much was needed in the area of prevention that could not be provided without the necessary resources. Typhoid and tuberculosis caused major health problems affecting the province in its early years. Typhoid swept the province many times and cases could be traced to the disposal of raw sewage in the streams and rivers. When a vaccine for the disease became available in 1913, it was offered free of charge to any municipality that required it. With the onset of World War I, new recruits for the Canadian forces from Alberta were given vaccines against smallpox and typhoid fever prior to their departure for the battlefront.[15]

Health education was increasingly seen as important, and a public campaign entitled "Swat the Fly" was initiated in 1911 in Edmonton to teach the populace about improving sanitary conditions in their homes to prevent the spread of scarlet fever. As there were no individuals readily available to do this, volunteers were sought, and in 1912 the Local Council of Women was asked to become involved in developing literature for school children to teach them basic hygiene and further the objective of improving home sanitation.[16] Nurses were the most numerous group of health workers, but they had not yet been employed in public health work, and nursing was not recognized as a profession with regulatory legislation until 1916.

WOMEN AND HEALTH IN THE COMMUNITY

The roots of public health nursing in Canada can be traced to the work of women in the settlements of New France in the seventeenth and eighteenth centuries. The concept of caring for the sick and the poor was central to Christian beliefs about the relationship between the body and the spirit and was reflected in the European missions in the new world. In particular, approaches to healing and Christianity employed by the Roman Catholic religious orders in New France were critical to their work with the native people of the colony established by their government in North America.[17] Women had been primary caregivers for the sick and needy in the community in France, and French religious orders, which attracted women of social standing to membership, offered nursing services in hospitals and in the community.[18] These services were developed in New France where "Intuitive concepts of community nursing may be recognized in the relationship between the persons giving and receiving care, in the attention given to people without community supports, and in the stark political and financial problems that had to be confronted."[19] Caring in the community for the sick and the poor had legitimately fallen within the scope of women's roles in society for centuries, and as hostels, hospitals and orphanages were developed, caregiving for those who required these services also became the domain of women.

The importance of class differentials in stimulating the development of modern public health services in Canada has been raised by Boutilier.[20] Philanthropy and helping were closely associated with the upper and middle class strata of society while the recipients of that assistance were clearly members of lower socioeconomic groups who needed basic essentials of life. From the time of Nightingale, the concept of selfless caring for the poor has been very much a part of nursing's ideology.[21] Women have been important in achieving societal goals involving philanthropic and altruistic objectives, a reflection of the belief that women had natural abilities to nurture and care for the young as well as those who were ill in the family. Consequently, philanthropy and altruism have been reflected strongly in nursing organizations. As nursing emerged as a profession for lay women in Canada from the 1870s onwards, mothering and domesticity remained the link from the home and the women's movement into the world of professional nursing.

Women's associations became key players in the public health crusade in Canada. When the National Council of Women approved the formation of the Victorian Order of Nurses in 1898, they embraced a professional standard of education for nurses in Canada. This standard recognized the need to acquire essential knowledge to practise nursing as well as the fundamental attributes of altruism, philanthropy and moral duty that nurses as women were believed to share with all women.[22] In the context of changing social roles for women, the transition from domesticity to professionalism was a process in which the acquisition of knowledge and increasing sophistication of practice were important in establishing and legitimizing nursing as a profession. As a result of the need for the service and satisfaction with its quality, nursing gained respect and legitimacy among the health disciplines and the general public. Although today the Grey Nuns are known primarily for their work in hospital nursing and administration, these nursing sisters are considered to be Canada's first visiting nurses. From the 1738 founding of their order in Montreal and continuing for more than a half century after their establishment in Alberta in 1859, they visited the sick in their homes. Until the discovery of antibiotics, health care centred largely on the care of those with infectious diseases that surfaced regularly in successive epidemics. Since there was no means of treating the physiological effects of these diseases until antibiotics became available, nursing offered the only possibility for alleviating symptoms and promoting comfort of the afflicted.

The worldwide epidemic of Spanish influenza following World War I in 1918 and 1919 drew attention to the importance of health in the well-being of the community and served as a catalyst for health consciousness on the part of women's groups.[23] Collins has referred to the United Farm Women's Association (UFWA) "as the social conscience of the farmers' movement in Alberta" and contended that it both reflected a mainstream of public opinion in Alberta and that its influence upon the United Farmers of Alberta (UFA) party policy platform was substantial.[24] Prior to the election of a United Farmers of Alberta Government in 1921, the party was able to exert sufficient influence upon the incumbent Liberal Government to pass legislation establishing public health services in the province. In the Speech from the Throne for the legislative session of 1919, the approach of the Liberal Government was clearly to support the establishment of preventive as well as curative services and assumption of public responsibility for the operation of health programs:

> This experience brings clearly to view the need of further health and sanitation laws and regulations throughout the province. To this end legislation will be brought before you for consideration, which will have the object of bettering the conditions generally common and in giving the matter of health administration a more prominent part in the public service of the province.[25]

Clearly the women in the UFWA presented a strong case for the development of health legislation and the impact was powerful in that the incumbent governments passed legislation for which the group had lobbied.

THE DEVELOPMENT OF PUBLIC HEALTH NURSING

Nurses were hired by the province to work in the public health field as early as 1916: "Early in 1916, the Department of Agriculture hired three women, two of whom were nurses" and they were "appointed to give courses in the Agricultural schools on personal and public health, and to lecture to Women's Institutes on health education."[26] Their work may have led to the organization of a Public Health Nursing Service in 1918 under the leadership of Miss Christine Smith as Director of Nursing and her staff of four nurses.[27] When The Public Health Nurses' Act came into force on 17 May 1919, a special register of public health nurses was established. The Act also contained details about the curriculum of a special course of study, duties of the public health nurse and regulations concerning the practice of midwifery in Alberta. When the first course in public health nursing was offered to the nursing staff members in the Public Health

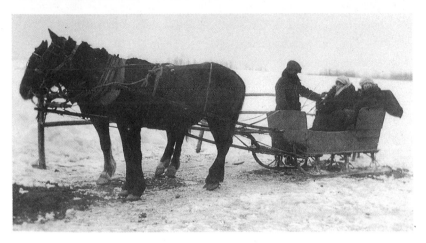

↜ *Kate Shaw Brighty starting out on a home visit at Onoway, pictured driving horses, circa 1919–1920. (AARN HN–28)*

Nursing Service by the University of Alberta in 1918, it became the first university course in nursing in Canada. A second course in 1919 produced eight graduates including Kate Shaw Brighty who later became the eighth President of the Alberta Association of Registered Nurses. These nurses were appointed to the public health nursing staff in June of the same year.[28] Later in 1919, Alberta became the second province to establish a separate Department of Public Health through the Public Health Act.[29]

The establishment of the Public Health Nursing Service occurred at a time when the Spanish influenza epidemic reached Alberta. Thus one of the first activities in which nurses became involved was caring for those who contracted the disease: "Miss Christine Smith, superintendent of public health nurses for the Province of Alberta, reports that since the beginning of the epidemic over two hundred nurses, V.A.D.'s and volunteers have been sent out through her department . . . to every part of the province."[30] However in an address to the United Farm Women's Association a few days later, she explained that "They had done little yet for child welfare, but she suggested that child welfare stations could be established in the country, where there might be clinics once a week, with a local doctor and a public health nurse in charge."[31]

Even though provincial initiatives to involve nurses in the growing public health program began in 1916, there is some evidence that municipalities

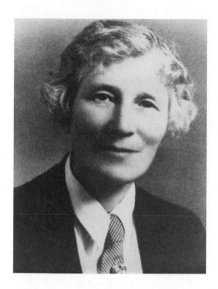

⟜ *Kate Shaw Brighty, Director of*
Public Health Nursing for the
Province of Alberta, 1929–1943,
pictured in public health
nursing uniform. (AARN P24)

hired nurses to develop and operate public health programs several years previously. Schartner reports that in Calgary "in July of 1913 a Pure Milk Station for babies was set up under Miss Mary Patterson . . . goal was to provide pure milk to undernourished infants. The babies were weighed each week and the mothers given advice on the care and feeding of their children."[32] Later that year an infant hygiene care home visiting program was initiated and visits made "to poorer families who could not afford the services of a trained nurse at the time of childbirth."[33] Because of mothers' needs for information about care of infants, the program was expanded to include visits to all new mothers as soon as possible after birth. This led to the establishment of a free well baby clinic under the direction of Miss Patterson. Following a move to drafty and thus rather unsatisfactory quarters in the General Hospital in 1921, Calgary city council directed that four regional clinics be set up. Unfortunately the facilities continued to be unsatisfactory and six months later, the central clinic was reestablished.[34]

The first provincial child welfare clinic was established in Edmonton in 1920 by Christine Smith, Director of the Public Health Nursing Branch[35] to support the health of children and to give mothers assistance in promoting health and preventing illness in their children. Blanche Emerson was appointed supervisor of the Edmonton clinic, a position she retained for 26 years. Similar clinics were subsequently opened in other centres includ-

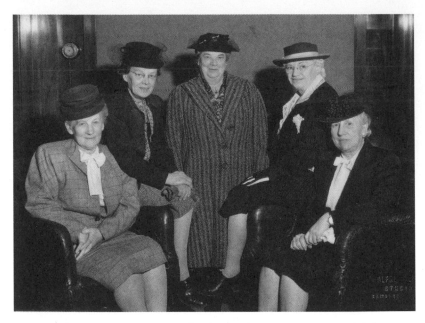

↬ *Public health nurses Marion Lavell, Olive Watherston, Amy Conroy, Isabel Hawkes and Blanche Emerson pictured at the Public Health Nursing Spring Conference, April 1946 when they celebrated 25 years of public health nursing service. (AARN HN–16)*

ing Medicine Hat, Drumheller and Vegreville with Blanche Emerson's assistance. Marion Lavell, a graduate of the Toronto General Hospital, and the second course in public health nursing offered by the University of Alberta in 1919, reported that at first the public had difficulty understanding the fundamental nature of public health:

> People didn't have an idea of what baby clinics were, or what they were for, and they needed them very badly at that time because doctors didn't have time and didn't have any public health training. Theirs was curing illness and ours was trying to prevent it, you see. Giving inoculations for diphtheria and smallpox and telling them how to feed. For a long time we had to go out and make the feedings for them.[36]

In these clinics, medical and dental care for children were provided and nurses carried out school health inspections and immunization of

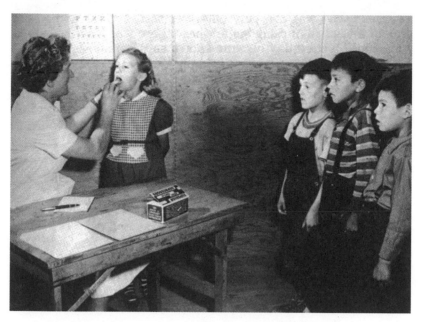

❧ *School health examinations in Slave Lake, 1953. (From* These Were Our Yesterdays, *p. 181)*

preschool children. The supervising nurses of the clinics were also responsible for inspecting private nursing homes and foster homes for infants. While they were provincial employees, other public health nurses comprising the staff of each clinic were employed by the city in which the clinic was located. Because of the prevalence of infectious disease, the health education aspects of the work of the clinics assumed considerable importance.[37] Public health nurses were front line professionals in all of the public health centres that were developed in many regions of the province.

Mary Watt joined the staff of the City Hall public health clinic in Calgary in 1928 when she was asked to relieve for a staff member. Interviewed in 1973, she spoke of the initial reluctance of people to seek inoculations and vaccinations: "In those days people weren't very anxious to be inoculated and it wasn't until after the wars that it was taken for granted that everybody should be done." She went on to explain that "people hadn't been used to it [immunization], you see. They didn't like the inoculations. Some of them thought it was poison."[38] Such views are still heard today when new vaccines become available for serious infectious diseases. Miss Watt spoke of the appointment of the first public health nursing staff to serve in Calgary in 1922 including Miss Lavell who was loaned to the city by the provincial government and Miss Effie Craig who was hired by the Calgary health department "to establish infant and preschool clinics."[39] Reflecting on her 34-year career with the Calgary health department, Miss Watt spoke of the tremendous effort required on the part of personnel to establish a wide range of public health services in a growing urban area such as Calgary.

Recognition of the high infant mortality rate in the 1920s led to the establishment of public health programs staffed by nurses throughout the province. These programs have continued to be a mainstay of health departments throughout the province to the present time. The occurrence of polio epidemics in the 1930s led to the involvement of health departments in attempts to prevent outbreaks. Bans on public gatherings and closing schools were variants of the quarantine measures that had been used with diphtheria and scarlet fever epidemics. However, these measures were largely abandoned by the 1950s in recognition of their limited value in preventing transmission of the disease. When Alberta became a site for trials of Salk vaccine in 1954, public health clinics were held to immunize children with the new vaccine.[40] The civil defence movement of the 1950s was an outgrowth of the Cold War and the development of a variety of nuclear weapons. This engaged the attention of public health authorities, including nurses, for about two decades. Many nurses received training at the federal centre in Arnprior and there was also public education for responding to nuclear warfare. Beginning in the 1960s, public health nurses became involved in other areas including venereal disease clinics where treatment and prevention of gonorrhea and syphilis were primary issues. These clinics were eventually referred to as sexually transmitted disease clinics and assumed new importance with the advent of new sexually transmitted diseases, such as that caused by the human immunodeficiency virus. In the 1970s public health nurses began to give birth control information to those who requested it. Also, a more comprehensive approach to preschool screening was initiated and nurses did assessments of vision and hearing, behaviour and physical and developmental status of all school age children.[41]

Voluntary Organizations and
the Development of Public Health Nursing

The outbreak of war in 1914 occasioned the enlistment of large numbers of young military recruits, and health emerged as an issue when a large proportion of new recruits were declared not fit to serve.[42] The death toll in the war also drew attention to the value of life and the need to take steps to preserve it. Following the war when the League of Red Cross Societies encouraged its member nations to facilitate the cause of public health worldwide, the Canadian Red Cross Society developed a peacetime program that would have substantial impact upon the health of people.[43] One of their objectives was to prepare nurses for public health work and grants were given to universities across the country in 1920 to develop courses in public health nursing.[44] Although it was reported that the University of Alberta was one of five universities receiving funding, the University could not confirm that it received a Red Cross grant for public health nursing courses.[45] The certificate courses in public health nursing of two and later three months duration, were offered in 1918, 1919 and again in 1921, and prepared public health nurses for the new roles opening up in their field. These courses began prior to the Red Cross grants and led to the development of a degree program in nursing at the University in 1923–24, and public health or community health nursing, as it is more often termed today, continued to be an essential component of degree programs at the University. With the establishment of a nursing program at the University of Calgary in 1969 and at the University of Lethbridge in 1979, public health nursing education was extended to growing centres of higher education in the south central and south areas of the province. As acute care shifted from home to hospital over the course of the twentieth century, community nursing gradually became defined as prevention of illness and promotion of health, even though acute care continued to be offered in the home by visiting nurses.

The Victorian Order of Nurses was an organization established in 1898 through the determined efforts of Lady Ishbel Aberdeen, wife of the Governor-General of Canada. This voluntary organization offered the services of its nurses in areas of home nursing, maternal and child health and development of cottage hospitals primarily in frontier areas where these

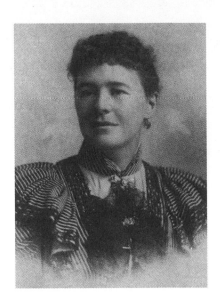

↝ *Lady Aberdeen, Founder and first President of the Victorian Order of Nurses for Canada. (From* The Victorian Order of Nurses for Canada 50th Anniversary, 1897–1947, *used with permission of* VON)

were needed. In Alberta this included five sites, all of which were transferred to the jurisdiction of other organizations after the work had been initiated.[46] A VON branch was established in Edmonton in 1907 under the leadership of the organization's first president, Emily Murphy, and with one nurse, a Miss McCulloch on its staff. The local nurses' association opposed the establishment of the Calgary branch, but a determined group of local women including Lady Lougheed as its first president persisted and the Calgary branch was initiated in 1909.[47] VON programs were planned according to the needs in a particular community and included both preventive and restorative approaches to meeting the health needs of their clients. The VON initiated prenatal classes in Edmonton and the Board of Health became involved in 1965, after which time the VON withdrew from offering this service. For decades in Calgary and in Edmonton, the VON was the sole provider of visiting nursing services. However, in both cities, the official public health agencies took over responsibility for visiting nursing services or home care. This process began in the 1970s and by the 1980s, the VON had withdrawn from offering visiting nursing services in the large urban centres in the province. However they have continued with programs to meet different needs including the meals on wheels program that began in 1968, adult day care centres, work in the crisis shelters for abused women and their children, and blood pressure and foot care clinics.

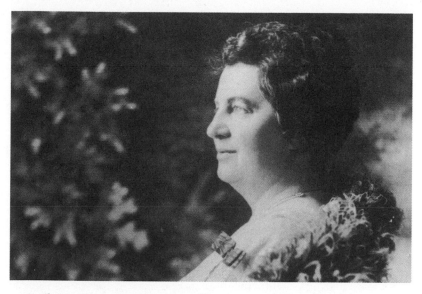

⤳ *Emily Murphy, founding President of the Victorian Order of Nurses
Edmonton branch in 1907. (City of Edmonton Archives EA–10–1970)*

VALUING PUBLIC HEALTH NURSES' WORK

The systematic neglect of the roles played by nurses in documented histories of health care organizations is evident in local histories of hospitals
and health agencies. This reflects values prevalent in society over time and
is not unique to the health field. However, the greater prominence given in
historical records to work performed by men over that of women seems
curiously inappropriate when viewed through the lens of contemporary
standards. Clearly there is a relationship here to nursing as a profession
that has historically attracted women to its ranks. With a few notable
exceptions, many of the histories of health care organizations focus upon
the work of physicians associated with the organization over time with little or no mention of those in other professions who provided some of the
primary services offered by the organization. Since nurses were key players
in nearly all of health agencies, the omission of discussion of their work is
somewhat striking. The status accorded physicians in the histories of organizations would seem to parallel their status in the health care field. As
Meryn Stuart has pointed out: "By 1900, physicians had ensured their control over hospitals, and were sending their patients there. They also moved

to dominate the field of public health."[48] In doing so they became the superiors of nurses and policy decisions were vested in their realm of responsibility. The manner in which gender conflict in public health in the 1920s became manifest and approaches which public health nurses in Ontario took to coping with it has been explored by Stuart.[49] It is likely that similar patterns developed in Alberta, but no research that might substantiate this has yet been undertaken. Stuart's analysis stands as a signal piece of historical research on roles, relationships and conflict in public health nursing and provides a unique description of how public health nurses functioned with considerable independence in an environment essentially controlled by medicine.

Although the undervaluing of women's work has undoubtedly contributed to a dearth of literature about public health nurses and nursing, it may also have been a factor in their relatively low profile in public health work and indeed the invisibility of nursing and nurses even though nurses were the front line professionals who carried out public health programs at the community level in health agencies. There are other barriers to documenting and discussing the role and contributions of nurses in public health and some of the factors referred to may well have influenced these as well. Lack of records and other sources of primary information about health department operations and in particular the work of public health nurses are serious problems for those who attempt to pursue historical questions of interest pertaining to public health and public health nursing. Even though histories of organizations and exploration of historical questions of professional work are undertaken by a variety of writers, the level of understanding of the mission of the organization and the work performed by its professional nurses has been seen to be critical to an objective and balanced portrayal of the organization.

Public health nursing clearly grew out of the charitable and philanthropic work of middle and upper class women with the sick poor in the community. As public health nursing became identified as a unique and specialized area of nursing, women's groups championed its legitimacy and stood up to opposition of the medical profession and to political parties to support the development of public health nursing services. The services of public health nurses were seen as vital to the health of the community in a society that was repeatedly devastated by epidemics of a variety of infectious diseases for which there were no effective treatments. Prevention through immunization and health education became accepted as the most useful approach to preventing the spread of infectious diseases and public health nurses were seen as the front-line professionals who could most successfully carry out public health programs targeted to these objectives. Nurses employed to carry out public health responsibilities have carried out their responsibilities with distinction over three-quarters of a century. As the community is emerging as the setting in which both major curative and preventive services will be offered in the future, the challenges are new and perhaps even greater than they have been in the past.

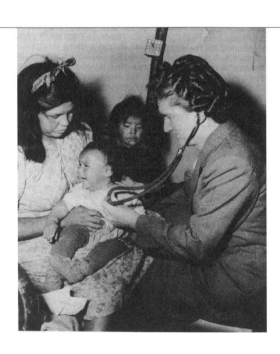

↬ *Laura Attrux making
a home visit and
providing treatment in
Slave Lake, 1953.
(From* These Were
Our Yesterdays, *p. 178)*

5

District Nursing on the
Alberta Frontier

District nurses left a unique and historic legacy on the Alberta frontier. Their practice was distinctive because they were legally permitted to function in a range of advanced roles including midwifery and emergency care further to Section 49 of the Public Health Nurses Act which came into force on 17 May 1919:

Notwithstanding the provisions of The Medical Profession Act, or any other Act or Ordinance, it shall be lawful for any nurse, who has taken a course in obstetrics, and who has obtained the consent of the Minister, to practice midwifery in any designated portion of the province where

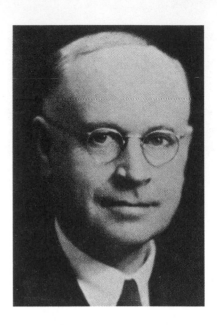

in the opinion of the Minister the services of a registered medical practitioner are not available, and to charge such fees as the Provincial Board of Health may decide are fair and reasonable.[1]

Health services offered by district nurses were widely accepted and endorsed by Albertans in an era when the population was small and scattered and services sparsely distributed. The primary impetus for the establishment of the District Nursing Service in Alberta came from women's groups who argued that there was an urgent need to assist women at childbirth at a time when health services had not been established throughout the province.[2] By virtue of the fact that no other health care was available to people in these areas of the province, district nurses became involved in areas of health other than midwifery and public health. In modern terms, district nurses could be described as nurse practitioners or specialists in advanced nursing practice. According to Dr. Malcolm Bow, Deputy Minister of Public Health in 1935, district nurses were:

> stationed in frontier communities in which neither medical nor hospital facilities of any kind are available. Some of these nurses are located in districts sixty miles from the nearest doctor or hospital. A district nurse

is often required in the course of her duties to assume the role of doctor, dispenser, bedside nurse and any other role the occasion may require. Her duties are, however, chiefly in maternity and first-aid work.[3]

He went on to say that "Such district nursing calls for women of courage, skill and sound physique, as well as a high degree of initiative and devotion to service."[4] The work of district nurses was highly valued in communities and plaques and other forms of recognition presented to these nurses in recognition of their professional contributions attest to the regard in which they were held.

THE DISTRICT NURSING MOVEMENT

In 1859, the same year the Grey Nuns established their first mission in Alberta, William Rathbone of Liverpool, a wealthy philanthropist developed a system of visiting nursing that served as a model for the development of district nursing in Britain. William Rathbone's efforts had the support of Florence Nightingale and offered an innovation in community care that influenced other countries. Nightingale recognized the importance of the environment in promoting health and preventing illness in an era when the industrial revolution dramatically transformed urban living. The slums, which developed in factory neighbourhoods, housed labourers who could not afford the services of the physicians of the time. These people needed health education, care and treatment, and the risks for childbearing women and young children were particularly great as slum conditions led to poor hygiene and nutrition and the spread of communicable diseases. Visiting nurses in the community offering a range of services to factory workers and their families offered positive and effective solutions to the considerable health needs of this group of people.

Linkages between the development of visiting nursing, health education and the industrial revolution are further supported by developments that took place in North America towards the end of the nineteenth century. Formal public health initiatives were first established in the industrialized areas of the continent. As in Britain, the initial intent was often to provide nursing care to the poor in their homes. For example, in 1877 the Women's Branch of the New York City Mission employed a nurse for precisely that purpose.[5] Significantly, during the 1880s and 1890s several visiting nursing societies were founded in highly industrialized urban areas in the United States. Early nursing leaders such as Lillian Wald and Adelaide Nutting espoused the cause of public health nursing and its importance as a focus of nursing practice. By the turn of the twentieth century, public health nursing in the form of district nursing had spread throughout the western world. In fact, the proceedings of the Jubilee Congress of district nursing held at Liverpool in May 1909 revealed that Australia, Britain, Canada, Finland, Germany, Holland, Norway, Sweden, Switzerland and the United States had developed various forms of district nursing.

Major social upheavals often tend to focus attention on the importance of health. World War I was such a period of time and in Alberta as elsewhere the war brought to light issues buried in complacency. The general health of the populace was one important issue that arose when young men's fitness for war service was examined. That many were declared unfit for service came as a profound shock to society. Further, the loss of so many young lives at war was further troubling as the impact on the future of entire families was a powerful one. A third coincidental factor was the impact of the worldwide epidemic of Spanish influenza in 1918–19 which took a great toll in an era when drugs to combat secondary bacterial infections were simply not available. In the Alberta legislature, the Speech from the Throne in 1919 reflected the demand for change:

> The war imposed a strain upon the extended and thinly staffed social services of the province. . . . A growing shortage of doctors, dentists and nurses eliminated many . . . of the scanty services that most had only begun to enjoy. War is a great solvent of old certainties, political as well as social, economic as well as moral . . .[6]

THE EFFORTS OF WOMEN IN ESTABLISHING PUBLIC HEALTH NURSING SERVICES

The case for social reform was argued articulately, persistently and ultimately successfully by national and local women's groups where their efforts led to the development of an infrastructure to support public health nursing. The importance of the health of mothers and children became the focus of concern for many of these groups, as these were powerful issues of the time. Suzanne Buckley has noted that "These efforts to reduce infant mortality were in fact part of the general progressive trend to clean up cities. An important factor in this trend was the establishment of social services designed to control urban ills" and it was thought that the institution of public health measures "would keep at bay the moral and physical decay that threatened the existing social order."[7] As the American Public Health Association celebrated its half century jubilee in 1921, Lavinia Dock, noted nursing historian and public health nurse, stated "Public health nursing, as it is to-day, in its still incomplete phase of development, has expanded slowly and naturally from that neighbourly office of visiting and attending the sick. . . ." She went on to note that it had moved in different directions: "As modern science has transformed the medical art, visiting nurses have become infused with a hopeful zeal for a corresponding transformation in the crude adjustments of our physical and social mechanism of living, such as may set free the higher spiritual forces."[8]

Women's associations were key players in the public health crusade in Alberta and across the country. Local organizations of Women's Institutes and women's wings of political parties such as the United Farm Women's Association requested better distribution of health care services particularly in remote areas where women had little opportunity to have assistance during childbirth. Irene Parlby, who was president of the UFWA in 1917, worked tirelessly to promote the health of mothers and children:

> Is it not right that we should endeavour to adjust conditions that every child born in the world shall at least have a fair chance of a healthy normal life; that every mother shall have the care *which is her right*, when she takes that journey into the valley of the shadow . . . ? *Is it more than justice* that every child of school age should be given a square deal in his battle for life . . . ?[9]

Infant and maternal mortality statistics at the time tended to justify the need for nursing assistance for women relative to childbirth and the care of infants and children. In 1921 the maternal mortality rate in Alberta was higher at 6.7 per 1,000 live births than in any other province with the exception of Quebec.[10] Interestingly infant mortality statistics in Alberta for 1921 were lower than in all other provinces at 56.5[11] per 1,000 live births. Notwithstanding the relative position of the Alberta statistics for maternal and infant mortality, they would be considered horrific by today's standards. Mrs. Parlby next suggested that health care was not only the right of the individual, but also the duty of government to provide.[12] The United Farmers of Alberta was a political party that had a profound influence on the liberal government in power until 1921. Paul Collins has stated that while the UFA and the UFWA jointly pressed for health reforms, "it was the UFWA which drafted most of the content" and that the UFWA was the social *conscience* of the farmers' movement in Alberta."[13] Irene Parlby, who was appointed to the cabinet in the UFA administration of 1921, stated that "at the end of the war, the UFA could not yet take direct political action, but a working understanding existed with the Liberal Administration."[14] The establishment of the Department of Health, the Public Health Nursing program and district nursing attest to the "strategic role played by the farm women prior to 1921."[15]

The efforts of the National Council of Women of Canada were also instrumental in arguing the case for urgently needed improvements in health care at the national level. Lady Ishbel Aberdeen, the wife of the Governor General of Canada, had the opportunity to travel widely across the country in the course of her husband's efforts to meet the people of Canada. She was particularly impressed by the rationale put forward by women in isolated areas of the west asking for health support during child-birth and with family health problems which had to be faced with very lit-tle assistance or support up to that point in time. When she assumed the presidency of the National Council of Women, she set out to seek solutions to the problems faced by women.

Perhaps Lady Aberdeen's most noteworthy accomplishment in the area of public health nursing was the creation of the Victorian Order of Nurses in 1897 patterned on the British district nursing system. Its establishment was no mean feat, for there was vociferous opposition from physicians, a powerful group that had to be convinced to support the scheme. Significantly, the Victorian Order nurses in the east embarked on tubercu-losis prevention and, from the outset, provided services to the poor of the cities. Meanwhile in the west, where curative services were not as well developed as in the east, the Victorian Order founded cottage hospitals in five sites, all of which were transferred to the jurisdiction of other organiza-tions after the work had been established.[16] A VON branch was developed in Edmonton in 1907. However when a branch for Calgary was proposed in 1908, John Gibbon reported that it was "opposed by [the] local Nurses'

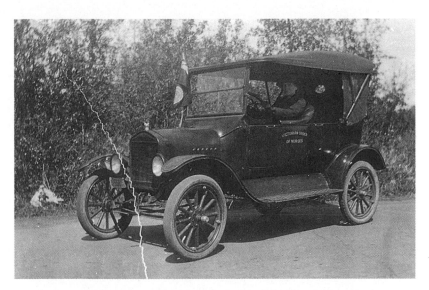

↪ *The first* VON *automobile, 1921, Victorian Order of Nurses, Edmonton.*
(AARN P440)

Association insisting that the VON would deprive them of a livelihood".[17] Opposition was overcome and the branch was established there the next year, 1909. VON visiting nursing services were thus available in the two major urban centres in Alberta when the cries from women's groups for health care were beginning to be heard. Since VON was well positioned to expand its operations to offer district nursing, the questions arises as to why it did not become part of the effort to develop midwifery services for women offered by district nurses since "midwifery had been proposed as a job for the order at the time of its founding."[18] There is some evidence that the VON removed itself from offering midwifery for some of the same reasons that prevented organized nursing from becoming involved in facilitating and promoting nurse midwifery by district nurses on the frontier.

Controversy Erupts Over District Nursing

Organized nursing was not involved in or in support of the movement to establish district nursing in Alberta. The minutes of the Alberta Association of Graduate Nurses (AAGN), revealed that it was preoccupied with ensuring that nurses who were practising were registered and with the development of standards for the registration of nurses. The AAGN had strong feelings about the establishment of midwifery in the province and at the meeting of 22 May 1917, the minutes refer to the appointment of L.M. Edy and L.C. Armstrong to serve as delegates to the Canadian National Association of Trained Nurses (CNATN) annual convention in Montreal in June, 1917 and to speak out "to disclaim any responsibility in regard to midwives being placed in the West."[19] The CNATN endorsed this position at their convention and opposed the practice of midwifery by nurses in isolated areas of the country as follows:

> That each province be asked to appoint a strong committee to interview the Government of each province, stating:
> (A) That the Canadian National Association of Trained Nurses considers the introduction of midwives into the sparsely settled districts as inadequate to meet the needs of the people.
> (B) That the nurses of Canada are willing to supply these needs if the Government supplies the hospitals in the needy districts and assures a living wage to the nurses.[20]

At the AAGN meeting of 7 May 1918 "A petition was read from the Calgary Association of Graduate Nurses asking that the Alberta Association of Graduate Nurses become affiliated with the United Farmers of Alberta."[21] The issue was put aside as "It was considered that this was too important a matter to be settled without an investigation as to the value or otherwise to the Association of such affiliation, and on motion it was decided to lay the petition on the table until further information was procured."[22] At a meeting two months later, members of the Council indicated that "they could not see from the information at hand that any particular benefit would accrue to the Association by such affiliation."[23] They further achieved consensus that "affiliation with the Women's Institutes might be of considerable help to the Association as it was stated that this organization had a membership of about 8,000 of the women of the province taken from all classes."[24] However, the issue of affiliation with women's groups was a troubling one over time, and the minutes of the meeting of 14 May 1920 reported that Miss Winslow was to "discuss the affiliation with other women's organizations at the national convention in Fort William."[25] The Association opposed the district nursing plan and the development of mid-

wifery services in the following resolution passed at the meeting of
16 October 1923:

> Resolved that we, as an association of registered nurses, realizing the
> needs of our outlying and sparsely settled districts, feel that we cannot
> feel that we should assume such responsibilities. We would respectfully
> recommend that small hospitals be established in the outlying districts
> with modern equipment and staffed by qualified nurses with special
> training in obstetrical work, and that some arrangement be made by
> which properly qualified medical men might be attached to these dis-
> tricts.[26]

Even though district nursing was established in 1919 and grew steadily from
that time on, it was clear that the AARN did not change its position and that
there was some animosity between women's groups and the organization.
This culminated in resolutions passed at the 1925 AARN convention:

> That the Association withdraw from affiliation with the National
> Council of Women, the Social Service Council of Canada, and the Child
> Welfare Council of Canada.

and

> That we approve of the action of the executive of the national
> Association in withdrawing their membership in these various social
> Service Organizations.[27]

The quest of Marion Cran, a trained maternity nurse from Britain, who
"came to Canada at the invitation of the federal government to check out
the lay of the land for British female immigrants"[28] was one in which she
identified the need for midwifery services for women on the Canadian
prairies. Moved by the hardships women experienced in childbirth where
there were no provisions for assistance for them, she travelled to each of the
western provinces to encourage the development of services under the auspices of government. In Alberta she met with the Minister of the Interior as
well as Premier Rutherford to attempt to persuade them to develop a cadre
of nurses with midwifery training under the auspices of the Government in

order to give assistance in childbirth to the settlers' wives.[29] She said: "Further I asked if it were not possible that such a body of maternity specialists be attached to the existing order of Victorian Nurses, acting as an endowed Government body, but incorporated with the present order."[30] The ideas and proposals she presented to the governments of each of the western provinces were ignored. She then decided to go to Ottawa and approach the Victorian Order of Nurses "determining to lay the matter before the committee and ask for consideration at its hands."[31] She states:

> I saw the committee and detailed my scheme once more, and knew directly I spoke to the matron that I had met prejudice. The pity of the whole position is this, that while the fully trained nurse is more than a trifle scornful of maternity work, she is violently antipathetic to the "half-baked" sister, the midwife who has taken only the short maternity training and is not qualified for all branches of nursing. I have noticed that prejudice over and over again, and always with resentment. They might scorn the maternity nurses to the crack of doom and welcome if they were willing to do the work themselves, but they are not. They oppose the idea of giving maternity nurses a definite status, and themselves leave the work undone. Meanwhile the mothers suffer. Any scheme for alleviating the distress, which none denied, was unwelcome to the Victorian Order of Nurses.[32]

It was interesting that within the VON, the issue was seen as one of maintaining standards, and Chief Superintendent Mary Ard MacKenzie

> told the gathering at the annual meeting [of 1917] that skilled, modern nurses were essential for the West, and that it was inconceivable that VON would offer substandard service in selected parts of the country. Certainly, she said, the situation was serious; but it was better to begin as one meant to go on, and lay a solid foundation for the future.[33]

This was in opposition to some members of the Board who wanted to "recruit British-trained midwives, through VON, for the West."[34] Controversy over the "practice of midwifery, which had been proposed as a job for the Order at the time of its founding"[35] would result in the resignation of the Chief Superintendent Mary Ard MacKenzie who "resigned, staying only long enough for a replacement to be found."[36] However, the nurses on staff maintained the position she had taken against midwifery becoming a major program of the VON through the boards of their local branches and the proposal to offer midwifery did not go forward at that time.[37]

THE WORK OF DISTRICT NURSES

Alberta was only the second province to establish a separate Department of Public Health through the Department of Public Health Act passed in 1919; New Brunswick was the first.[38] The passage of this legislation followed the establishment of the Public Health Nursing Service in the Department of the Provincial Secretary in 1918, and the passage of the Public Health Nurses Act early in 1919. Through the latter a special register of public health nurses was established. According to Mary Conlin Sterritt, one of the first two district nurses appointed in 1919:

> The history of district nursing in Alberta begins on October 15, 1919 when the first two District Nurses were sent to the Peace River Country by the Department of Public Health, in answer to urgent petitions from women's organizations in the area. These were visiting nurses with special training in obstetrics. Stationed in districts where there were no doctors or hospitals, these nurses were qualified to accept full responsibility for all cases of illness, emergencies and maternity cases, the latter being the most important aspect of their work.[39]

She went on to describe a number of aspects of her work in very isolated areas: "During the flu epidemic there were forty cases of flu in my district. Never before or since have I appreciated my bed so much. I was constantly 'on the go'. It was like a relay race; only the nurse was the only thing not 'relayed'. One would hear where I was and pick me up to take me a bit farther on, and so far into the night."[40] The potential dangers of the circumstances in which these nurses found themselves were very real threats which were always there. Miss Conlin recalls one such situation:

> I remember one night I had a call many miles to the north of my district where fences or road allowances did not exist. The man who came for

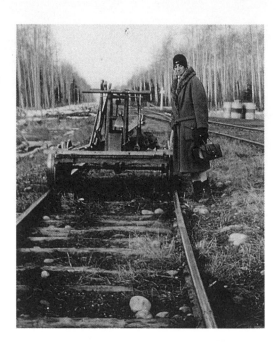

✎ *Miss Mary Conlin at Jarvie about to leave for a case by means of a railway hand car, circa 1920.* (AARN HN–3)

me had been able to find the trail out, but on his way back with me, the road vanished and we seemed to be in a desert of snow.

He "gave the horses the rein" and after wandering for a considerable distance in circles, their feet at last struck the ruts and this was all they needed. They immediately got on the road that took us to the patient's home.[41]

The provincial travelling clinics emerged from a clinic organized in the summer of 1923 by Olive Watherston, a district nurse for a small district nursing station at Halcourt southwest of Grande Prairie. She made arrangements for a physician to come to Halcourt in order to allow children who needed tonsils removed to have this done at a clinic in the town. The arrangement was successful and led to the development of another such clinic the following year, and then to the organization of similar clinics on a provincial basis beginning in the late summer of 1924. These clinics had a somewhat broader focus than the original clinic, offering physical and dental examinations as well as minor surgical procedures in many centres over the summer period. The clinics provided a means of offering health care to the rural population that was scattered over a wide geo-

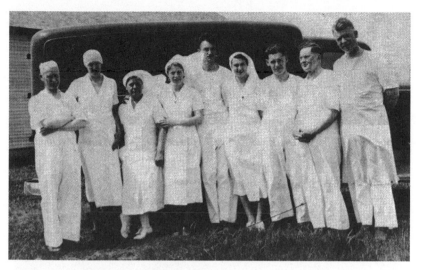

↬ *Provincial travelling clinic staff of 1935. Left to right: Dr. Heacock (Dentist), Dr. Owens (Anesthetist), Miss Watherston (Charge Nurse), Laura Allyn (Surgical Nurse), Thornton Wood (one of the drivers and a fifth-year medical student), Mrs. Caffrey (Nurse), Arch. McEwan (other driver and a dental student), Dr. Gilchrist (Dentist), Dr. Bridge (Surgeon). (From* These Were Our Yesterdays, *p. 68)*

graphical area and served people who often travelled considerable distances over difficult roads. According to Jane Stewart "The travelling clinic was very popular and provided a much needed service in the outlying parts of the province from 1924 to 1931 and 1934 to 1942, and never had a fatality."[42] Over this period of time many thousands of examinations were conducted and treatments given to children and adults who needed care. Local organizing committees involved school board members and women's groups who made arrangements for the selection and preparation of a suitable site for the clinic. Public health nurses came to the centres which had requested visits by the travelling clinic to meet with organizing committees "giving them instructions regarding the necessary arrangements for the clinic."[43] During this preparatory visit, the nurse "also made a preliminary examination of all school children and recommended to the clinic all children who should be examined by the doctor and dentist."[44] Isabella Thyne Ranche recalled her work as a district nurse "visiting schools, lumber camps, delivering babies, pulling teeth, stitching cuts inflicted by saws and

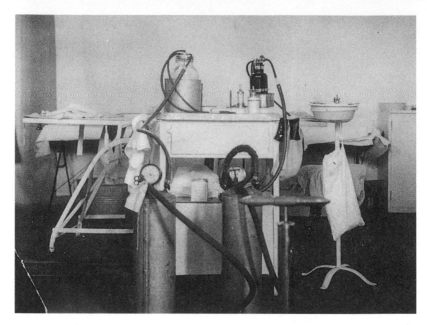

↝ *Makeshift operating room set up for a travelling clinic.* (AARN HN–18)

axes, setting bones, treating general illness and disease and giving inoculations" and

> In May 1927 came another challenge. I was asked by Miss Clark, our Public Health Nursing Director, to join the Travelling Clinic for the summer. . . . We travelled to all the northern towns that did not have their own medical assistance, and as far south as the Alberta-Montana border. I was sent ahead to meet the school trustees who kindly transported me from one school district to another by wagon or buggy, or an old Ford which frequently became bogged down in the mud.[45]

Marion Lavell, a graduate of the Toronto General Hospital School of Nursing came to Alberta following service with the Canadian Army Medical Corps during World War I. She completed the course in public health nursing at the University of Alberta after which she was assigned to hold clinics, set up exhibits at country fairs and give health lectures in many locations of the province. In recalling her journeys to northern Alberta to give clinics, she facetiously referred to the journey on the E.D.

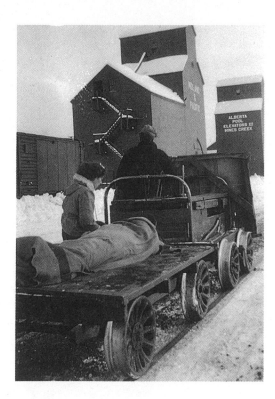

◦ Taking patient by speeder to Fairview.
(AARN HN–24)

and B.C. Railway (Edmonton, Dunvegan and British Columbia Railway) which she said they renamed the Extremely Dangerous and Badly Constructed Railway. This apparently was improved when it was later taken over by the Northern Alberta Railway. In 1922, she was assigned to establish a Child Welfare Clinic in Calgary and she talked about "opposition to immunization, but gradually the mothers were educated to the need for children to be protected against communicable diseases at an early age."[46] By 1923, total clinic attendance in Calgary for the year was 5,312.

That the cost of health care was an issue for the settlers is confirmed by district nurse, Philippa Chapman, who served from 1935 to 1953, primarily in Breton west of Leduc, and also in Valleyview, for two periods of time. She recalls: "The District Nursing Service really started because of the maternity needs of the homesteaders' wives. No one had any money and so they would seldom call a doctor. If they went to a hospital with no money, they would be put on relief, and it became a charge against their land."[47] She referred to poverty amongst the settlers:

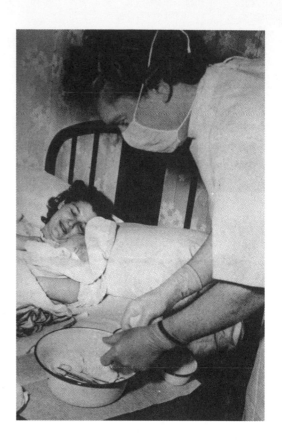

Laura Attrux attending a home delivery in Slave Lake, 1953. (From These Were Our Yesterdays, p. 179)

Other charities remembered the hard-pressed settlers in the Peace River and we often received quantities of used clothing and very nice layettes. You can't imagine what these gifts meant. The people had nothing, literally nothing. Many of them had come from the dried-out regions of southern Alberta after years of crop failures. They came into a new, unbroken land, with their few belongings, rickety conveyances and often leading sickly, half-starved cattle. The Peace River promised a fresh start where there were trees and an abundance of good land, but a harsh climate and no civilized comforts.[48]

Like other district nurses, Philippa Chapman developed a deep respect for the pioneer homesteaders describing them as "fine, brave people" who experienced "struggles against loneliness" and "the cold and primitive living conditions."[49]

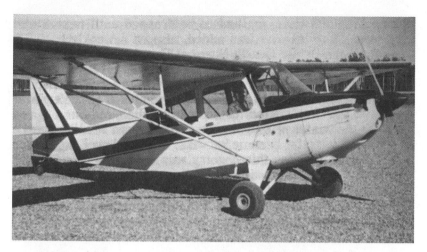

↬ *Laura Attrux pictured inside the Cessna 150 she purchased in 1967 to assist her in her work. (From* These Were Our Yesterdays, *p. 190)*

Laura Attrux had a 35-year career as a district nurse from 1939–1974, and served the communities of Whitecourt, Smith, Swan Hills, Slave Lake, Wabasca, Paddle River, High Level and Rainbow Lake over this period of time. In an interview six weeks before her death in September 1987, she stated that she had delivered 1032 babies over her career and although she "had a fair number of abnormal obstetrics," she never lost a mother.[50] The approach she used would appear to be very close to the modern one of assisting the public to care for their own health. She observed that people "didn't come for any little thing, . . . You trained people to look after themselves at this work."[51] In the interview she discusses the other kinds of work she did aside from midwifery: "Lumber camps produced a lot of emergency work. It may be a cut with a saw, an axe, broken legs, squashed legs . . . I could only hope to render first aid and get them out. I have stitched ligaments and tendons at times. If you didn't do it, you knew very well some patients would not go out."[52] One particularly difficult case she recalled:

> was an accident in the bush in winter. They brought this man in the back of a truck to my office. Oh he was a mess! A log had fallen on him. The log caught his head a bit on the side and sort of glanced off. He

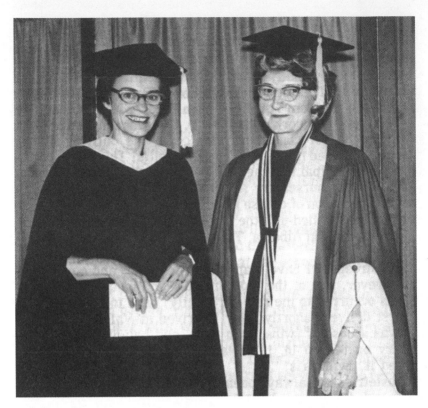

✧ *Dr. Laura Attrux with Ruth McClure, Director of the School of Nursing, University of Alberta, at the University of Alberta convocation ceremony in May 1970. An honourary Doctor of Laws degree was conferred upon her in recognition of her devoted service in remote areas of Northern Alberta. (From* These Were Our Yesterdays, *p. 192)*

received a skull fracture and before I stitched him you could see the cracks in the skull. He was conscious, but a mess with blood, hair, bark, all over the top of this head. I worked on that man two and one half hours; first of all to remove foreign bodies. After I got it cleaned, I stitched it. That was a job too. I kept him overnight in my living room on quite a long table. . . . The next day I phoned the doctor in Edmonton to notify him I was bringing in this man. . . . About a week later I was sending another patient to the same doctor. I asked how the first patient was doing. He said, "Just fine. He is going home tomorrow, we never touched him . . . no sign of infection."[53]

Laura Attrux was always alert to ways in which she could improve how she served the communities to which she was assigned as a district nurse. When she was 58 in 1967, she decided to learn to fly a plane and proceeded to buy a Cessna 150. This allowed her to fly her plane to hold clinics in Rainbow Lake: "It was a real blessing. I started out using my car, but it was a long and tortuous road. Sometimes you just couldn't get there. It took three hours at least. In the plane it took less than one hour."[54] Laura Attrux's work brought her not only the respect of the communities she served, but also of her profession. In addition to a number of other honours, the University of Alberta conferred an honourary doctor of laws degree upon her in 1970.

Although the district nursing program was gradually discontinued as communities developed health facilities and engaged the services of physicians and nurses to staff them, this period in the life of the province was an important one. Just as the Grey Nuns had earlier provided the only health support available to citizens in the St. Albert and Edmonton regions, district nurses provided the only care available to those in remote locations who experienced illness and accidents and to mothers in childbirth. District nurses were knowledgeable and had completed a course in public health at a university as well as a program of nursing education. Most also had considerable experience prior to obtaining advanced preparation in public health. Numerous accounts of the work of these nurses with the people they served give an indication of the nature of the service provided often under extremely difficult conditions. These nurses were highly regarded and respected for their knowledge and skills and for their commitment and concern for the populace.

Photo of Rossie Crowe and Nettie Garfield taken at Currie Barracks Hospital, Calgary in 1942. Both were assigned overseas duty during the war; Rossie Crowe served for a long period on the hospital ship The Lady Nelson and Nettie Garfield saw active duty at Taplow. (Photograph courtesy of Nettie Garfield Pedlar)

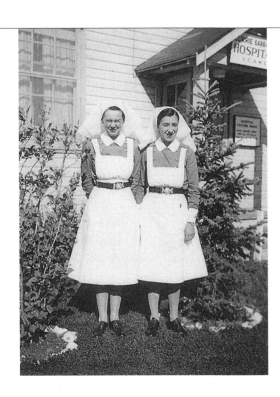

6

Alberta Nurses in
the World Wars

Modern nursing may be said to have emerged from the demonstration of nurses' effectiveness during a period of war. It was Florence Nightingale's single-handed determination to establish nursing as a legitimate and respected profession for women that led to the request from the British Government for her to lead a party of 38 nurses to tend wounded British soldiers during the Crimean War. Conditions when she arrived at the battlefront shocked and angered her and she wrote in 1856: "I stand at the altar of murdered men."[1] Although the British Army had physicians in the Crimea, there had been little attention paid to sanitation or cleanliness, and soldiers were dying in scores. Nightingale waged her

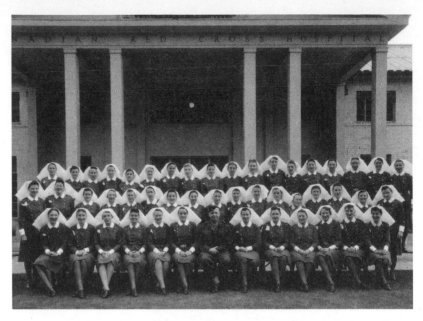

↦ Canadian nurses staffing No. 11 Canadian General Hospital at Taplow. Helen Wilson (Matron) is seated to Col. C.A. Watson's right, while Nettie Garfield (Assistant Matron) is on his left. (Photograph courtesy of Nettie Garfield Pedlar)

own war with the bureaucracy of the medical establishment of the British Army. It was a war of wits, determinations, and politics. Nightingale reflected in a letter to Sidney Herbert, Secretary at War in the British Cabinet that: "There is not an official who would not burn me like Joan of Arc if he could, but they know that the War Office cannot turn me out because the country is with me. That is the position."[2]

Although Nightingale drew her inspiration from other nurses, principally the German deaconnesses trained by Theodore Fliedner and the French nursing orders, she was the first to focus the attention of the world media on the need for well-prepared nurses to care for the wounded and the sick. There were also other nurses who worked tirelessly on behalf of British soldiers in the Crimea including Mary Seacole. Nightingale was not alone in drawing attention to the need for a humane approach to meeting individual needs. It became widely known that Nightingale and her staff of nurses made every possible attempt to make the wounded comfortable and to care for them in ways that would foster their recovery. These nurses were able to achieve dramatic reductions in morbidity and mortality through application of principles of cleanliness to the care of the wounded and accounts of Nightingale's work were distributed to the British press by a reporter covering the war. This successful demonstration of the work that could be carried out by nurses through care provided to wounded soldiers in the Crimean War had a remarkable impact on attitudes towards the acceptability of nursing as a career for women and the respect that was accorded those who took up nursing as a career.

NURSES IN MILITARY CONFLICTS IN CANADA

Nurses have played pivotal roles during military conflicts throughout Canadian history. The bipartisan role played by the nursing sisters of the Hotel Dieu hospitals in Quebec and Montreal during the hostilities between the French and English from 1756 to 1763 was exemplary. During the Northwest Rebellion of 1885, a military request for nursing services shows the influence of Florence Nightingale and the experience gained during the American Civil War: "No volunteer nurses. If you can send an organized body under a trained head, they will be welcome."[3] Two groups of nurses responded to the call, one headed by Mother Hannah Grier from the Anglican order of St. John the Divine in Toronto; the other by Miss Miller, a head nurse at the Winnipeg General Hospital.[4] In 1898, nurses with the Victorian Order of Nurses were attached to the Yukon Military Force and accorded considerable praise for their efforts.[5]

In 1899, an offer of a Canadian contingent of nurses for the Boer War was made by the Canadian government to Mr. Joseph Chamberlain. The first group of four nurses was sent to assist in South Africa under the leadership of Georgina Fane Pope, a Bellevue Hospital-educated nurse from Prince Edward Island. She described the conditions she experienced as follows:

> We nursed in huts and found the work at times very heavy, often times having our dinner between nine and ten p.m. We received our first convoy of wounded a few days after the Battle of Maggersfontein and Modder River when the beds were filled with men of the Highland

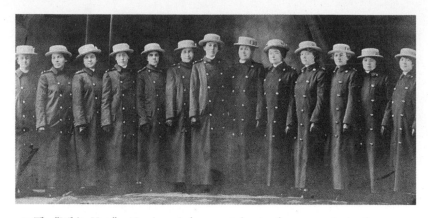

⊕ The "White Hats"—Nursing reinforcements leaving for overseas in April, 1915. The white straw hats were a mandatory part of the uniform and had been worn in the South African war. They were supported strongly by Matron Georgina Pope, but Nicholson reports that they were not universally popular amongst the nurses, some of whom managed to lose them overboard during the Atlantic crossing. (NAC)

Brigade. We remained at Wynberg for nearly a month, when No. 3 General Hospital of 600 beds was pitched under canvas at Rondesbosch, a few miles away—Here we arrived on Christmas Day and remained almost six months, having at times very active service; sometimes covered with sand during a "Cape South-Easter"; at others delayed with a fore-runner of the coming rainy season, and at all times in terror of scorpions and snakes as bed-fellows.[6]

Nurses in World War I

The South African nursing experience was sufficient to persuade the Canadian Army Medical Corps that an army nursing service ought to be an integral part of the permanent corps.[7] Georgina Pope and Margaret Macdonald were appointed to the staff on a permanent basis in 1906. When World War I broke out, the Army Nursing Corps consisted of five nurses. However, within three weeks of the declaration of war, thousands of nurses had volunteered for service overseas. Margaret Macdonald, who was appointed Matron-in-Chief of the Army Nursing Corps, described the first group of volunteers:

The selection, from coast to coast, of over one hundred nurses from thousands of applicants, the vast majority of whom were entirely unacquainted with Army Life and regulations, constituted somewhat of a problem. However, when all the formalities incident to the appointment of these as Nursing Sisters were concluded, it was astonishing how quickly and naturally in becoming military minded they fell into place. Their example and esprit de corps became the pattern for the many hundreds that followed.[8]

There are many accounts of the nature of service rendered by Canadian nurses during the war, all of which make note of the flexibility and devotion to duty that was required. Matron Macdonald described the introduction of the first group of nursing sisters to field nursing:

Their first introduction to Field Nursing began at Salisbury Plain in 1914; patients, many seriously ill, poured into huts that were ill-equipped to receive them. Cold, damp weather with continuous rain prevailed, adding much to the general discomfort. The sisters literally ploughed their way through mud and water from hut to hut; their living quarters left much to be desired. In the matter of rations, assuredly, vitamins were not the order of the day.[9]

The number of Canadian nurses who joined the Canadian Army Medical Corps in World War I was 3,141, and of these 2,504 served in the Overseas Military Forces of Canada.[10] In total, 46 nurses lost their lives in military service during this war. Nurses' war service was distinguished as evidenced by the number of honours bestowed upon them. Nurses earned such honours as Commander of the Order of the British Empire, Officer of the Order, the Royal Red Cross, first class, Royal Red Cross, second class, the Military Medal, the Royal Victoria Medal as well as foreign decorations of various kinds. As G.W.L. Nicholson noted:

In four years of war, nursing sisters from Canada had earned a high reputation while making their special contribution to the cause of humanity, justice and freedom. They had established a noble precedent that would inspire those who were to prove themselves worthy successors in another world conflict.[11]

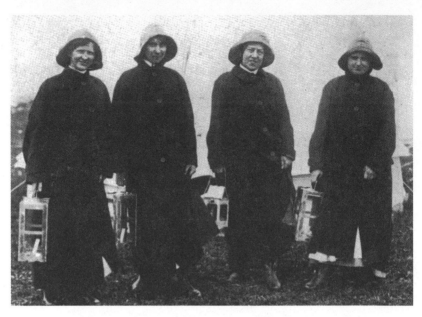

↬ *Four Victorian Order Nurses who enlisted in the Canadian Army Nursing Service, 1914–1918. (From* The Victorian Order of Nurses for Canada 50th Anniversary, 1897–1947, *used with permission of* von)

The recruitment of nurses in Alberta for World War I occurred prior to the legal recognition of nursing as a profession in the Registered Nurses Act of 1916. It was a period of time when nurses were just becoming organized in the province and beginning to press for legislation for registration. The war effort enhanced this quest and also their image of altruism, competence and dedication. Historically, nursing has tended to move forward in terms of its goals during times of great social upheaval, and the first World War was no exception. The war effort may have been an important factor in the willingness of legislators to bring forth legislation incorporating nursing in 1916. The professional organization in nursing was established under the Act, the Alberta Association of Graduate Nurses becoming the Alberta Association of Registered Nurses under the terms of the Act.

The schools of nursing were the focus of the recruiting effort for war service, possibly because they were the only organizations with lists of graduates and addresses for contacting them in the absence of a provincial

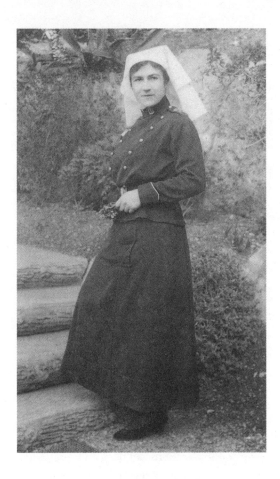

↪ *Ellen (Nettie)*
MacRae Chinneck,
first graduate of the
Royal Alexandra
Hospital School of
Nursing, circa 1915,
during service in
World War I.
(AARN P546)

organization that registered nurses. Graduate nurses were recruited from each of the schools. The first school to be established in the province, the Medicine Hat General Hospital, sent 15 nurses to war.[12] From the Calgary General Hospital School of Nursing, 14 nurses went overseas and 12 were stationed in Canada. From Calgary also, seven Holy Cross Hospital nurses saw war service. In Edmonton, four graduates who had completed the program at the Edmonton General Hospital School and seven from the Royal Alexandra Hospital School were recruited. One graduate from each of the Lamont School, the Galt School and St. Michael's Hospital School served in the armed services during the war. In all, there were approximately 65 nurses from Alberta schools of nursing who served in the war effort.[13]

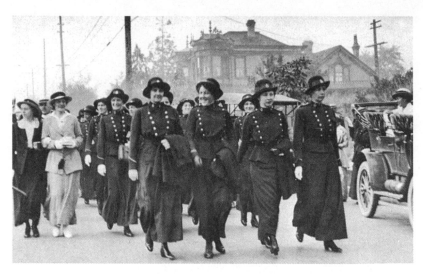

↪ *Nursing sisters of No. 5 Canadian General Hospital marching to the train at Victoria, B.C. in August, 1915 en route to Salonika.* (NAC)

WAR SERVICE UNITES NURSES

The war had the effect not only of uniting the country, but also of uniting nurses. Provincial and national nursing organizations were in a very early stage of their development. Prior to the war there had been no impetus and little opportunity for nurses in various parts of the country to meet and learn about nursing in different regions of Canada because transportation and communication were in an embryonic state. As Nicholson noted: "For the first time since nursing was organized as a profession in Canada, nurses from hospitals in the East met and mingled with their opposite numbers from the West, submerging local loyalties in a newly found adherence to a nation-wide service."[14] This was one of the first occasions which drew nurses together for a common purpose, and it would not be the last. Indeed, the war effort unified nurses and enhanced commitment to the profession. The organizational efforts of nurses to achieve important professional goals would be enhanced by the nurses who had served with the Canadian troops during this war. Indeed many nurses who gained experience in war service and leadership would go on to become leaders in the profession upon their later return to civilian life.

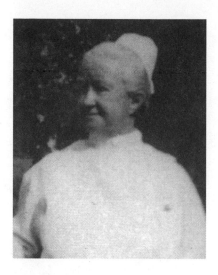

*⇨ Jean I. Gunn spearheaded the
drive for a Canadian nurses war
memorial in the Houses of
Parliament. (TGH Alumnae
Archives, used with permission)*

The contribution of nurses who gave their lives in war service was recognized by their colleagues in a war memorial. Plans for this memorial
were developed under the auspices of the Canadian National Association of
Trained Nurses (CNATN), an organization that became the Canadian Nurses
Association in 1924. A committee was established at the national meeting of
the CNATN in Vancouver in 1919 with Jean I. Gunn, Director of Nursing at
the Toronto General Hospital, appointed to chair the committee. It was
decided that a national memorial would be commissioned and displayed in
Ottawa and nurses groups across the country were asked to raise money to
underwrite the design and construction of the artwork. Alberta nurses
contributed $1,800 to support the cost of the National Memorial Fund
against the total projected cost of $35,000.[15] A sculptured bas-relief of
Carrara marble by the artist whose design was selected for the memorial,
G.W. Hill, R.C.A., depicted the history of Canadian nursing from its
French-Canadian origins to the First World War. It was installed in the Hall
of Fame in the Parliament Buildings outside the entrance to the
Parliamentary Library. On 24 August, 1926, it was unveiled by the Acting
Prime Minister Sir Henry Drayton with Matron-in-Chief Margaret
Macdonald and hundreds of nurses, guests and members of the public in
attendance.[16] A provincial war memorial was also developed for the nurs-
ing sisters of Alberta who served overseas: "The memorial was to be in the
form of a 'tablet' and designs were called for from amongst the member-

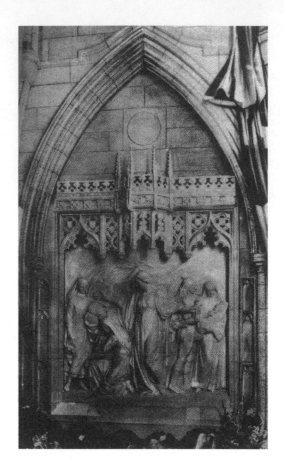

↬ *Nurses' War Memorial, a sculptured bas-relief of Carrara marble by artist G.W. Hill. Situated on a wall in the Parliament Buildings in Ottawa, just outside the parliamentary library, Ottawa. Picture was taken prior to application of Canadian Nurses Association crest in the medallion space over the sculpture. (From* Canadian Houses of Parliament: A Souvenir Book of Views, *Ottawa: Photogelatine Engraving Ltd.)*

ship. The memorial for Alberta nurses was eventually developed and hung in the medical building at the University of Alberta."[17]

The first Overseas Nursing Sisters' Association was formed in Edmonton in April, 1920 by a group of nursing sisters meeting at the Macdonald Hotel.[18] They elected as their first president, Alice Blackwell Turner who had seen service "with No. 2 Canadian Stationary Hospital at Etaples and No. 15 General at Taplow."[19] They worked hard to develop their membership and after recruiting Alberta nursing sisters, they had 39 on the membership roster. Other groups organized across the country, next in Montreal, then in Calgary where an organization was formed on 26 January 1922.[20] The Canadian organization was formed in 1929 and

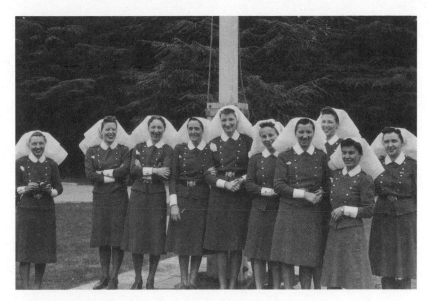

↝ *Nurses in uniform during overseas service during WWII. Nettie Garfield is fourth from right. (AARN)*

became the umbrella group for all of the local groups in operation. At the outset membership was restricted to those who had served overseas, thus preventing those who had seen war service in military installations in Canada from joining the organization. This restriction was to be removed some years afterward when the word "overseas" was removed from the name of the organization.[21]

Nurses in World War II

Margaret Macdonald, who was given the rank of major, was succeeded by Edith Rayside as Matron-in-Chief of the nursing service. The total number of nurses who served during World War II was approximately double that of World War I, at 4,000. Matron-in-Chief of the nursing service of the Army Medical Corps from 1940 to 1944 was Elizabeth Smellie. In civilian life, Miss Smellie had been chief superintendent of the VON; she became the first Canadian woman to achieve the rank of colonel. The significant service provided by nursing sisters during World War I led to the establish-

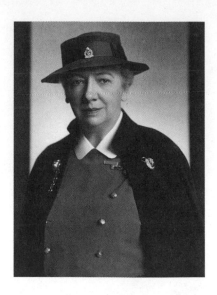

↦ *Elizabeth L. Smellie, Matron-in-Chief, Nursing Service of the Royal Canadian Army Medical Corps, 1940–1944. (Photograph by Yousuf Karsh, AARN)*

ment of a permanent corps of nursing sisters by the Royal Canadian Army Medical Corps (RCAMC), as well as a registry of nurses who could be available for active service in the event of war. Twenty-four Canadian general hospitals were established to care for the wounded during World War II, compared with sixteen during World War I. In addition, there was a convalescent hospital in France, a neurologic and plastic surgery hospital in England, and casualty clearing stations, totaling 34 overseas hospitals. Sixty hospitals were maintained in Canada, as well as two hospital ships. All were staffed with nurses.[22] In response to a request from South Africa, nurses under the leadership of Matron-in-Chief Gladys Sharpe were sent to care for wounded British soldiers.

For the major part of the war, Canadian nurses staffed the military hospitals in England and Canada and did not see service under battle conditions in Europe until 1943, when they were sent to assist after the invasion of Italy:

Canadian nurses were the first to reach Sicily after the invasion. . . . The unit was recruited largely from Winnipeg, and other Western cities, but the first girl ashore was Lieutenant Elizabeth Lawson of St. John, New Brunswick . . . Lieutenant Trennie Hunter, of Winnipeg, was a close second. The Matron of this hospital is Miss Agnes J. MacLeod, of Edmonton. They were described as a "group of grimy, tin-hatted girls, perspiring in the terrific heat and burdened with cumbersome equipment."[23]

Conditions were described by one Red Cross officer: "Comfort was a rarity to them that first winter. Often casualties were heavy, and they were on duty in the wards night and day."[24] Gladys Sharpe, describing conditions in South Africa and the response to the arrival of Canadian nurses, stated:

Our beds filled rapidly, the first convoy via hospital train brought casualties from Burma, Madagascar, the Middle East and Singapore, at the rate of 257 admitted in just two hours—the highlight was the official opening ceremony at which Field Marshall Smuts took the opportunity of publicly thanking "Canada" for sending nurses.[25]

It is reported that, up to this point, nurses in military service held the relative rank of officers, but did not actually have the official status of officers or the authority that accompanied the rank. This was changed, about half-way through the war, by order of the Privy Council, who granted nurses commissions equivalent to those of other commissioned officers. By contrast, nurses in Britain and the United States did not achieve this status until the end of the war.[26]

A total of 3600 nurses served in the Canadian armed forces and Canada loaned another 300 nurses to the Union of South Africa. Others volunteered for Red Cross activities to support the war effort, and still others kept the hospitals and community health agencies in Canada operating throughout the war.[27] Many Alberta nurses were among the Canadian contingent and served with distinction. Two Alberta nurses served as important nursing leaders during the war. The first was Agnes MacLeod who had graduated from the first class to enter the baccalaureate degree program in nursing at the University of Alberta and was Director of the School of Nursing at the University of Alberta at the time she enlisted for active duty. She became principal matron with the Canadian armies in Italy and was wounded in service. Following the war she was awarded the Royal Red Cross and later became the chief nurse in the Department of Veterans' Affairs in Ottawa. Ann Fuller enlisted in the American army and

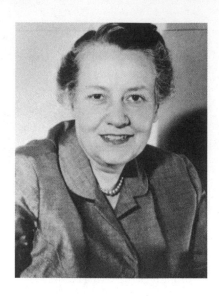

↪ *Agnes MacLeod, principal matron in Italy with the Royal Canadian Army Medical Corps, who had earlier served as Director of the School of Nursing at the University of Alberta (1937–1940). (Faculty of Nursing, University of Alberta)*

when she retired in 1965, she did so as Chief Nurse of the United States Army Nursing Service.[28]

Service by Alberta Nurses

The Alberta nurses who signed up for war service were able to do so in Calgary and Edmonton and began as second lieutenants, "being assured of a promotion to first lieutenant in six months."[29] Enlisting in the air force or the navy "was a little more complicated. The RCAF had a three-week induction course at the Institute of Aviation Medicine in Toronto and the navy had two weeks of lectures in Halifax followed by a familiarizing sea run."[30] Nurses who volunteered for South Africa were recruited to the Canadian army, then loaned to South Africa. Emily Mayhew, who had graduated from the Royal Alexandra Hospital School of Nursing in 1940 signed up for the South African forces, and later transferred to the Canadian army where she served on hospital ships throughout the war. Another Royal Alexandra graduate, Frances Ferguson, who became President of the AARN in 1950, served with a casualty clearing station in France following the landing in Normandy and recalled the workloads the casualty clearing stations handled. A station was to handle a maximum of 200 casualties with a staff of eight nurses who would also have to staff the operating rooms. This con-

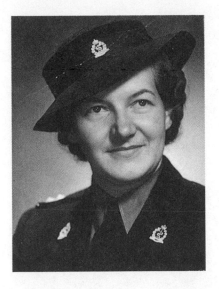

⊹ Frances Ferguson, graduate of the Royal Alexandra Hospital School of Nursing, who served in France following the landing in Normandy. (AARN P803)

trasted with conditions in England where there were normally two nurses working 12-hour shifts for a 50-bed ward with some extra staff available if needed.[31]

Nurses reported that their work was satisfying, even though it was very hard work. Irene Greenwood Henderson, who served with the Edmonton Unit at Vasto on the Adriatic coast, recalled being posted to work in the Field Dressing Station for surgical units:

> We had three wards of very severely wounded men; one was mostly head injuries, another chest, both had amputees too. I had a gas gangrene ward and most so massively injured with amputations that required general anesthesia to change any dressings. . . . The patients were stoical, co-operative, and considerate of each other which served to alleviate our stress.[32]

Beatrice Cole Hunter wrote the following of her experience during the conflict:

> Walking into those long, 45-bed wards of battle-hardened soldiers was, at first quite unnerving for this novice Nursing Sister. I shall always remember being asked by a young corporal if I would wash his feet, as

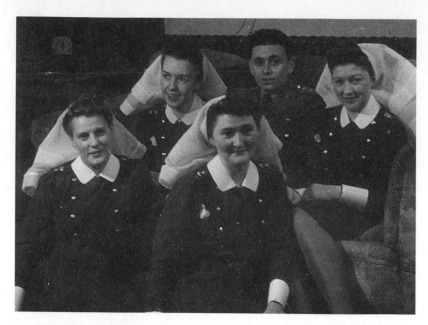

⊕ Beatrice Cole Hunter, an Alberta nurse and Regina General Hospital School of Nursing graduate of 1943, saw active duty at No. 19 Canadian General Hospital at Marsden Green, England. Pictured in 1945, second from left with (left to right) Leila Monroe, Margaret MacLean, Capt. (M.O.) I. Perlin and Elsie Barr. (Photograph courtesy of Beatrice Cole Hunter)

he couldn't reach them. "Certainly," I replied, then gasped as I pulled back the covers. He had no legs.[33]

Writing about her experiences some 50 years following the war on her thoughts about the experience during those years, Jessie Morrison, a distinguished Alberta nurse, reflected on the past:

The thoughts that came to me were, "This is it. The reason for my being here. It has finally all come together." I am sure I prayed something like this: "Dear God, may right prevail. May the horrors of war be the least possible. May I be equal to what lies ahead." This I do know, the faces of the boys who had been patients over the years flashed before me—army, navy and air force—so young, so vulnerable.[34]

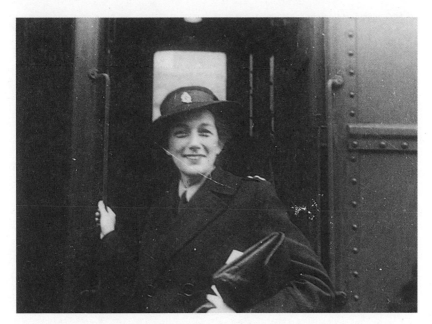

❧ *Jessie L. Morrison, Royal Alexandra Hospital School of Nursing graduate, saw active service at No. 10 Canadian General Hospital in Yorkshire.*
(AARN P804)

Nettie Garfield Pedlar who graduated from the University of Alberta with a B.Sc. in Nursing in 1938, had a background of service with the VON in Winnipeg and Calgary prior to enlisting for military service. Her disappointment at being stationed at Currie Barracks in Calgary for what seemed to her to be a very long time was overcome when the unit at Calgary was mobilized and became the No. 11 Canadian General Hospital. Upon arrival in Britain she served in several locations to which the wounded were evacuated from the battlefront, and later in the war she was sent to a hospital in Holland that served as a casualty clearing station. She talked about the influence of penicillin which had just become available on those with serious wounds:

Penicillin I'm sure saved many, many lives. When I was in training, if you had punctures in the abdomen, peritonitis set in and the patient always seemed to die unless he had a wonderful source of resistance. But

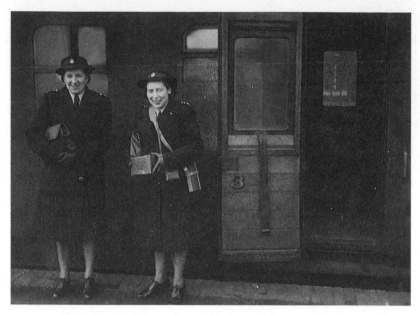

⤙ *Nettie Garfield with Mae Deana Freeman, en route home from Holland in 1945. (Photograph courtesy of Nettie Garfield Pedlar)*

with penicillin these patients were saved. I've seen many patients come in with eight or nine gunshop wounds or shrapnel wounds in the abdomen—and you'ld think they would never make the grade, but they did and it was just wonderful . . . that so many people did recover.[35]

Following her return from war service, Nettie Pedlar went on to Columbia University to study for her master's degree in public health nursing which she completed in 1947. Many nurses who had been posted overseas during the war also went on for further education upon their return to Canada. They did this not only because returning veterans were offered educational scholarships to improve their educational status, but also because these nurses had become deeply committed to nursing through their war service and wanted to become as well-prepared as possible for their future work.

The Second World War often is seen as the beginning of women's emancipation in the world of work, and there are compelling statistics to support this argument. More women were employed during this period of time than at any other time prior to this. By June of 1943, over 255,000 women were engaged in the war industry. These were the women who, when there was a shortage of men to keep the industries of the country in operation, aided in the production of materials necessary to the war effort. Many have argued that this was the first step in the recognition of women's equality and right to work. Women were allowed to penetrate what had previously been a man's world of work. However, the fact that the gains were made during the war, but lost immediately afterward, points to the fact that these were not gains at all, but simply a temporary substitution to accomplish certain national goals. As Ruth Roach Pierson has noted: "Canada's war effort, rather than any consideration of women's right to work, determined the recruitment of women into the labour force."[36] These civilian roles were essential to the country during wartime, and without the efforts of women, the industries producing services and products in which women were engaged could not have been productive.

Even though there were positions for nurses in private duty, hospitals and public health agencies before wwii, for most of the decade preceding the war there had been widespread unemployment among nurses. When war broke out their efforts were badly needed by their country, both at home and overseas. Nurses did not fail to respond to the patriotic calls to duty. Many had just undergone a decade of economic hardship, and jobs opened up in great numbers. Despite the risks involved with serving with the armed services, nurses volunteered their services willingly and served with distinction under very difficult conditions in many areas of the world where Canadian forces were engaged in battle. The shortage of nurses became the predominant issue of the war years, and there simply were not enough nurses to supply all of the needs of the country. Since civilian women were generally told to leave the positions they had filled so well during the war, one might think that this happened for nurses as well. However it did not, for the postwar period was a time of great expansion in health care, and with the advent of medicare, the demand for nurses was greater than it had been during the war years. As well, nursing was a sex-segregated profession and it was not seen as an acceptable profession for men at this time. Thus, unlike other women, nurses were encouraged to fill the available positions upon their return to Canada, and those who had

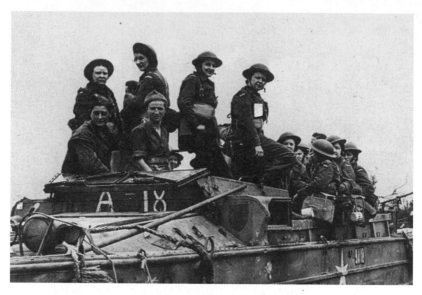

↝ Nursing sisters of No. 10 Canadian General Hospital landing in Normandy coming ashore at Arromanches in amphibious DUKWS. (NAC)

seen domestic service were encouraged to continue their work. Because women were largely viewed as the only ones who could perform nursing roles, this stereotype was advantageous in many ways to this group of working women, for they did not suffer the rejection that occurred to women who performed other kinds of work when the war ended.

Although there have been successions of conflicts between various countries of the world since World War II including the Korean Conflict, the Vietnam War and the somewhat short-lived Gulf War, Canada's involvement was peripheral and relatively minimal in the first two cases and quite brief during the Gulf War. However, Canada has been invited many times by a various countries to serve in peacekeeping missions around the globe and has developed an excellent reputation for its work abroad. Nurses have been a part of these official military efforts, some of which have involved considerable risk to life. Nurses have also served in peacekeeping roles with international organizations such as the Red Cross to help civilians in need when there is ongoing conflict in an area. There have been numerous examples over time of the risks taken by these volunteer nurses. Perhaps the most rivetting and horrifying of these was the January, 1997 murder of several Red Cross nurses, one of whom was a Canadian nurse, in cold blood in Rawanda. Peacekeeping efforts by the Canadian military in Bosnia over a period of serveral years were fraught with danger for those who served, some of whom were to lose their lives as a result of the conflict around them.

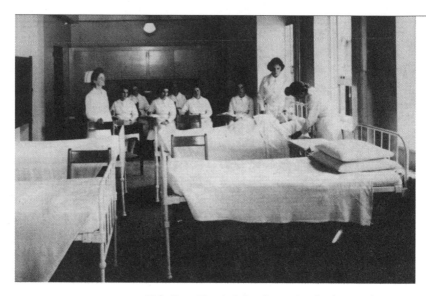

Holy Cross Hospital class in nursing fundamentals with Miss Huck, Instructor. (Photograph from Nurses and Nightingales)

Nursing Education Becomes
Synonymous with Nursing Service

The Development of Training Schools

PAULINE PAUL

Although there had been a long tradition of nursing within religious orders, the movement to establish nursing as a profession for lay women in modern times essentially began with the worldwide publicity focused upon nursing and the work of Florence Nightingale. Although there were other groups of nurses who advocated reform, Nightingale's decision to undertake nursing as a career and her widely-publicized and successful demonstration of the work that could be carried out by nurses through care provided to soldiers wounded in the Crimean War had a remarkable impact on nineteenth century society both in Britain and elsewhere in the world. Unsolicited donations to the

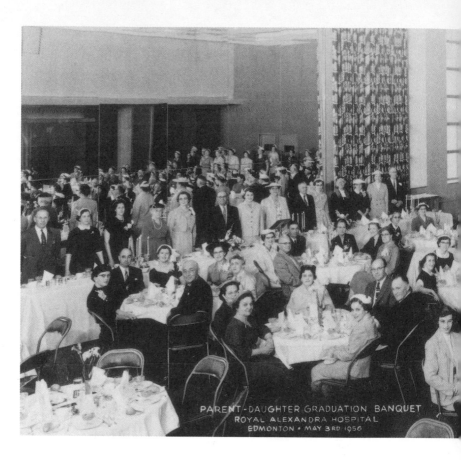

PARENT-DAUGHTER GRADUATION BANQUET
ROYAL ALEXANDRA HOSPITAL
EDMONTON • MAY 3RD 1956

Nightingale Fund from grateful families and enthusiastic supporters streamed in and Florence Nightingale decided in 1860 to use the proceeds to establish a School of Nursing in association with St. Thomas' Hospital in London, England. The heightened interest in the Nightingale school was reflected in considerable publicity about its operation and a desire on the part of other jurisdictions to develop schools based on a similar model. The idea soon swept the world and many hospital training schools for nurses were subsequently established throughout Europe and North America.

"THE HISTORICAL ACCIDENT"

The "historical accident" as Esther Lucile Brown termed it, referred to the failure to apply the fundamental philosophy of the Nightingale model to

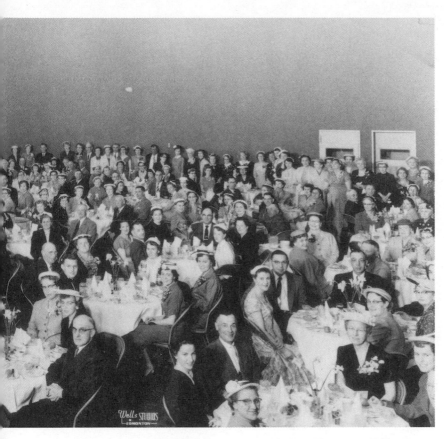

↬ *Parent-daughter graduation banquet, 1956, Royal Alexandra Hospital School of Nursing, Edmonton.* (AARN P265)

the new schools.[1] The educational orientation of the Nightingale school made possible by independent financing was all but forgotten as the new schools sought to care for the needs of hospitalized patients through care primarily given by students who had insufficient opportunity for instruction and learning. Students thus provided a service of considerable value to the hospital for which they received little in the way of compensation. The establishment of schools of nursing was a definite asset to hospitals because the students recruited to the schools provided the means by which the nursing service of the hospital could be rendered at minimal expense. The rush to establish hospitals in the early part of the twentieth century was undoubtedly reinforced by the financial incentive offered by the establishment of schools of nursing in association with hospitals. The problems of operating the early hospitals were difficult and complicated by the fact that "many hospitals offered free services to the sick who were poor"[2] as well services to those who could pay. Thus it became a matter of necessity to provide services to attract paying patients to the institution. As Susan Young has observed:

> With evidence demonstrating that trained nurses were more effective than untrained aides, paying patients were more likely to enter a hospital which employed trained nurses. However, trained nurses were in limited supply and one way to guarantee a supply of nurses was to operate a training school.[3]

The financial advantage to the hospital of operating a school of nursing was clear and this led to the need for hospitals to establish schools of nursing to give them a competitive edge relative to other institutions to which paying patients might turn for care. Operating a training school also provided security against incurring a financial loss if the number of paying patients was to drop at any point. Therefore, the education of nurses became closely associated with hospitals at a developmental stage in the establishment of both hospitals and schools of nursing not only in Alberta, but also across the country. As late as 1965, the Canadian Nurses Association found that 105 out of the 161 hospital schools of nursing that participated in what was known as the School Improvement Program, reported that the selection of clinical assignments was not based on the students' educational needs, but on the service needs of the patient care units.[4] Many persistent problems were identified by those who surveyed nursing education in Canada. Surveyors such as Weir, in 1932, and Mussallem in 1965, found that hospital schools of nursing used their students as a workforce, that hours on duty were too long, that nursing instruction in the classroom was limited and insufficient, and that the teaching personnel were ill-prepared and too few in number.[5] There was some noticeable improvement between the time at which each survey was published. However, it is remarkable that the key issues had remained the same and that the lack of financial independence of schools of nursing dictated the norms. The entrenchment of the hospital-based system of nursing education would carry with it certain features that nurses considered to

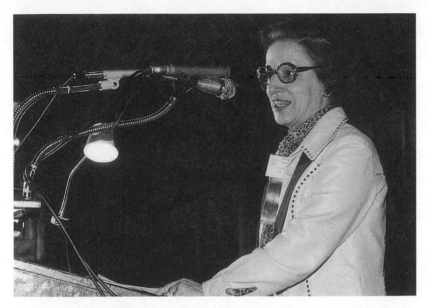

↦ *Helen K. Mussallem, Executive Director of the Canadian Nurses Association, whose studies of nursing education in Canada in the 1960s were important in guiding strategies to improve the system of nursing education.* (AARN P802)

be undesirable, and it would be working towards improving standards of education in the schools which would become a primary preoccupation of the professional association for many decades.

As the preferred method of instruction, hands on experience had the potential of introducing the students to most activities that took place in a hospital. However, the possible benefits of this form of learning were often lost because of the conditions that existed in the hospital. Lack of variety of clinical experiences was a regular problem in the schools operated by small hospitals, and in larger institutions it was not uncommon for students to remain for a very long time on a few units in order to satisfy the staffing needs of the hospital. Those who considered the hospital school of nursing to be a sound form of education often argued that apprenticeship was the best method for learning nursing procedures. However, for most of the century, the lack of nursing instructors and of other graduate nurses on patient care units meant that there were few role models for students for observation, questions and general discussion. In most cases senior students were left in charge of teaching junior students and this with very limited supervision. It can be argued that nursing students were not under a true apprenticeship program since there were no masters guiding the novices.[6]

Monitoring Diploma Nursing Education

Until 1921, hospital based programs in Alberta functioned independently and there was no coordinating body overseeing standards of nursing education. Beginning in 1921, the monitoring of diploma nursing education became the responsibility of the University of Alberta. Although the establishment of the Committee on Small Hospitals was an important step towards the establishment of basic standards, Young found that the committee played a very limited role until the late 1940s, when a position of advisor to schools of nursing was established.[7] Yet, even after the creation of this position it was found that even though many rural hospital schools of nursing did not meet the established standards, they were permitted to continue to operate. Political reasons undoubtedly influenced the lack of action. In 1953, Dr. Andrew Stewart, the Chairman of the Committee on Nursing Education and also President of the University of Alberta, stated: ". . . the only disciplinary measure available to the University for the discipline of schools that contravened the training regulations was to close the school. This would put the University of Alberta in a bad light in the eyes of the public."[8] It is apparent that the Committee on Nursing Education and the Alberta Association of Registered Nurses, which repeatedly lobbied for changes had little power and that hospital administrators through associations such as the Alberta Hospital Association were able to control the situation. Considering how long it took to effect changes in nursing education and the difficult conditions under which nursing students were educated in the hospital, nursing students who persevered in the system can be described as committed and devoted to nursing and to their hospital school of nursing.

The Educational Experience

The establishment of the Medicine Hat General Hospital in 1890 was followed by a training school for nurses in 1894. Even by that time, the idea of establishing a school for nurses had become synonymous with sustaining hospital operations. In the annual report of the medical superintendent of the Medicine Hat General Hospital two years prior to the establishment of the school, the following statement exemplifies this:

> The time has also come when a training school for nurses should be started. We are constantly receiving applications from young ladies who are anxious to acquire a nurse's training. This could be done with very little additional outlay. There are few ways in which the hospital can benefit the public more than by being able to supply a nurse's training to those who are anxious and willing to acquire one and who are often willing to give their time and work gratuitously for the sake of the information they receive.[9]

The talents of women were being solicited in order to provide the care needed in the hospital. However, they were also subject to an array of rules and regulations governing their conduct:

> The nurses are enjoined to observe carefully at all times, the ethics of nursing, and to cultivate the professional spirit which includes a cheerful, willing obedience to authority. Dignity, decorum, and quietness of manner must be observed and the entire time of duty devoted to the welfare of the patients. When off duty nurses should participate in only wholesome recreation, and at all times must guard against anything that would bring dishonour to their school or their profession.[10]

They were nevertheless expected to work for little remuneration—in other words to subsidize the operation of the hospital almost as volunteers. It is unlikely that this situation was unique in western Canada or in North America, as the new schools were established based on the service that could be provided by women.

Individual histories of Alberta's hospital schools of nursing show that there were great similarities from one school to another. The hours of work were gruelling in most of the schools of the 1910s. At the Edmonton General Hospital School of nursing students worked 78 hours a week, with their Sunday afternoon free.[11] Mrs. Breggen, a graduate of the class of 1917 of the School of the University of Alberta Hospital, stated:

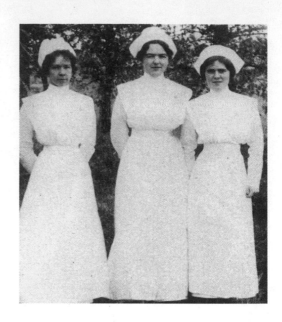

↝ *Elizabeth Patteson (right), Class of 1913, Galt Hospital School of Nursing with (left to right) Lillian Donaldson and Lucy Hatch at their graduation. (From* White Caps and Red Roses*)*

I was a big healthy girl in those days. Good thing too or I wouldn't be here to tell about it. Annie Baird, the matron, was a hard nut. We weren't coddled. Duty was seven to seven and seven to seven we were supposed to get a half-day off a week. If there was an admission just when you were ready to go off duty you had to stay there listing clothes and jewellery. Fifteen-cents rings and the likes and you were lucky if you got off at two o'clock. [. . .] We learned our nursing techniques by being "apprenticed" to a senior nurse [senior student].[12]

The reminiscences of Elizabeth Patteson a 1913 graduate of the Galt Hospital School of Nursing are also similar judging by her description of classes being held in the evening after a twelve-hour day.[13] Twelve-hour shifts were the norm since the graduates of the Royal Alexandra Hospital and the Holy Cross Hospital also recalled the same type of work schedule.[14] An early graduate from the Lamont Public Hospital School of Nursing wrote:

We worked twelve hours a day, often they ran over, minus any time off . . . more than one girl went to bed crying with sore feet, as most of us could not afford special shoes. We often specialized very sick patients,

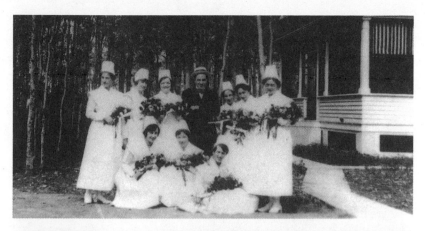

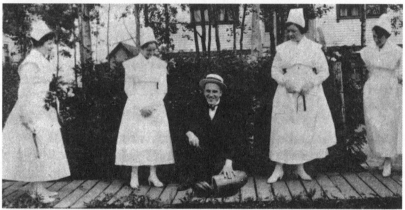

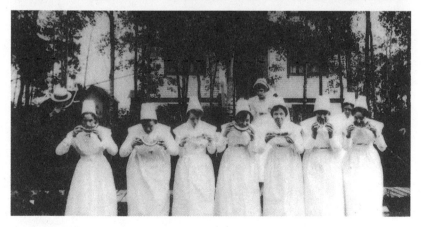

↬ *Lamont graduates celebrating their success in 1922. (AARN P146a and P146b, and from Florence Love's* The Lamp Is Golden: Lamont and Its Nurses 1951–1962, *Edmonton: The Archer Memorial Hosptial School of Nurses Alumnae Association).*

fresh postoperatives or accident cases until 1:00 a.m. having been on duty continuously from 7:00 a.m.[15]

Students at the beginning of the century were regularly sent to the wards prior to having received any form of instruction. This is how Dorothy Jackson, a graduate from the Holy Cross Hospital School of Nursing described her first day:

> I well remember being sent to St. Anne's, a male medical and surgical ward. I was put under the supervision of a classmate who had been there three months, in the ten bed solarium at the east end of the ward. She told me to bath a man at one end of the ward and I asked, "How do I do that?" I was given a basin of water and told how to proceed and how far to bath, etc., and was left on my own.[16]

The experience of Marion Moodie, the first graduate of the Calgary General Hospital School of Nursing, the second school to be established in Alberta in 1895, consisted of an even more rapid immersion in 1895:

> As first pupil nurse, I entered on St. George's Day, April 23, and was sent to get what sleep I would in a vacant ward upstairs, as I was to commence my probation by taking charge at night while the Matron and Head nurse, who had been having a very busy time, got a chance to rest.[17]

Histories of Alberta schools of nursing revealed that for most of the first half of the century, nursing students attended the few lectures provided to them after twelve hours of work on the wards. During his investigation, George Weir, recorded observations about students' behaviours at evening lectures. He wrote: "A few who have been long hours on ward duty, yield to the weariness of fatigue: first a condition of passive attention, then the glassy stare of mental torpor, reaching its culmination when Morpheus claims the victim!"[18] If hospital administrations had seriously taken the educational needs of the students, time could have been found for instruction, and cleaning tasks could have been delegated to other individuals. As Scollard who described the situation at the Calgary General observed: "Like

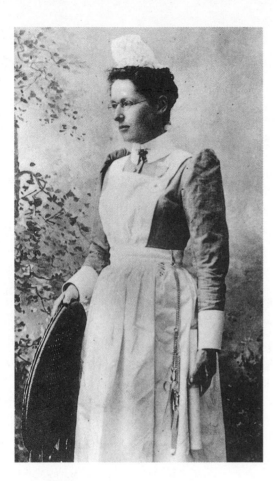

↝ *Marion Moodie, the first graduate of the Calgary General Hospital School of Nursing, 1898.*
(AARN P267)

elsewhere they not only performed the bulk of the nursing tasks in the hospital, they performed a host of menial tasks that could never be termed educational and which could as well have been done by untrained personnel."[19] Not surprisingly, the health of nursing students was often affected by their too long hours of work and illness was a common cause of withdrawal from nursing programs.

It would be wrong however to conclude that none of the schools or none of the nurses who taught in these schools had showed interest, creativity and vision relative to nursing education, or that none wanted to provide the best possible experience to nursing students. For example, in 1917 the Grey Nuns organized a three-day meeting for schools of nursing run by their order in the west that was held at the Edmonton General Hospital. The purpose of this assembly was to discuss nursing and nursing education. Proceedings of the conference clearly showed that the sisters believed that theory and practice were related and should be arranged concurrently and that a holistic approach was needed for patient care. They further gave credence to the view that nursing students were learners who needed to develop a spirit of inquiry and that the application of scientific principles in nursing was important.[20] The presence of a determined leader could also bring positive change. For example, Fannie Munroe, Assistant Superintendent at the Royal Alexandra, and President of the AARN from 1932 to 1936, fought for shorter hours and encouraged the students to establish self-government.[21] It has been seen that it was often much more difficult for lay nurses to bring about changes in nonreligious schools of nursing operated by men and physicians, than in a Roman Catholic hospital such as the Holy Cross or the Edmonton General, where the sisters were totally in charge of the entire institution.

The life of early nursing students was strictly controlled and ladylike behaviour was expected at all times. The memories of Harriet Gerry, a graduate of 1922 of the Royal Alexandra Hospital School of Nursing, are probably typical. She stated:

> The living, four to a room, the rising bell, the lights out, rules and regulations—kept, broken or ignored—the long hours, the absolute necessity for self-discipline to become nurses, the immersion of one's self in the life of the hospital to the exclusion of family and friends, and the joys and sorrows shared, all gave a deep sense of accomplishment and satisfaction and with the passing years only the funny and kindly memories remain."[22]

Curfews were imposed in every school and students had to be imaginative when they wished to maintain a social life. For example, at the Misericordia Hospital in the late 1920s: "The students coped with their long hours and strict discipline in a variety of ways. One way was to sneak out after 9:30 p.m. and go dancing at a dance hall located on 110 Street. The escape route was through the power plant via the tunnel which connected it to the main building."[23] At the Galt Hospital, the common escape and re-entry route of the same decade consisted of the ladder of the fire exit of the hospital, and even the removal of the two lower rungs of the ladder did not stop adventurous students.[24] At face value these descriptions are amusing and show that students took initiative, if not considerable risk in pursuing a life outside the hospital and the school. However, one has to wonder about the values in a system in which young women were required to hide their absences.

Appearance was also under strict scrutiny. Nursing uniforms were a status symbol and the stage at which a student had reached in her program could often be identified by the variations. For example, in some schools senior students could replace black stockings with white ones. Uniforms of the early decades were anything but comfortable. A description of the uniform used at the Medicine Hat General School of Nursing in 1914, provides a good example of the dress code:

> The uniform for student nurses, and rigidly enforced, was dresses and aprons nine inches from the floor, no less and certainly no more, with MHGH embroidered on the left arm. The bib crossed over the back and was fastened with safety pins underneath the apron band. A very stiffly starched, modified Eton collar, the cap worn well forward on the head, no puffs or curls unless natural. With black stockings and high black boots, the uniform was complete.[25]

Hairstyle seem to have been the subject of considerable regulation. At the Holy Cross Hospital some members of the 1926 class were dismissed from the school because they had "bobbed their hair."[26] The same year, some students from the Royal Alexandra also adopted this new style and the school attempted to reprimand them. The episode has been described in the history of the school:

> During this period of time the windblown bob became fashionable, and the nurses, so regimented in nearly all other aspects, were eager to be in style. For those who had their hair cut, the veil was introduced as a sort of punishment and they were not permitted to wear their cap. The veil, however, proved all too popular and others bobbed their hair just for the pleasure of wearing it.[27]

Regulations often reflected the religious values of the time. For example the Lamont students of 1910 as students in a hospital operated by the Methodist Church were forbidden to dance or attend dances and no doubt the same prohibition would have been in place in Catholic schools of nursing.[28]

For many years students had no forms of organization through which they could have brought forward suggestions about discipline. One must wonder if there was active disapproval of this on the part of hospital administrations, or whether students simply did not consider that they had a voice in the system. In 1924, the Lamont students were granted the privilege of establishing a student council.[29] It appears that they were the first to be able to do so and that student associations became commonplace well into the 1930s and 1940s.

The crash of the stock market in 1929 had a profound effect on the west and greatly affected Albertans. Thus, unemployment was high and the social safety net almost nonexistent. The hardships of the day played a role in the recruitment of nursing students. The records of the Edmonton General Hospital showed that enrolment increased during the 1930s.[30] The words of Alvine Cyr Gahagan, a graduate of 1932, suggest why:

> The crash of 1929...affected many of our parents. Edmonton being a farming district, these people found it hard; they could not sell their products. Skilled people could not find jobs in their chosen professions. We in training felt that we were lucky; we worked hard and studied hard, but the sisters fed us well. I can still see those tray-like table tops, with gallons of cream and milk for all the cereal that we wanted. I remember puffed wheat and rice, yes, the famous porridge, "oatmeal". Then for lunches, they would put out a whole pound of butter at a time, with two or three kinds of jam; sometimes the whole can was there, and the same with peanut butter. I remember making sandwiches with all these in them—was that ever good. These were our lunches in the morning at 10 o'clock and the evening snacks. These were beside our three full meals. No wonder when I would come to the lunch counter I would say, "no potatoes, please, Sr. Chauvin..."[31]

During the Depression, the Calgary General School of Nursing "... was flooded with applicants as worried parents grasped at the opportunity for

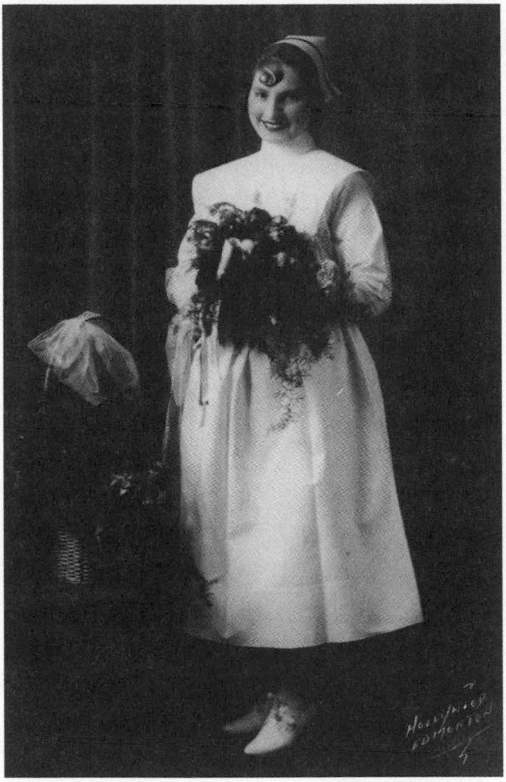

Graduation picture of Alvine Cyr from the Edmonton General Hospital School of Nursing, 1932. (Photograph courtesy of Alvine Cyr Gahagan)

free room and board along with nursing training for their daughters."[32] A graduate from the Royal Alexandra confirmed that she had come to nursing because her financial situation did not permit her to think of anything else at the time and that at least training ensured room and board.[33] In summary, it may be suggested that nursing schools became quite attractive during the depression years, since they offered shelter, food and some education.

However, the schools were not exempt of financial difficulties. It has been estimated that if it had not been for the assistance provided by its Alumnae and by the hospital Women's Auxiliary, the Royal Alexandra School would not have been able to maintain its standards. It is remarkable that the Alumnae provided the funding required to purchase the equipment needed for the teaching of dietetics. One has to admire the fact that so many of the nurses who gave money made sacrifices for their school.[34] Although it is impossible to know exactly how much nurses supported

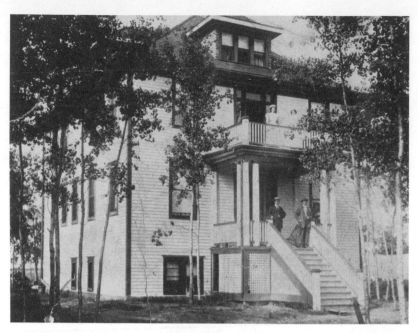

☙ *The Lamont Hospital, Lamont, Alberta in 1912.* (AARN P614)

their schools, it is likely that alumnae members of other schools assisted their *alma mater* since nurses in general showed great generosity during this difficult era.

Although it would have been interesting to provide detailed information about the small hospital schools of nursing of the province, it was difficult to find information on them.[35] The fact that small schools were located in rural areas, the limited data about them, and findings of the Weir Survey suggest that conditions were particularly harsh in the hospitals where they were located. Most of them were in operation before running water and other commodities reached rural areas. By virtue of their size, the small rural hospitals could not offer varied learning experiences. In fact the size factor created so many problems that it was recommended in the Weir Survey that hospitals with fewer than 75 beds should be prohibited from operating nursing schools. Young has pointed out that through the efforts of the Alberta Association of Registered Nurses, the standard in Alberta had been raised to a minimum of 100 beds to operate a nursing school just prior to the publication of the Weir Report.[36]

In 1915, a school opened at Vegreville General Hospital (later known as St. Joseph's Hospital). This school and the Lamont School were the only two rural schools that survived for any length of time. The continual growth of Vegreville probably explains why the school managed to outlive other rural schools. However, a description provided by Cashman confirms the extent to which living conditions were harsh during its first years of operation:

> There was no running water. The kitchen was in the basement and the students had to carry boiled water from the kitchen to the second and third floors. [. . .] One Spring, Sister Josephine and some students [. . .] came down with typhoid. It was traced in the hospital's well, behind the building, and the water had to be hauled three blocks from the convent.[37]

The Brett Sanatorium School of Nursing was also opened during the 1910s. However, it closed in 1922 soon after the death of Dr. Brett.[38] The High River Hospital School of Nursing which operated between 1921 and 1934 also had a short existence. However it did have one claim to fame in that its first two graduates received their diplomas from the hands of the Prince of Wales who was passing through the area at the time of graduation.[39] St. Mary's Hospital School of Nursing, Camrose, lasted from 1922 until 1935 and Mrs. E.W. Snider, one of its first graduates, recalled a high dropout rate.[40] This was not unusual in nursing schools but it is likely that conditions in rural schools made attrition even more prevalent than in the city schools.

CHANGE IN NURSING EDUCATION

The postwar years brought many changes in nursing education. Several influences became apparent in society and in the nursing profession. The nursing profession became stronger and more influential, there were acute and increasing shortages of nurses, and liberalization in society in general and of women in particular was apparent. Undoubtedly these and other factors played important roles in shaping the hospital schools of the era. More educational options than ever opened up to young women and it became necessary to modify the schools in order to attract a sufficient number of recruits. Immediately after World War II, hours of work per week were still long but they had been reduced to 48 in a number of nursing schools. It nevertheless took until the 1960s for the 40-hour week to become the norm. There is no doubt that the battle between the needs of the students and the needs of the hospital came into play whenever innovative change was proposed.

One of the most significant changes of the era was the introduction of the block system of education. The Holy Cross Hospital School of Nursing, which adopted this system in 1947, was probably the first one in the province to implement it.[41] Commonplace in the 1950s, the system had the advantage of increasing the number of hours spent in the classroom. It was also a compromise that ensured the availability of students in clinical areas since blocks of lectures alternated with blocks of clinical practice. The words of Nora Tennant, a nurse who taught at the Galt School of Nursing in the 1950s, show however that the compromise was difficult for some:

Students were taken off wards for a period of time to develop through education, a realm of knowledge. On completion of their classroom experience, students returned to the clinical areas to apply the knowledge gained. This put a burden on hospital schools of nursing as the students were out of service and staffing and budgets had to be adjusted to meet the needs of patient care.[42]

Soon after the implementation of the block system, schools of nursing found it advantageous to establish master rotations. Again the needs of the hospitals were taken into account as indicated by records of the Edmonton General Hospital School of Nursing: "This plan assures a stable number of personnel in the clinical field and guarantees that each student is certain of the experience in each area for a proper length."[43]

Another milestone of the era was the restructuring of the nursing department of most hospitals. The most significant outcome of this remodelling was that schools of nursing became officially separate from nursing service departments. The Calgary General Hospital was likely the first hospital to engage in this type of restructuring. In 1952, Gertrude Hall became the Director of Nursing of that hospital and she brought with her impressive experience that was bound to lead to changes. As former

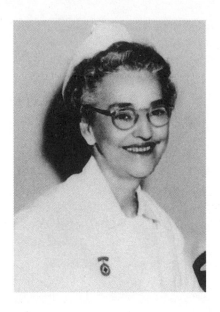

↝ *Gertrude Hall, Director of Nursing of the Calgary General Hospital in 1952 and formerly Advisor of Nursing and General Secretary of the Canadian Nurses Association.*
(GAA NA–2600–26)

National Advisor of Nursing and General Secretary of the Canadian Nurses Association, Miss Hall was well prepared and could convince others of the need to separate education from service. It is likely that her ability to artic- ulate the belief that patients deserved specialized nursing care given by graduates rather than by students played an important role in her ability to implement new administrative arrangements that simultaneously favoured the learning needs of the students. The words of D. Scollard reflect the magnitude of the changes brought by the new Director: "Dealt with sepa- rately, patient care and education of student nurses—the two chief func- tions of the department—were restructured in a way that was unrivalled even by the changes in the physical plant [a new hospital opened the same year]."[44] Significantly, she found a strong ally in the person of Margaret Street, an important nursing leader in Alberta, who was given the responsi- bility of reorganizing the clinical component of the nursing program.[45]

Although progress was made, the balancing act between service and education continued to take place. For example, in 1959, the students of the University of Alberta Hospital School of Nursing were asked to leave their classes and return to their assigned nursing units if they were needed there.[46] The statement made by Geneva Purcell about the conditions that existed in the 1960s at the University of Alberta Hospital School of Nursing

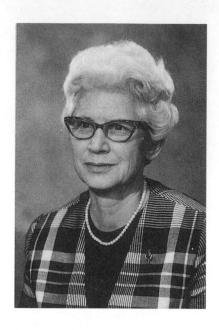

*⏤ Geneva Purcell, Director of
Nursing, University of Alberta
Hospital, 1962–1975 and
President of the AARN,
1969–1971. (AARN P806)*

is indicative of the fact that reforming the system took time. She stated: ". . . the needs of the hospital came ahead of the student's learning experience."[47]

DIPLOMA SCHOOLS SHIFT TO
THE GENERAL SYSTEM OF EDUCATION

In Canada, the 1960s were a period when traditional values and approaches to the health care system were questioned. In particular, the advisability of providing health insurance under the auspices of provincial and federal governments and the educational preparation of health professionals were scrutinized. In general, professional associations and nursing leaders advocated that the education of nurses should be transferred to educational institutions. After the publication of the Report of the Royal Commission on Health Services, provincial governments gradually embarked on the transfer of nursing education from the hospital to educational institutions. The transfer was most rapidly achieved in Ontario and Quebec, while Alberta and British Columbia were much more reluctant to alter the status quo. In Alberta, consensus was far from present, for while the nursing leadership and many nurses endorsed the national position, the government supported by a number of nurses, physicians and administrators, contended that hospital schools remained the best option for nursing education. In 1963, the Alberta Department of Health published a report on nursing education in which it was clearly ascertained that hospital schools of nursing should continue to be the providers of diploma nursing education.[48] It appears that cost was the most important deterrent for the surveyors. They took the position that two-year college programs would be more expensive because hospitals would have to hire more graduates to replace the substantial workforce made up by the third-year students.[49] They also specifically stated that the separation of nursing education from the hospital was uncalled for since: " . . . the trend in medical education is to closer integration with the hospital. . . ."[50] The use of such a premise reveals the extent of the surveyors' bias. Indeed, if they had really endorsed the position they were advocating, they would have proposed that medical education be transferred from the universities to hospital schools of medicine.

The position of the Alberta government was made very clear when it allowed the opening of a hospital school of nursing at the new Foothills Hospital in Calgary in 1965. From inception the school adopted policies that reflected the new norms in nursing education. For example, the ratio of students per clinical instructors was set as one to ten, and the school abolished " . . . the stipend, that relic of apprenticeship servitude. . . ."[51]

Nonetheless the creation of that school was against national trends in nursing education and indicates the extent to which it would not be easy to normalize the education of nursing students. However, those who believed that colleges should be responsible for diploma education did not remain idle. Two years later, Mount Royal College in Calgary developed the first diploma program outside of a hospital.[52] Sister Marguerite Letourneau, a Grey Nun who was a member of the committee formed to plan a strategy for the implementation of the Mount Royal program described the climate which existed at the time: "Political forces exalting changes, persistently parallelled by equally strong opposing forces, were frequently interlocked with pressures to transfer responsibility for the prescription, maintenance and control of standards in nursing education."[53]

Although the first college program was established in Calgary, it was in Edmonton that the first hospital elected to transfer its school of nursing to a mainstream educational institution. In 1967, the Edmonton General Hospital School of Nursing and the Misericordia Hospital School of Nursing (which later abandoned the project) began negotiations to affiliate with Collège Saint-Jean.[54] Beginning in the fall of 1968, the nursing students of the Edmonton General Hospital began taking general education courses at Collège Saint-Jean while nursing courses and clinical experience were provided at the hospital. However, in 1970, Collège Saint-Jean became part of the University of Alberta and a diploma program in nursing was out of the question since a degree program was already offered by the University. Other arrangements therefore had to be sought for the nursing program.

Believing that the affiliation with an educational institution had proved beneficial, the Grey Nuns of the Edmonton General Hospital completely transferred the program to the new Grant MacEwan College in 1973. It is evident that some opposed the new program. In 1973, G.L. Pickering, Executive Director of the Edmonton General Hospital, stated that the closure of the school did not mean that the hospital was no longer interested in nursing education but that on the contrary:

> it was because of our desire to improve nursing education and to bring it in line with advanced thinking on the subject that we made the decision, five years ago, to make such changes as were considered necessary to achieve those objectives [. . .] We took note of the fact that nursing educators and nursing associations had been advocating a change in the education of nurses for many years and that these changes were well advanced in many Canadian provinces. We could not escape the conclusion that if it is the policy of our society to permit professional groups generally to have overall discretion and control of the direction of their membership then this policy should have uniform and equitable relevancy, including its application to the nursing profession. It seems somewhat ironical that the majority of those who are opposing changes in nursing education belong to other professions in the health field which enjoy the very privileges that they are advocating should be denied to the nursing profession. [. . .] To the hospital which insists that it is financially advantageous to operate a school of nursing, I will only say that either they are not conducting an educational program in the best interest of the students, or the individuals making their financial studies are not providing them with proper information, or their situation may be a combination of both.[55]

Even though hospital programs only phased into the college and university system in 1995 in Alberta, the development of a number of college programs and the expansion of university programs which offered alternatives for those aspiring to become nurses had occurred some years prior to this. Also the strong belief of nursing educators working in the hospital programs in the need to develop a learning environment for students, which would facilitate their development, created such a climate for change that hospital administration eventually had to abandon the practice of using nursing students as primary workers over a period of years. Throughout the 1960s and 1970s the province continued to be reluctant to change. A good indicator of this caution is that it was only in 1983 that the government finally took measures to transfer the funding and administrative responsibility for hospital schools of nursing from the Departments of Hospitals and Medical Care and Social Services and Community Health to the Department of Advanced Education.[56]

After World War II when the hours of work on the nursing units began to be significantly shortened, nursing students became involved in more social activities in which they often competed with students in other schools of nursing. For example, in Edmonton, Glee Club competitions and sporting events were organized between the four hospital schools of the city. Similarly, in 1954 in Calgary, intramural basketball games were played between the Calgary General and Holy Cross students.[57] The late 1960s brought the end of curfews and compulsory residence living was gradually abolished. These changes reflected the fact that nursing students were increasingly permitted to live like any other group of college students. In the 1970s when it became acceptable for women to wear pants, schools of nursing permitted the introduction of pant uniforms. In contrast with the 1920s, the fashions of the day entered the nursing schools which again reflected a greater alignment with society.

Making the baccalaureate degree the point of entry to the profession had also been a goal of the Alberta Association of Registered Nurses since the publication of The Report of the Alberta Task Force on Nursing Education in 1975.[58] In the 1980s nursing educators became increasingly united toward reaching this goal by year 2000. In 1985, the University of Alberta Faculty of Nursing and Red Deer College began planning for the implementation of a collaborative model for a four-year baccalaureate program in nursing. Starting in 1990, the resulting collaborative program

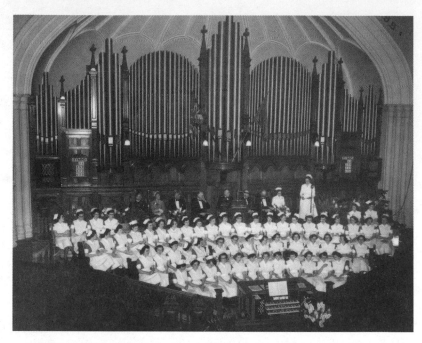

♦ *Choral Club, Royal Alexandra Hospital School of Nursing at graduation, McDougall United Church, circa 1950–1955. (Photograph courtesy of Royal Alexandra Hospital School of Nursing Archives)*

between a university and a college was the first of its kind in Canada. In 1991, the collaboration was extended to include all diploma schools of Edmonton: the University of Alberta Hospitals, Grant MacEwan College, the Misericordia Hospital and the Royal Alexandra Hospital. In 1993 similar arrangements were made between the University of Calgary Faculty of Nursing and the two diploma schools in Calgary at Mount Royal College and Foothills Hospital.[59]

Motivated by economic constraints the government of Alberta announced in 1994 that all hospital schools of nursing would be closed. However, it should be remembered that the authority for the financing of hospital diploma schools had been transferred to the Department of Advanced Education some years earlier in 1983. This would make the transition to the colleges and university somewhat easier, as would the fact that in the Edmonton, Red Deer and Calgary regions, collaborative/conjoint programs (in which all students received a common curriculum and the university was responsible for all teaching in the final years of the program) had been operating for a period of a few years prior to the announcement. Consequently, colleges and universities have become the only institutions offering nursing programs and all students entering a school of nursing have the opportunity to proceed to a baccalaureate degree in nursing.

For most of this century the majority of nurses in Alberta have graduated from hospital schools of nursing. Nursing educators and leaders have fought long and hard to improve the conditions that existed in nursing education. For too many years, nursing students were asked to serve the hospital at the expense of their own development. Even if this arrangement was far from ideal, it is evident that young women who selected the field of nursing were dedicated to the welfare of their fellow citizens. In many instances they showed true heroism considering the responsibilities they were given even when they were still students. The students of today are confronted with new challenges. They enter nursing at a time when the health care system is in transition and when the roles played by nurses are being transformed. Not unlike their predecessors they will have to take responsibility for the shaping of the future. However, their broader preparation will be their best asset and it is foreseen that they too will in time contribute to building a more humane Alberta.

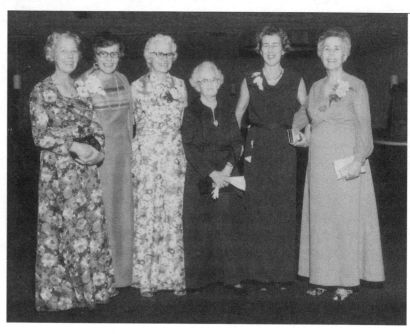

↬ *Former leaders gathered to attend the 50th anniversary of the University Schools of Nursing, (left to right) Helen Penhale, Ruth McClure, Geneva Purcell, Ethel Fenwick Cooper, Jeanie Clark Tronningsdal and Margaret Street (keynote speaker). (Photograph courtesy of Ruth McClure)*

The Emergence and Growth
of University Nursing Education

The struggle for social equality, which became a rallying cry for women in the first quarter of the twentieth century, also took hold on the prairies where the energies of women and men alike were required to work the land and to provide the services that were necessary in a frontier milieu. Women in western Canada became seriously involved in commenting on needs in health and education and developed organizations to put forward their ideas. Five Alberta women pressed forward with "the persons case," petitioning the Supreme Court of Canada and ultimately the Privy Council of Great Britain to declare that women were "persons" and as such could be elected to public office. Education had long been viewed by women as a means of surmounting perceived inequities in society. This was also true in nursing as expressed by Alice Baumgart and Rondalyn Kirkwood "Nursing within the university metaphorically represents the struggle of women to have their experience and knowledge validated and legitimized, and their professional expertise recognized as a university discipline."[1]

After World War I, the Canadian Red Cross Society became a partner in the formation of the League of Red Cross Societies and in planning an international program for peacetime activity in public health:

> It was decided that there should be a great worldwide public health organization to help bring up the standards of physical and mental fitness of the world . . . the promotion of health, the prevention of disease and the mitigation of suffering throughout the world.[2]

This organization served as a catalyst for the development of university programs in nursing across the country. The stimulation of the Canadian National Association of Trained Nurses, later the Canadian Nurses Association, was critical in this development, for the national professional organization invited the Society "to co-operate in a sweeping programme to improve and expand the country's nursing services."[3] A national committee was formed with representatives from the CNATN, the Canadian Red Cross Society and the St. John Ambulance Association and they endorsed the following resolutions on 10 September 1919:

> That the Central Council of the Canadian Red Cross Society should approach the universities with a view to the establishment of Nursing Departments, and that this action should be followed up by the Provincial Branches which should receive copies of the correspondence between the Head Office and the university; . . .
>
> That the adoption of the above policy should entail grants-in-aid to the universities establishing such courses. . . .[4]

This was followed by three-year grants from the national organization of the Canadian Red Cross Society to Canadian universities for the development of postgraduate courses in public health nursing. Although it has

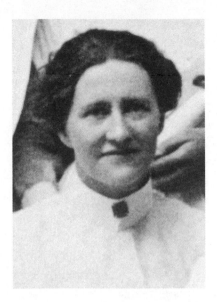

↝ *Victoria Winslow, first President of the Alberta Association of Graduate Nurses, 1916–1921, later to become the AARN. Photo taken in 1913 upon her graduation from the Medicine Hat General Hospital School of Nursing. (AARN P406)*

been reported that the University of Alberta received a Red Cross grant in 1921, the University had no record of receiving such a grant.[5] In any case it had become involved in offering a course in public health nursing in 1918, two years prior to the Red Cross grants to universities.

The passage of the Registered Nurses' Act in 1916 set the stage for the developments in postgraduate education in public health nursing and established the Alberta Association of Graduate Nurses, forerunner of the Alberta Association of Registered Nurses. At the first annual convention of the AAGN in December, 1917, President Victoria Winslow put forward the following objectives for the fledgling organization:

> That there be legislation to bring nursing education under the University of Alberta. . . .
>
> That there be a summer school for nurses established at the university similar to that established for teachers, which would enable nurses to learn the latest methods of treatment.[6]

When the Minister of Education appointed a Board of Examiners for setting uniform registration examinations, the Association was invited to appoint a member to the Senate of the University of Alberta.[7]

University Courses in Public Health Nursing

In Alberta, as elsewhere in the country, the catalyst for the introduction of nursing programs to the university was the perceived need for additional and highly capable nursing staff for public health work. In the aftermath of World War I, the impact of casualties and disability led to new value being placed upon promoting and maintaining health. The devastating consequences of the war along with those of the worldwide influenza epidemic of 1918 and 1919 led to support for public health programs and new patterns of health care delivery to prevent disease and improve the health and well-being of the Canadian populace. The health of mothers and children was seen as particularly critical to the nation because nurturing the health of the young was believed to raise the likelihood that the adult population of the future would be healthier than that of the past. In the new movement to promote health in the community, nurses were seen as central players with a need for additional, university-level preparation for their work.

When the first course in public health nursing was offered in 1918 shortly after the establishment of the Public Health Nursing Service, it became the first nursing program offered by a university in Canada:

> The appointment of Public Health Nurses was a prominent item . . . on the above mentioned programme. Miss Christine Smith being appointed as superintendent, and four graduate nurses—Misses Sargent, Davidson, Clark and Thurston—were engaged as field nurses. These, after receiving special training at the University, and from specialists along public health lines, were placed at different points through the province."[8]

This course was of two months duration and began on 1 April 1918.[9] A second course was held in 1919, again from 1 April to 31 May. The third time the course was offered was in 1921, this time for three months from January through March. The Public Health Nurses' Act, passed in 1919, designated the University of Alberta as the institution offering the course, specified that it would lead to a certificate or diploma, and authorized the graduate to "affix after her name the letters 'PH'."[10] The Act provided that:

(1) There shall be established in connection with the Provincial University a special course of study for nurses. (2) The said course shall include sanitation, personal hygiene, bacteriology, public health, examination of eye, ear, nose throat and teeth, the pre-natal period, infant welfare, child welfare, inspection and instruction of school children, communicable diseases, preventive medicine and methods, and such other studies as from time to time the Senate of the University may prescribe.[11]

Although such detail in an act of a provincial legislature would be highly unusual today, the fact that it was seen as important to set out matters of curriculum in a statute designed to ensure knowledgeable nurses for public health duties in the province is fascinating. That legislators felt compelled to do so may have been based on some uncertainty about whether the provincial university would offer the configuration of subjects believed to be consistent with sufficient public health nursing knowledge to ensure quality practice, or it simply may have been a reflection of the enthusiasm and commitment of the Hon. A.G. MacKay, Minister of Health and Member of the Legislative Assembly for the frontier area of Athabasca. The interest of the Acting Director of the Provincial Laboratory and Associate Professor of Medicine at the University of Alberta, Dr. Heber Jamieson, in public health nursing was also high.[12] Following a trip to Manitoba in 1917 to study a district nursing plan which was in operation there, he recommended that a similar plan be developed in Alberta: "He convinced Mr. MacKay and Alberta's district nursing service became official policy."[13] According to Cashman, the election of the United Farmers of Alberta government in 1921 led to the cancellation of the public health nursing courses that had received direct funding from the Government, even though they were *bona fide* courses offered by the University of Alberta.[14]

THE DEGREE PROGRAM IN NURSING AT THE UNIVERSITY OF ALBERTA

Because the early degree programs in both Canada and the United States established the pattern of university jurisdiction over those courses taken at the university and hospital jurisdiction over the theoretical and clinical nursing education gained within the affiliated hospital, diploma programs were often established at the same time degree programs were approved. This occurred at the University of Alberta where degree and diploma programs in nursing were established simultaneously. In 1924 the University of Alberta Senate approved a diploma course of 36 months, and a program in Nursing leading to a B.Sc.[15] It was undoubtedly fortuitous that the degree program in nursing at the University of Alberta was approved in the mid-1920s when economic conditions were highly favourable and prosperity seemed endless. Following the stock market crash on 29 October 1929, Canadian universities suffered an enormous shortfall in economic resources over the following decade and a subsequent decline in operations resulted. This was particularly true on the prairies where there was tremendous hardship because of the sharp loss of revenues in the provincial economies. The lack of growth at the University of Alberta through the Depression is seen in the decline in general revenues from $1,070,148 in 1930–31 to $877,396 in 1940–41, a drop of approximately 18% over a 10-year period.[16] In the context of such conditions, the University made the decision that it could not offer the final year in the nursing degree program. Students were sent to complete the final year of university courses in the program at the University of British Columbia (UBC) where economic conditions were more favourable than at the University of Alberta.[17] Designed as a temporary arrangement, this situation prevailed until 1937.[18]

Concern over Nursing Education

Disquieting deficiencies in the education of nurses were well understood by leaders in the nursing profession from the establishment and subsequent entrenchment of the diploma system of education in schools associated with hospitals. Education for entry to professional practice within this system was fraught with shortcomings, not the least of which was the lack of proper educational standards, Because the developing degree programs for nurses constituted a new system for preparing a basic practitioner, there were difficulties in ensuring that the programs were not just slightly better versions of a bad model. Nursing leaders thought at first that the solution was the development of a standard curriculum for the diploma schools, and enormous amounts of energy were directed to developing a series of these standard curricula to serve as models for schools over a period of years from the 1920s to the 1940s.[19] In that the problems were complex and

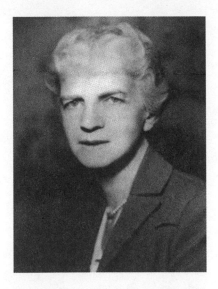

⊸ *E. Kathleen Russell, Director of
the School of Nursing,
University of Toronto, 1919–1952
(From* A Divine Discontent:
Edith Kathleen Russell,
Reforming Educator*)*

systemic, it is not surprising that publishing a standard curriculum did not solve them. The financial incentive for maintaining a nursing workforce composed of students in a school of nursing was unmistakeable. Since the primary function of the hospital was to provide health services to patients, the availability of nursing students to provide care at very little cost allowed an institution to maintain an economically viable operation in an era where hospitals were not supported by funds from taxation. University schools were, for the most part, inextricably linked to the problems relating to standards in the diploma schools, because with one notable exception in these formative years, most followed a "nonintegrated" pattern in which two or three years of university courses in the arts and sciences were "sandwiched" around a hospital diploma program.

At the University of Toronto, a three-year national Red Cross grant in 1920 stimulated the development of a course in public health nursing, a development similar to that occurring at other major universities across the country. However at the conclusion of the Red Cross grant in 1923, the Director of the School of Nursing, E. Kathleen Russell, expressed dissatisfaction with the results obtained by preparing public health nurses in this manner:

from the standpoint of educational procedures, the whole arrangement is indefensible except upon the ground of emergency need. If we consider the product in relation to the time and energy expended . . . this same product is sadly inadequate to meet the requirements of public health nursing and the result is most unfair to the student who had spent so much time upon an ill-arranged programme of studies.[20]

Although the public health courses continued to be funded by the University, in 1926 the first version of what was to become the basic degree program was implemented at the University of Toronto. It involved two years at the university studying public health nursing and a two-year component of nursing education in a hospital setting, for which graduates received diplomas from both institutions.[21] Soon after, the first in a series of substantial Rockefeller Foundation grants allowed further experimentation in the design of a basic degree program in nursing and culminated in the introduction in 1942 of a basic degree program in nursing. This program was the only one of its nature in North America and established a new "integrated" model of basic degree education in nursing where courses in the arts and sciences and were pursued along with nursing and where the university retained control over the complete education experience of the student. This new and innovative pattern of university education for nursing was an important development in Canadian nursing and was viewed with considerable interest by nursing educators in Alberta.

When the Strathcona Hospital was transferred to the University of Alberta in 1922, the University was given the responsibility for administering the Hospital.[22] However, a legislative change in 1929 transferred jurisdiction for the hospital from the University to the Hospital Board, which reported to the provincial government. Two *ex officio* representatives from the University to the Hospital Board were named at this time, the president of the University and the dean of Medicine.[23] Although the University may not have been troubled by the separation of university and hospital operations and its resulting loss of control over the administration of nursing in the Hospital, this development nevertheless had later ramifications for the operation of the nursing programs of the Hospital and the University.

Despite the fact that the University had offered courses in public health nursing in 1918, 1919 and 1921, the development of a degree program coincided with the introduction of a diploma program at the hospital. Although the first diploma class was admitted in the fall of 1923, formal approval of both the 36-month diploma program and five-year degree program by the Senate of the University did not take place until 1924.[24] The first baccalaureate class of four students was admitted in July, 1924. All came with previous university work and were given advanced standing in the program.[25] Agnes MacLeod had already earned a bachelor of arts degree from the University and graduated in 1927 with her B.Sc. in Nursing degree. She went on to graduate study at Columbia University and earned a master's degree prior to returning to Alberta to become director of the University of Alberta School of Nursing.[26] This work was interrupted by service in World War II following which she resigned as director upon her return to Canada to become matron-in-chief for the Department of Veterans' Affairs.[27]

NURSING EDUCATION THROUGH THE DEPRESSION AND WAR YEARS

The decision of the Canadian Medical Association in 1926 to appoint a committee to study nursing education led to a demand by nurses that such a study be conducted jointly in which nursing and medicine were equal partners. The study conducted by Dr. George Weir that resulted from this initiative yielded hard data on a wide range of matters in nursing education so that he was able to draw hard-hitting conclusions and make strong recommendations for action.[28] This report had a major impact upon the thinking of nurses about their profession and was the first investigation of conditions in nursing and nursing education in the Canadian context. Dr. Weir's conclusions were backed by data and his recommendations supported much of what nursing leaders in Alberta and elsewhere had been recommending for some time. The appalling state of nursing education applied as much to degree as diploma education since the diploma program was a building block around which the degree program was arranged. Recommendations of the study focused upon developing educationally sound programs in which the student's learning, health and general welfare were considered to be of paramount importance. An early response to the Report in Alberta was the appointment of an inspector for schools of nursing to monitor and report on conditions in the schools. As Eleanor McPhedran was one of the most respected of Alberta nurses, her appointment was viewed highly favourably by nurses.[29] It took decades for some of the Weir recommendations to be achieved, such as that authority for operating schools of nursing should rest within the general educational system. Nevertheless the impact of the Report was consequential and it had a wide-ranging impact upon nursing education in Alberta at all levels. It was arguably the most important external report on nursing education to be conducted in the twentieth century and its data and findings reverberated throughout the province for the remainder of the century.

The 1930s were difficult years for Canadian universities. The growth and expansion reflected in university operations of the 1920s were out of the question as the deep economic crisis took hold in the 1930s. Since the University of Alberta did not offer the final year of the degree program in nursing until towards the end of the decade, nursing program costs were minimized until there was more optimism about the future. As things began to stabilize, some growth was evident, and in 1940, the University reported a total of 89 students pursuing the degree option, or approximately 18 students in each year of the program. Faculty data indicates that in that same year, there were no nursing faculty who held academic appointments in the University, even though there were three faculty members listed who were assigned to teach in the program.[30] While this was not an uncommon finding across the country, of the six universities in Canada offering nursing programs in 1940–41, the University of Alberta was one of three in which nursing faculty members did not hold continuing academic appointments. The three members of faculty were listed as sessional instructors.[31]

INTEGRATED BACCALAUREATE DEGREE PROGRAM EMERGES

Although enrolment declined in some fields in the 1940s because young men went off to serve in the war, education in the health sciences became an area of national priority with the realization that health professionals were critical to the war effort and were also essential to care for the civilian population. Enrolment in the degree program in nursing was relatively stable at 85 at mid-decade, but by 1950–51, this figure had climbed to 113.[32] When the oversupply of nurses in the Depression years gave way to severe shortages, there was pressure to educate more students. The enlistment of nurses for war service and the resulting vacancies in civilian health agencies exacerbated the problem. However, as public recognition was accorded to nurses and nursing, the low standards which had plagued the profession for so many years and which Professor Weir had decried, slowly began to rise in both service and education. University schools of nursing began to reap benefits in the form of direct institutional grants as a result of new federal interest in higher education. In an accounting of grant disbursements in 1948 under the Dominion-Provincial grants program, the federal government reported distributing $12,945.47 to the University of Alberta School of Nursing over the three years of the funding program—1942, 1943 and 1944.[33]

The postwar boom brought an awakened interest in nursing and nursing education and university nursing programs began to thrive across the country. The availability of external funding from organizations such as the W.K. Kellogg Foundation for fellowships in nursing allowed faculty members in university schools to enhance their academic preparation through graduate study. To this end, between 1949 and 1954, the Kellogg Foundation reported giving grants amounting to $10,862 to Alberta nurses.[34] However, there were serious problems in the prevailing model of university nursing education across the country. In the Report of the Royal Commission on Health Services of 1964,[35] universities were castigated for continuing to espouse a model that was educationally flawed. However in the period between the inception of the University of Toronto program and the Royal Commission Report there were only two integrated nursing programs to be established. The first was at McMaster University in 1948 and the other in western Canada at the University of Alberta, where an important attempt was made to establish an integrated degree program in nursing in 1952.

The Structure and Operation of the School of Nursing[36]

The appointment of Helen Eileen Marie Penhale as Director of the University of Alberta School of Nursing followed the resignation of the former director, Agnes J. MacLeod. Miss Penhale came to Alberta from the University of Western Ontario where she had been a faculty member in the Institute of Public Health. She was a graduate of the Mount Sinai School of Nursing in New York and held bachelor's and master's degrees from Teacher's College, Columbia University. The announcement of her appointment in the 9 March 1946 edition of the *Edmonton Bulletin* noted "She is well known in Edmonton, having taught for two seasons at the university summer school for graduate nurses."[37] Prior to Miss Penhale's appointment, an item on the agenda of the 14 September 1945 meeting of the University of Alberta Hospital Board was entitled "Letter from Dr.

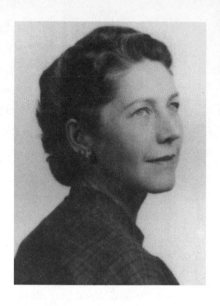

Newton Re. Organization of Training School."[38] In it, Dr. Robert Newton, President of the University and a member of the Hospital Board, proposed that the Director of the School of Nursing "should have complete jurisdiction over the instruction of students both in the University and in the University Hospital, while the Superintendent of Nurses in the hospital should have supervision of service, duties, discipline, et cetera."[39] Dr. Angus McGugan, Medical Superintendent of the Hospital, appeared to have some concern about this as he acknowledged the University's jurisdiction in granting "degrees to degree students . . . diplomas to diploma students,"[40] and authority in the direction of subjects basic to the science of nursing such as physiology, anatomy and others. He inferred that the Hospital should have control over the clinical subjects in the nursing program, citing the Canadian Nurses' Association's standard curriculum to support his argument: "one should be careful not to take any steps which would divorce the Art of Nursing from the Science of Nursing and vice versa."[41]

Apprehension about the possibility of losing the services of senior nursing faculty who were heavily committed to providing nursing supervision in the hospital appeared to be at the root of a concern expressed about the adequacy of University Hospital representation on the Council of the School of Nursing since the Council held responsibility for curriculum and policy in the School.[42] Although the Board decided that representation was

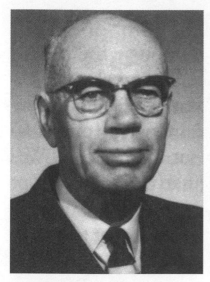

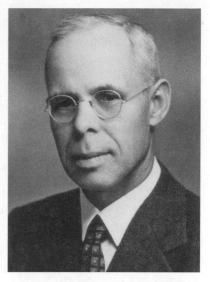

↬ Dr. Angus McGugan, Medical
Superintendent of the
University of Alberta Hospital,
1942–1960. (From More Than a
Hospital)

↬ Dr. Robert Newton, President of
the University of Alberta,
1941–1945. (UAA 69–12–6)

adequate, the concern over the issue was perhaps a signal that the value of services provided by staff and students would be watched very carefully in the structure and operations of the School of Nursing.

The proposal continued to be the subject of discussion for several meetings of the Hospital Board and despite any lingering doubts, approval was granted unanimously upon Dr. Newton's motion ". . . that a Director of the School of Nursing of the University of Alberta be appointed and that such Director have charge of the instructional services both on the Campus and in the hospital."[43] The concern did not end there however, and Dr. McGugan maintained that there was a need to clarify the duties of the Director of the School of Nursing and the Nursing Superintendent of the University Hospital to avoid misunderstandings. In that Miss Penhale had not yet arrived to take up her duties, the Board decided to wait until her arrival to clarify the roles in question.

A matter considered at the 13 September 1946 meeting of the University Hospital Board drew attention to the vesting of administrative authority for the School of Nursing. The Minister of Health had questioned the need for senior matriculation as a requirement for admission to the School of Nursing and was informed that "the Training School comes under the administration of the University."[44] However, in questioning the Hospital's conclusion, the Minister "contended that the University of Alberta Hospital Act of 1929 placed the authority for the education and training of medical students and nurses under the Hospital Board: Section 7, Subsection c."[45] This was an issue that would be revisited at a later date.

At the bimonthly meeting of the Board on 10 January 1947, Miss Penhale was invited "to make representations regarding the organization and operation of the School of Nursing."[46] Presumably the purpose of this presentation was to clarify the roles of the Director of the School of Nursing and the Superintendent of Nurses. Miss Penhale noted that: "The position of the Director of the School of Nursing, Associate Professor of Public Health Nursing and Health Education is not sufficiently clear to make for good working relationships. I have outlined two plans which might be considered. A third was presented to the body on 12 October 1945.[47] Here Miss Penhale referred to the plan submitted to the Board by Dr. Newton some five months prior to her appointment. This suggests that the reorganization requested by Dr. Newton had originally been raised by Miss Penhale as a condition of her employment. The two plans outlined by Miss Penhale on the occasion of her appearance before the Board on the 10 January 1947 included an arrangement known as Plan A where the Director of the School would be a campus official to whom the Director of Nursing Service and the Director of Nursing Education would report. She noted that if there was a conflict or problem between those holding these positions, the Director could mediate or if necessary refer the matter to the Council of the School of Nursing for discussion and resolution.[48] Plan B was a proposal in which the Director would simply be "in charge of nursing education on the campus and in the hospital".[49]

The Board approved Plan A following a three-hour meeting in which the administrative organization of the School of Nursing was the only item on the agenda. This was undoubtedly a controversial matter. Although both plans extended the authority of the Director of the School of Nursing, Plan A went further than Plan B because control of the sizeable nursing service component given by students would be necessary to implement a new program model, and Plan A stipulated that the Director would have this control. Plan B was closer to the plan Dr. Newton had originally proposed in 1945 and would have had the effect of ensuring that the Director of the School of Nursing would have control of both nursing education in the hospital and in the university, but she would have no responsibility for nursing service in the hospital. Miss Penhale was asked to bring a more detailed document to the Board to identify how the plan that had been approved would be implemented.[50]

When Miss Penhale's plan entitled "A Proposed Plan of Organization and Operation of the School of Nursing" was considered, she was called before the Board "explain several details."[51] Dr. McGugan recommended that the report be submitted to the Superintendent of Nurses and the Hospital Medical Advisory Board for their information and recommendations.[52] Finally, and more revealing, Dr. McGugan "also indicated that the plan proposed to delegate considerable responsibility and authority for nursing education and nursing services to the University either directly or through the Council of the School of Nursing, and referred to Section 7, sub-section c of the University of Alberta Hospital Act."[53] It is clear from this reference that the earlier interpretation of the Minister of Health that the Hospital held the responsibility for the three-year diploma School of Nursing by virtue of the provisions of the University of Alberta Hospital Act, had been accepted by Dr. McGugan and the Board. The Superintendent also "pointed out that the proposed plan would mean a material increase in the cost of the School of Nursing."[54] Following further discussion, Dr. Newton moved: "That the Board approve Miss Penhale's plan in principle and ask her to begin putting it into effect as may be practicable."[55]

Unresolved Issues

It seems likely that the Board and the Superintendent, Dr. McGugan, were not completely satisfied that the new directions in nursing education were either necessary or desirable. This was not the end of the discussion of Miss Penhale's organizational plan. Although the plan was approved at the meeting of 24 January 1947, the first item on the agenda of the regular Board meeting of 13 February 1947 referred again to this and a "revised draft of the organization of the School of Nursing, University of Alberta," was presented for consideration. The draft was considered at length. It was moved by Dr. Ower, seconded by Dr. Newton, that the revised draft, with certain alterations, be approved. Carried."[56] Perhaps significant is that all of the motions on the reorganization of the School of Nursing at University Hospital Board meetings were made by the University President, Dr. Newton. It seems apparent that Dr. Newton's support for Miss Penhale's desire to establish an integrated degree program in nursing was unwavering despite opposing arguments put forward by Hospital Superintendent Dr. McGugan.

It is difficult to know the influence of the prevailing educational philosophy of members of the Hospital Board in relation to the issues here. However, an item on the agenda of the 12 December 1947 meeting underscores the importance of student services to the Hospital. Dr. McGugan commented on the withdrawal of two first-year and one second-year student noting that attrition "represented a loss of a very material sum of money to the hospital in the training of these individuals and that an attempt should be made to devise some safeguard for the prevention of withdrawals in the future."[57] Thus, students were seen primarily in an economic light since hospital operations were subsidized by the substantial contribution they made. It seemed that curriculum concerns and educational needs of students were secondary to economic considerations.

HELEN PENHALE'S VISION OF NURSING EDUCATION

The new Director of the School of Nursing stepped into a leadership position where the lines of authority and responsibility between the University and the Hospital were unclear. It is evident that the Director had a vision of the directions that needed to be taken in university nursing education. In a keynote address delivered at a Canadian Nurses Association Convention, Miss Penhale asserted that: "Encouraging students to master a body of knowledge and certain skills is not enough; we have a responsibility to start them on a program of self-education and to give them the fundamental insights and ways of thought that will enable them to draw the maximum profit from their later education in the school of experience."[58] Her concept of education as self-directed and as a lifelong process, was one that educational philosophers espoused in decades to come. Miss Penhale described the integrated baccalaureate nursing curriculum that she and her colleagues implemented in the following way:

> The objective of the integrated academic and basic professional program is to select well-qualified young women and prepare them for

community nursing service in hospitals and public health agencies; at the same time, to give them a perspective on the opportunities for professional women and needs of communities for their active participation as citizens.[59]

Some two decades later, Miss Penhale referred to the uniqueness of the integrated program she and her colleagues had developed:

the type of program we attempted to design was one with a much broader base [broader than previous programs], especially in the social science area. It would require more courses in this discipline as well as requiring nurse-teachers qualified to help students utilize the concepts they had learned in the classroom.[60]

Miss Penhale was particularly concerned by duplication of learning experiences in the clinical learning environment. While she believed that some repetition was valuable in learning, she deplored repetition that did not contribute to learning.[61]

Miss Penhale earned the respect of her peers as she became involved in activities of the nursing profession soon after her arrival. She became acting President of the Conference of University Schools of Nursing, a national organization of university schools of nursing. She was also elected President of the Alberta Association of Registered Nurses in 1953 and served in that capacity until 1955. Two years following her appointment as Associate Professor and Director of the School of Nursing, Miss Penhale was promoted to the rank of Professor and awarded tenure.[62] It seems reasonable to conclude that her performance was deemed to be highly commendable, if not distinguished within the University. Her professorial appointment was a significant step forward for the Faculty of Nursing, for just five years earlier, no nurse had even held a continuing academic appointment on the staff of the University.[63] Universities of the 1940s and 1950s were relatively small institutions and nursing education a modest undertaking in comparison to other disciplines. A review of the situation across Canada revealed that few nurses held continuing academic appointments in universities at the time.[64] In the case of Miss Penhale's promotion to professor, it is likely that final decisions were vested in President Newton.

The New Structure and Its Problems

Following the approval of the new administrative structure for nursing education and service, the arrangement seemed at the outset to be satisfactory. The first indications of discord were sounded at the 13 May 1949 meeting of the Hospital Board in the reference to a special committee that had been appointed "to consider the matter of nursing services in the hospital."[65] The only issue described in any detail related to a submission from Miss Penhale, who wrote:

> In reply to your request to bring suggestions to the meeting in writing in order to expedite discussion may I present the following:—
> 1. A Director was appointed on March 8, 1946. The specific duties of the Director were tabled and have probably never been too clearly defined.
> The new set-up has been in operation almost three years and has obviously not worked. Is it wise to continue the present organization or revert back to the former set-up?[66]

It appeared that Miss Penhale was unhappy with the division of responsibilities and had raised the matter for consideration. The Board "directed that the questions raised in Miss Penhale's letter be considered at the two June meetings of the Hospital Board" when Miss Penhale was to be invited to the first meeting and the Superintendent of Nurses, Miss Helen Peters, to the second one.[67] The issues were to be aired before the Board with separate appearances by Miss Penhale and Miss Peters.

Miss Penhale appeared as directed at the next regular meeting of the Board to discuss the organization of the Department of Nursing,[68] and reported to the Board that although the organization was satisfactory, the operation of the organization was not.[69] She explained that a problem was that Miss Peters continued to carry out duties belonging to the Department of Nursing Education and did not accept the responsibility for some nursing service duties. Here she referred to "the matter of making rounds in the hospital."[70] During Miss Peters attendance at the second meeting, she reported to the Board that she believed that the existing organization was satisfactory and that some conflict might be expected between those interested primarily in either nursing education or nursing service.[71] She appeared to suggest that the problem was not as acute as Miss Penhale had

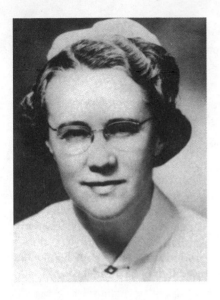

~ *Helen Peters, Superintendent of Nursing Services/Director of Nursing Services, University of Alberta Hospital, 1928–1954.* (UAA 69–90–186)

suggested, stating that "differences of opinion and problems arising there-from might be readily adjusted at conferences of the interested parties."[72] Miss Peters recommended "that the duties and responsibilities of the Director of the School and the Superintendent of Nursing Services should be clarified further, and specified in as much detail as possible."[73] She also indicated that it was her opinion that the day-to-day operation of the plan for organization approved by the Board was working much more smoothly now than previously. Further downplaying the problem, she stated that "the most acute problem at present is the scarcity of graduate nurses."[74]

Approval of the Integrated Program

In the meantime, Miss Penhale moved forward to revise the curriculum of the degree program. Her plan was to eliminate the five-year nonintegrated program in favour of a four-year integrated degree program, patterned after the University of Toronto model. The latter was approved as indicated in a letter from President Newton to Miss Penhale on 20 June 1950:

> The Board of Governors at a meeting June 16 approved the proposal of the School of Nursing, which came forward with the support of the Faculty of Medicine and the General Faculty Council, that beginning September, 1951, there be instituted an integrated course leading to the

degree of Bachelor of Science in Nursing and that after September, 1950, no initial registrations in the present B.Sc. course in Nursing be accepted.[75]

Although the intent had been to introduce the program in the Fall of 1951, this was delayed a year because it took longer to prepare the curriculum plan and secure the necessary support and approvals from the relevant councils and boards.[76]

At the 23 February 1952 meeting of the University Hospital Board, Miss Penhale sent a memorandum recommending "the introduction of the block system of ward training and the reduction of the Degree course from a five to a four year course." She pointed out that "the actual number of months spent in training in the Degree course essentially be unchanged."[77] The matter was deferred until Miss Penhale could be called before the Board for discussion, at which point "The Superintendent indicated that he questioned the advisability of any innovation at a time when there will be a very material problem in the matter of obtaining staff for the entire new wing."[78] However Dr. McGugan went on to say that "in the opinion of Miss Peters, upon whom the responsibility for staffing the hospital rests, the proposed block system would facilitate nursing services in the hospital."[79] The matter was tabled until the next meeting when it was approved on the motion of President Andrew Stewart.[80] The programs were considered by the University Hospital Board at the 28 March 1952 meeting when "Miss Penhale presented a brief in the matter of proposed changes in the basic programme leading to the degree of B.Sc. in nursing."[81] After "prolonged" discussion, Dr. J.W. Scott,[82] Dean of the Faculty of Medicine, moved approval of the program. The proposals for the program had been approved at a special meeting of the Council of the School of Nursing held on 21 March 1952. The motion included direction for the secretary to inform the General Faculty Council of the University that approval was forthcoming from the University Hospital Board.[83]

Following approval of the final version of the curriculum, the four-year degree program in nursing was implemented in September of 1952. Early the following year at a meeting of the Council of the School of Nursing, the number of classes admitted to the School of Nursing was considered: "It was pointed out that with the change of the Degree course, there will now be three classes of pre-clinical students admitted each year."[84] Concern was

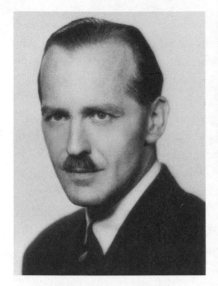

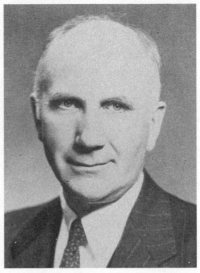

↬ *Dr. Andrew Stewart, President*
of the University of Alberta,
1950–1959. (UAA 69–12–18)

↬ *Dr. J.W. Scott, Dean of the*
Faculty of Medicine, University
of Alberta, 1944–1959.
(UAA 69–90–214)

expressed over the problems arising from the need to teach so many students simultaneously, and it was suggested "that the January class be eliminated."[85] Perhaps more revealing was the statement that "the loss of diploma students in this class might mean a serious loss of graduates from this school who will be available later as graduate nurses for the staff of this hospital."[86] Again, the service needs of the Hospital carried more weight than what might be best for students from an educational standpoint. These concerns foreshadow the difficulties which ensued.

Moves to Terminate the New Program

Later that same year that the Superintendent of the Hospital, Dr. McGugan, delivered what was the death knell of the new integrated program. At a special meeting of the University Hospital Board called on 9 November 1953, the sole item on the agenda was "Organization Department of Nursing."[87] The minutes state ominously that "Dr. McGugan, Superintendent, reviewed the present organizational chart and outlined the difficulties created by the Director of Nursing having dual responsibility to the University Hospital

Board and the University Board of Governors."[88] Dr. McGugan indicated that his need to make recommendations on the matter now had been precipitated by the illness of Miss Peters, Superintendent of Nursing Services.[89] He recommended the following:

That a Director of Nursing be appointed in charge of all nursing service in the University Hospital and that the University Hospital School return to the arrangement in existence prior to 1945. The Degree nurses would receive their training on an internship basis but during the course of their three years in the hospital, would be under the supervision of the Director of Nursing of the University Hospital. The Director of Nursing of the University of Alberta would continue to indicate the subjects to be taught and the amount of time each nurse is to receive in each subject and would periodically require a report of each nurse concerned.

The Hospital Board approved the Superintendent's recommendation on the motion of Dean J.W. Scott, indicating that it was:

in concurrence with the opinion of the Superintendent, that the question of divided authority as represented by the present position of Director of the University of Alberta and the University Hospital School of Nursing has created problems and would prefer that a separate school of nursing be established by the University Hospital and it is hoped that this school could operate in collaboration with the University of Alberta.[90]

At the Executive Committee meeting of the Board of Governors of the University, "The President referred to administrative changes proposed by the University Hospital Board which would, in effect, remove responsibility for training and nursing service within the Hospital from the Director of the School of Nursing."[91] Further, Dr. Stewart reported that: "The Director would still be responsible for the University's B.Sc. program, but Miss Penhale is not willing to stay on the University staff if the changes, to be effective January 1, 1954, are made."[92] The nature of the response of members of the Executive Committee of the Board of Governors is unrecorded in the minutes, save for the notation that "any such change, affecting the position of a member of the University, could not be made during the academic year, i.e., before May 15."[93] At the next meeting of the University Hospital Board, the response of the University Board of Governors was reported, indicating that they would be: "agreeable to terminate the present arrangement as of May 15th, 1954."[94] The Board of Governors also made it clear that candidates would be accepted from other diploma schools of nursing as well as those from the University Hospital in the future, and that "it would not be possible to present diplomas for University Hospital graduates at University Convocation."[95]

What is somewhat surprising in this situation was the acquiescence of the University's Board of Governors to the proposed changes in the programs that came from the Hospital Board. Further, since it was Dr. Andrew Stewart, Dr. Robert Newton's successor as President of the University, who moved that the University Hospital Board "proceed with the organization of its own school of nursing, to be effective May 16, 1954,"[96] one is led to conclude that Dr. Stewart had been convinced by Dr. McGugan of the need for taking such drastic action. The University thus failed to provide support for the four-year degree program offered by its own School of Nursing. The program was summarily terminated on the recommendation of the Superintendent of the Hospital and the Hospital Board with the concurrence of the President of the University and the University Board of Governors. On 23 March 1956, the Board of Governors of the University of Alberta was informed that Miss Penhale's resignation would take effect on 31 August 1956.[97]

Opposition to the Integrated Degree Program

The strongest opposition to the integrated program clearly came from the University Hospital, in particular its Medical Superintendent, Dr. Angus McGugan. Dr. McGugan wrote in 1964:

> With the appointment of the Associate Professor of Nursing of the University, Miss Helen Penhale, as the Director (August, 1946), the school became known and was in fact the University of Alberta School of Nursing (January 1947). This change was made against the advice of the hospital administration. Objections were based on the opinion that the principle of authority without corresponding responsibility is administratively unsound.[98]

The extent to which the Superintendent of Nurses of the Hospital, Miss Helen Peters, supported the new program and the change in the organization of the School of Nursing is not known, although prior to the point at which she became terminally ill with cancer in 1953, Miss Peters had appeared to downplay problems. Dr. McGugan was very supportive of Miss Peters and wrote later that she ". . . pioneered in the establishment of the recognition of nursing as a profession. She was definitely resistive to any attitude of condescension or patronage, or any attempt at domination directed at either herself, any particular nurse, or at the profession in general by the nouveaux riches or noveaux [sic] eleves."[99] There was also evidence that the new Dean of the Faculty of Medicine, Dr. John W. Scott, did not support the program.[100] He also reflected later that he fully supported the Board position and that: "The thing that concerns me today is that nurses are becoming more and more 'doctors' and the people who do the *nursing* are the nursing aides. I'm sure there still are dedicated nurses, but a great many of them only come around as executives and keep records."[101] Dr. Scott maintained some twenty years after the division of the two schools of nursing in Dr. McGugan's time "was a good thing."[102]

Despite their differences, it appears that on the surface Miss Peters supported Miss Penhale's plans for the degree program, and that her influence was sufficiently strong to overcome Dr. McGugan's objections to the program at the time it was proposed. When Miss Peters became terminally ill, whatever support she had provided seemed to disappear when Miss Jeannie Clark, who took Miss Peters's place, was not able to convince the Hospital Board and its Superintendent to allow time for the program to become established. Problems in the relationship between Miss Penhale and Miss Clark may be inferred from events described in Miss Penhale's memorandum to President Stewart on 16 September 1954. Miss Penhale states: "In my telephone conversation with Miss J. Clark, University Hospital, this morning, I was given to understand that the way in which I had handled two specific problems presented by two degree nurses, was considered as 'interference'."[103] These problems appeared to be "turf battles" over control of the clinical educational experience of the student, battles predicated upon the financial value of the service to the hospital provided by students. For Miss Penhale, who had already lost her integrated degree program and much of her authority and responsibility through the actions of the Hospital Board and the University, this situation must have been difficult.

Long after the events in question, Miss Clark attributed the failure of the degree program to the additional teaching load it placed upon members of the University Hospital teaching staff and the shaky financial basis upon which the program was proposed: "The concept was excellent but it was not developed with an adequate supporting budget."[104]

Many factors weighed against Miss Penhale and the timing of the introduction of the four-year integrated degree program in nursing at the University of Alberta. In this postwar period, there was an extreme shortage of nurses, which consumed and diverted the attention of hospital and nursing service administrators alike.[105] Students were looked upon as a workforce of considerable value to the hospital, and their illness and/or attrition was seen as a money-losing proposition for the hospital. Since there were only two integrated university programs in nursing in the country at the time, both of these in Ontario, understanding of this model of nursing education may have been limited. The Faculty of Medicine at the University of Toronto had been quite supportive of its own School of Nursing and Director Kathleen Russell's goals. The lack of equivalent support at the University of Alberta was undoubtedly an important factor leading to the failure to sustain an integrated baccalaureate degree program in nursing.[106]

Diminished authority and negligible influence wielded by university nursing administrators in this era have been attributed to administrative structures unfavourable to women by both Kirkwood and Kinnear.[107] Because of the low status of nursing in universities, support of more powerful male colleagues was essential for progress. Gender stereotyping and bias conditioned processes and outcomes. In the situation faced by Miss Penhale, the roles of the key players were critical and one wonders whether the outcomes might have been different if the presidency of the University had not passed from Dr. Newton to Dr. Stewart, if Miss Peters had not become terminally ill, or if Dr. McGugan and Dr. Scott had held more liberal ideas about nursing and nursing education. It is clear that the principal stakeholders here, namely physicians and hospital administrators, wielded significant power over nursing education and nursing service. When these powerful players did not support the goals and directions advocated by key nurses, the balance of power turned against the nurses, who were outnumbered and who were not present at the table where critical decisions about their discipline were made.

Since Helen Penhale was well-known and respected in her field, one may wonder why concrete support did not come from other nurses who shared her views. Support could have come from an organization known as the Conference of University Schools of Nursing (later the Canadian Association of University Schools of Nursing). However, circumstances within this new national organization were far from normal for a number of reasons. Member university schools of nursing struggled with shortages of qualified faculty as well as the large postwar influx of military nurses to university nursing programs. Further, "for much of the period between 1948 and 1951, Helen Penhale (Alberta) struggled [as acting president], with the help of the past-president, Kathleen Ellis (Saskatchewan), to keep the organization afloat while the president, Evelyn Mallory (British Columbia), and the vice-president, Sister Françoise de Chantal (Ottawa) were away on study leave."[108] After 1948 the organization lost much of its strength and unity of purpose when Kathleen Russell and Alma Reid, directors of the two integrated university schools of nursing in the country, objected to an independent role for the organization, believing it preferable to work through the Canadian Nurses Association in furthering the interests of university nursing education. The failure of the most prestigious schools to support the organization rendered it virtually powerless to fulfil its mandate until the latter part of the 1950s.[109] Finally, working relationships between Helen Penhale and other leaders in university nursing education may not have been sufficiently strong to engender support for the new integrated baccalaureate program in nursing.

Why the Alberta Association of Registered Nurses did not mount a campaign objecting to terminating the new integrated degree program at the University of Alberta is a matter of interest and one about which little information is available. Since Helen Penhale was the President of the organization during the time of the program transition, the Association may have believed that its objections would have been futile since its primary spokesperson was Miss Penhale herself. The AARN had made many representations about improving standards of nursing education over the years to the University, since by virtue of The Registered Nurses Act of 1916, authority for monitoring standards of nursing education was vested in the Senate of the University of Alberta. According to Young,[110] AARN concerns had been ignored over a period of several decades and the University consistently failed to fulfil its mandated responsibility to ensure that appropriate standards of nursing education were maintained in the diploma nursing schools of the province.

Divisions within the profession over the development of integrated programs may have also made AARN intervention in the dispute difficult. The integrated program model was viewed by some within the profession as usurping the power and authority rightfully belonging to the major program model in nursing education at the time, the diploma program and its sponsor, the hospital. Some nursing leaders who were involved in teaching and administration in the diploma schools were disinclined to promote the development of an integrated degree program since this was in some sense a competitive model. The question of whether nurses needed to be educated in universities was one in which there were overtones of gender bias relative to the value of higher education for women as compared with men. Since the University of Alberta program was the first of its type in Western Canada, hospitals and universities may not have been sufficiently prepared to accept this new development. There were inherent dilemmas for a society in which education for women was not valued as highly as that for men in such questions as whether or not to elevate the status of nursing to the university from the diploma level, to allow women to attend university for four years when two was the norm for a post-R.N. nursing degree in many centres, and to forego the considerable revenues that accrued to hospitals from the nursing service provided gratis by diploma nursing students.

Ironically, slightly more than a decade after the termination of the integrated degree program introduced by Miss Penhale, a new four-year integrated program was established at the University of Alberta by her successor, Ruth McClure. The recommendations of the Royal Commission on Health Services of 1964 were clearly influential as they resulted in closure of all nonintegrated degree programs in Canada within a decade.[111] As the forerunner of the integrated program established in 1966, the earlier program with two classes of graduates, undoubtedly created a climate for eventual acceptance of the idea that the university should assume primary responsibility for the entire education of the student in a degree program in nursing. Many Alberta nurses were deeply influenced by ideas and directions advocated by Miss Penhale. When those who held the reins of control in the dispute over the program were succeeded by others, it became possible to make the case for developing an integrated degree program in nursing at the University.

The termination of the program before the first class was even half way through the program of studies was perhaps not significant in the total scheme of things, for students graduated from an integrated degree program offered by the University Alberta thirteen short years later. Failures are an important, if painful, means of learning. Examining such episodes is useful to gain a greater appreciation of the complexity of change in large organizations, the nature of gender discrimination in health and educational settings and the need for effective communication and true collaboration of all interested parties in order to implement new program models successfully. What is instructive here is that this was a dramatic and well-documented episode in the history of university nursing education that illuminates the interplay of forces facilitating and thwarting progress in curriculum innovation. Underscored are professional goals including improving standards of university nursing education, achieving credibility for nursing as an academic discipline and extending equality for women in the university. The termination of the first integrated baccalaureate nursing program is also a well-documented example of a situation in which a leading nursing administrator was prevented from acting in ways designed to serve the public and the profession better. Such situations are not unusual even at the present time for all of the reasons that have been put forward in the analysis of this case. There are other examples of difficulties experienced by university nursing administrators cited that in many ways run parallel to the Penhale episode. However, no other incident can be assessed to the extent that is possible in the University of Alberta situation because of the existence of original records to support the analysis.

CONSOLIDATION AND GROWTH IN UNIVERSITY NURSING EDUCATION

The appointment of Ruth McClure as Director of the School of Nursing at the University of Alberta in 1956 led to two decades of consolidation and progress in university nursing education in the province. The new Director was appointed to an academic unit in which the roles of university nursing faculty and hospital nursing administrators had been clarified, however painful that process might have been. The separation of the two nursing programs allowed each organization to pursue its primary objectives and to move in directions that may not have been possible prior to the conflict

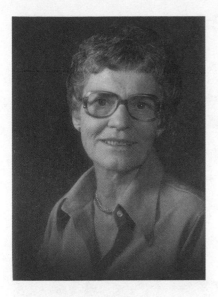

⊷ Ruth McClure, former Director and later Dean, Faculty of Nursing, 1956–1976. (Photograph courtesy of Ruth McClure)

over the form of the university degree program. For the School of Nursing at the University of Alberta, this meant that it could grow and develop as an academic discipline without responsibility for supporting the nursing service of the hospital. In the transfer of responsibilities from Helen Penhale to Ruth McClure, the role of the director had been clarified and consolidated within the University. Ruth McClure and her staff were given full authority over the degree program in nursing, even though there were lingering tensions for a time relative to the separation of the two schools. The passage of time, the rising status of women in society, the changing context of health care, issues of concern in the nursing profession, changes in higher education generally as well as other societal factors ensured that the energies of all were focused squarely on the challenges of the future.

The support given to the development of integrated degree programs by the Royal Commission on Health Services in 1964 led to almost overnight closure of five-year nonintegrated degree programs in nursing across the country.[112] At the University of Alberta, the first class entered the new four-year integrated program in 1966. Ruth McClure highlighted the approach she took as follows:

It was our belief that a university program in Nursing should be as similar as possible to other professional degree programs on campus.

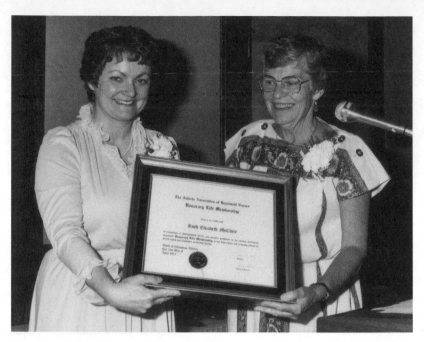

⤳ *Ruth McClure receiving honourary membership in* AARN *from President Janet Ross-Kerr in 1983. (*AARN P226*)*

Students should be mingling all the time with those of other disciplines. In the past, nursing students had been rather isolated . . . In retrospect, the transition occurred fairly smoothly. A great deal of time was spent by faculty members in interpreting the new program, developing affiliation agreements with health agencies and establishing sound working relationships with professional and administrative colleagues.[113]

The post-R.N. baccalaureate program established at the same time as the earlier four-year baccalaureate program had been introduced by Miss Penhale continued to take in students who had a diploma in nursing and wanted to study for a B.Sc. in Nursing. However, the certificate programs in teaching and supervision and in public health nursing were discontinued because the content had been consolidated within the degree programs, a development that was consistent with trends across Canada.

The School of Nursing operated on a more autonomous basis from the Faculty of Medicine following Ruth McClure's appointment and gained

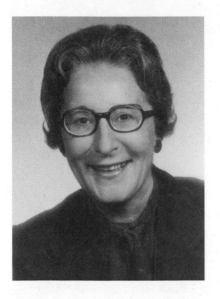

↝ Dr. Shirley Stinson was given responsibility for the new Master of Nursing program when it was initiated in 1975; pictured here as President of the Canadian Nurses Association, 1980–1982. (AARN SS4a)

formal autonomy as an independent unit within the University's administrative framework in 1966[114] under the new Universities Act when "The Schools of Home Economics, Nursing and Rehabilitation Medicine were authorized to have their own councils . . ."[115] In that these were all academic units comprised predominantly of women, this was a step towards structural equality within the administrative framework of the University. A change from School to Faculty status in 1976, at which time the Director became the Dean was a further move in this direction. With greater autonomy to enunciate its goals and to take new directions in its programs, the Faculty of Nursing began to develop plans to offer graduate programs in nursing.

A Master of Nursing program was approved under Dr. McClure's tenure and Dr. Shirley Stinson was given responsibility for the direction of the new program to which the first students were admitted in 1975. The development of a master's program was an important development in Alberta as only UBC in Western Canada offered a master's degree program in nursing. With the establishment of the first graduate program in nursing in the province and indeed on the prairies, the importance of research in nursing as a basis for graduate education began to be recognized. Nurses involved in graduate education realized that there was much work to be done to develop a research thrust in nursing to support graduate programs.

The movement to university-based education for nurses and to transfer responsibility for schools of nursing to the general educational system recommended four decades earlier in the Weir report began to take hold in the 1960s. The pioneering and very well-educated Grey Nuns whose mother house was in Montreal continued to have an important influence on nursing education in Alberta. They had, after all, taken steps to join forces with the University of Montreal and the school of nursing they had established, l'Institut Marguerite d'Youville, became the Faculté des Sciences Infirmières of that University offering a four-year integrated degree program. In keeping with trends in nursing education and their philosophy of teaching and learning, the sisters first reduced the length of their diploma program at the Edmonton General Hospital to two years. They then took steps to ensure that authority for the program was vested in the general education system when they made an arrangement in 1968 to transfer responsibility for the school to Collège St. Jean, a French-language community college in Edmonton. Their proposal to transfer the School was endorsed by the Alberta Association of Registered Nurses in June, 1967, in December, 1967, the Deputy Minister of Education agreed to consider the transfer proposal, and in 1968 the transfer took effect.[116] When, a short time later, discussion took place to transfer Collège St. Jean to the jurisdiction of the University of Alberta, there were discussions about the possibility of a French-language program in nursing. However, under the agreement concluded in 1970, the Faculté St. Jean could no longer be involved in professional programs. The Edmonton General Hospital attempted to convince the University to continue the program, but to no avail and the nursing program was transferred to Grant MacEwen Community College in 1970. It was ironic that despite this agreement, just a few years later, Faculté St. Jean became involved in offering a French language professional program in cooperation with the Faculty of Education.[117]

An Integrated Degree Program at the University of Calgary

In the meantime, nursing education began to develop within the new universities in the province. In 1966, the University of Calgary gained independence from the University of Alberta. The institution had previously been a branch of the University of Alberta. There was optimism within the new

University in a community that had fought the case for independence. It moved rapidly to develop programs in a wide variety of areas. The Alberta Association of Registered Nurses had recognized the need for a second university degree program for some time in Calgary, and found support in the recommendation of the *Report* of the Royal Commission on Health Services (1964) "that there be established as quickly as qualified personnel can be recruited at least ten more university schools to expand the annual output of university graduate nurses."[118] The *Report* further elaborated that "We believe these ten schools can be established in about five years. Among the Universities where these might be provided as additional faculties are:... University of Alberta (Calgary)."[119] The Alberta Association of Registered Nurses commissioned Sister Marguerite Letourneau, Director of Nursing of the Grey Nuns' Holy Cross Hospital in Calgary, to develop the case for such a development at the University of Calgary. The brief prepared by Sister Letourneau put forward a convincing case for the expansion of university nursing education in the province and recommended that: "a four year basic integrated baccalaureate nursing program be established at the University of Calgary with the greatest possible expediency."[120] The recommendations in the report were detailed and stressed that the program should be developed on the integrated model, that the faculty should be well-qualified for their responsibilities and should engage in research and scholarly activities, and that a graduate program in nursing should be considered as soon as possible. The advice of the profession was heeded by the University of Calgary and a second basic integrated degree program in the province was developed following the establishment of the School of Nursing in 1969 under the directorship of Dr. Shirley R. Good. After a year of planning the curriculum, gaining the requisite approvals, and establishing agreements for clinical experiences for students, the first students were accepted into the new Bachelor of Nursing degree program in 1970. Although there was pressure to develop a post-R.N. degree program along with the basic degree program, such a program was not offered at the outset, but was initiated within the first decade.

Leadership Crisis in the Formative Years of the New Program

The University of Calgary School of Nursing faced an unfortunate leadership crisis early in its history with the forced resignation of its first director, Dr. Good in 1972.[121] Factors which weighed heavily in the situation were largely external to the Faculty, and appeared to rest primarily with the President of the University, Dr. A.W.R. Carruthers. Dr. Carruthers had commissioned three reviews of the program and operations prior to his decision to terminate the appointment of Dr. Good. These included a review by Dr. W.R.N. "Buck" Blair, Professor of Psychology at The University of Calgary and author of the provincial "Blair Report" on mental health in Alberta; a review by the Advisor to Schools of Nursing in the province, Margaret Steed; and a review by Dr. Muriel Uprichard, Director of the School of Nursing at the University of British Columbia. The first two reports were positive, and indeed Dr. Blair advised the University to allow the School time to develop and consolidate its operations. The last report by Dr. Uprichard was unfavourable and recommended the dismissal of the Director.

Dr. Good, who had been appointed in 1969, had been recruited to the directorship from a senior consultant's position with the Canadian Nurses Association. The latter post was the position she held following completion of her doctorate at Columbia University, and her appointment in Calgary was her first appointment at the university level in Canada. When she was appointed as Director of the program, she was not offered an accompanying academic appointment in the University. Failure to offer her such an appointment carried strong overtones of gender bias. Even though there were relatively few women who held professorial appointments in the various departments and faculties of the University at the time, failure to grant such an appointment to an incoming director or dean constituted highly unusual practice. What this meant was that when Shirley Good resigned as Director of the School of Nursing, albeit under pressure from the incumbent President, she did not hold a professorial appointment in the Faculty to allow her to continue on the teaching staff of the School. The approximately 15 faculty members and 110 undergraduate students in the developing program found themselves without warning and overnight without the leadership of the woman who had undertaken the design and implementation of the program.

Although the Director of the School of Continuing Education, Dr. Fred Terentiuk, was appointed Acting Director of the School of Nursing and proved to be a capable administrator, the disruption to faculty and students at a critical time in the development of the new School was clearly a setback. Dr. Terentiuk called upon the faculty and students to work through the crisis and effectively held the program together during two

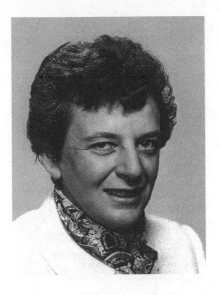

Dr. Shirley R. Good, Director of the School of Nursing, University of Calgary, 1969–1972. (Photograph courtesy of Shirley Good)

difficult years. Because of the situation surrounding the departure of Dr. Good, the climate was not conducive to the recruitment of a new director with the educational and experiential background for the position, and few who met these requirements were willing to take on the responsibility. Thus, the search for a new leader took two years, and in 1974 Marguerite Schumacher was appointed to the position of Dean since all "schools" had become "faculties" at the University of Calgary in 1973. Miss Schumacher's background as a past president of the Canadian Nurses Association, former chairperson of the Nursing Department at Red Deer College, and, prior to that, Advisor to Schools of Nursing in Alberta, gave her a strong background in the profession. Over the five years of her tenure as the chief administrator of the Faculty, there was consolidation and growth.

Graduate Education in Nursing at the University of Calgary

The appointment of Dr. Margaret Scott Wright as Dean of the Faculty in 1979 brought a new dimension to university nursing education in the province. Her background at the University of Edinburgh, where she headed up programs in nursing in the Faculty of Social Sciences, and later at Dalhousie University in Halifax was complimented by her background of service to the profession as First Vice-President of the International Council of Nurses. Under Scott Wright's leadership, the Faculty of Nursing

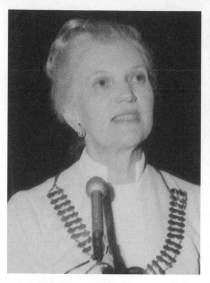 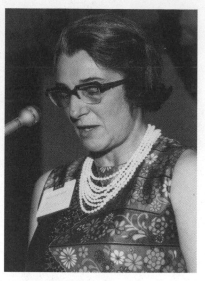

↪ *Marguerite Schumacher, Dean*
of the Faculty of Nursing,
University of Calgary,
1974–1979, pictured here as
President of the Canadian
Nurses Association. (AARN P30)

↪ *Dr. Margaret Scott Wright,*
Dean of the Faculty of Nursing,
University of Calgary,
1979–1984 and Acting Dean of
the Faculty of Nursing,
1989–1990. (AARN P720)

moved into graduate education and research. Beginning plans for a master's program in nursing had been formulated in 1976 with approval by the Faculty of Nursing Council of a motion to offer a master's degree program. Development of the proposal and approval of the program by the University was a process that lasted several years. At the outset, a special case arrangement for one student was approved by the Faculty of Graduate Studies.[122] This allowed an individual program at the master's level to be developed for a student of outstanding calibre and gave the Faculty of Nursing an opportunity to gain experience in offering graduate work prior to the approval of its master's degree program. Following approval of the proposal for the master's program, the first students were admitted in the Fall of 1981. A key disappointment to the Faculty at the time the program was approved was that a thesis option was not approved at the outset. This was a issue for which Dr. Scott Wright and her colleagues argued very hard at the time. However, the Dean of the Faculty of Graduate Studies recommended that the program start out as a course based program. Therefore, the program approved by the University and funded by the provincial government was a course based master's program.[123] This situation did not change for more than a decade when the thesis option was integrated into the existing program. Without a thesis option, the strong stimulus to research seen in programs requiring the completion of a thesis was absent. Leadership by Dr. Scott Wright and her successors who were well-versed in higher education and the affairs of the profession over the next five years was important, but the stimulation provided by the thesis requirement in the graduate program was delayed by more than a decade.

A Second Leadership Crisis

Dr. Joy Calkin succeeded Dr. Margaret Scott Wright as Dean upon her retirement in 1984 and when she left the deanship to become Vice-President (Academic) of the University in 1989, Dr. Janet Storch was appointed Dean. Dr. Storch was reappointed in 1994, but her leadership also became the subject of controversy when a conflict arose with university administrative officials leading to her resignation as Dean when it was clear to her that she had suddenly lost the support of senior administration. The circumstances surrounding the incident were not made public by the President's Office. A loss of support was highly unusual and quite unexpected given that Dr. Storch had been reappointed as Dean just a few months previously. However, this was not the only leadership crisis within an academic unit in nursing in the province and it may be that certain fundamental issues were common factors in this and the other situations.

Degree Program in Nursing
at the University of Lethbridge

In 1979 when program funding was granted by the provincial government, the University of Lethbridge developed a post-R.N. degree program in Nursing under the directorship of Dr. Joanne Scholdra. Although the program at the University of Lethbridge was relatively small in size, nurses in the southern part of the province had been asking for better access to university-level education in nursing. The size of the institution and its relatively modest student complement meant that it struggled for the first few years to recruit faculty with the necessary skills to mount the courses. There was also a leadership crisis in this small developing academic unit

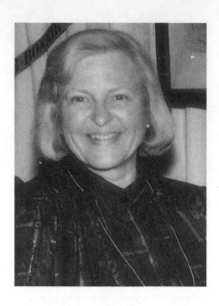

↜ Dr. Joanne Scholdra, formerly Director, School of Nursing, University of Lethbridge. (Photograph courtesy of Joanne Scholdra)

when the director, Dr. Joanne Scholdra, a respected member of the Alberta nursing community, found that her administrative appointment as director of the academic unit was summarily terminated by the university administration. Indeed, the University was later held accountable for wrongful dismissal in a civil suit over the matter. The appointment of Dr. Leslie Hardy to succeed Dr. Scholdra and the addition of several new faculty positions helped to offer some stability and the opportunity to develop depth in a variety of areas of clinical nursing. Discussions in the 1990s between Medicine Hat College, Lethbridge Community College and the University of Lethbridge have led to a collaborative integrated degree program similar to programs developed at the University of Alberta and the University of Calgary, and from which the first class graduates in 1998. This will undoubtedly facilitate further development of program offerings within the Nursing Department at the University of Lethbridge.

Distance Programming in University Nursing Education

Athabasca University was established in 1970 as an institution in which courses and degrees were offered using alternate delivery methods. This was an important development for the nursing profession as Athabasca

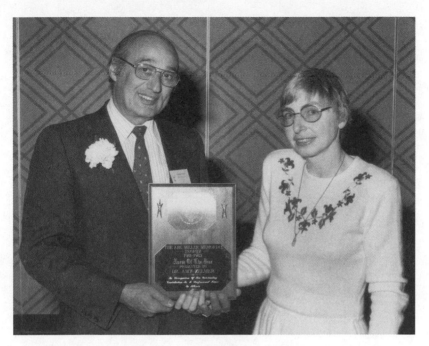

↪ Dr. Amy Zelmer, Director of the School/Faculty of Nursing, University of
Alberta, 1976–1980, receiving Nurse of the Year award from Mr. Justice Tevie
Miller at the 1982 AARN Convention. (AARN)

University soon became involved in developing distance programs in the
arts and sciences to support nursing programs at the three other universities in the province. In 1979, Dr. Amy Zelmer, Ruth McClure's successor as
Dean of the Faculty of Nursing at the University of Alberta, prepared a proposal to expand admissions to the first year of the post-R.N. baccalaureate
program from 72 to 144 students. Half of this expansion was to be offered
via distance delivery to off-campus students. Zelmer also developed an
agreement with Athabasca University to offer required arts and science
courses as well as to develop several courses including physiology, teaching
and learning for health care professionals, and nursing research for distance delivery pending government funding. The Government of Premier
Peter Lougheed failed to provide financial support for the expansion at the
time it was considered by the cabinet, and this provoked outrage from the
Alberta Association of Registered Nurses as the needed financing had been
promised by the Minister of Advanced Education and Manpower, Dr. Bert

Hohol. A few months later, a vigourous lobby for the needed funds met with success when the Government created a fund for professional schools that was given to the universities to support programs such as the expansion of the post-R.N. degree program in nursing.

The initial collaboration between Athabasca University and the University of Alberta in supporting the University of Alberta's off-campus post-R.N., program was significant as it facilitated the development of the resources to offer the baccalaureate degree in nursing on an entirely off-campus basis. It involved arts and science courses that could be taken by all distance students and several nonnursing courses required for the University of Alberta B.Sc.N., which were developed by Athabasca University with funds extended to it by Dean Zelmer from the funds for the expansion of the University of Alberta post-R.N. program. Even though several other institutions in Canada such as the University of Victoria and the University of Ottawa were highly involved in offering courses by distance delivery that carried credit in their degree programs in nursing, in 1984 the Faculty of Nursing at the University of Alberta became the first university in the country to offer an entire post-R.N. baccalaureate degree program in selected off-campus sites. Since Athabasca University offered a full range of arts and science courses at a distance, this enabled the University of Alberta post-R.N. program in nursing to operate entirely on an off-campus basis. The University of Alberta program was offered on a rotating basis over four years in four regions of the province, Red Deer and environs, the Grande Prairie area, Fort McMurray, and the northeastern (St. Paul, Vegreville) Alberta region. The program thus had all four years operating at the same time, each in a different region. The arrangement allowed many Alberta nurses in off-campus locations to complete their B.Sc.N. degrees. The program was offered for several years in this form. However, as Athabasca University developed, it found that an increasing number of the students taking the support courses it offered were nurses. Thus, the development of a post-R.N. degree program for post-R.N. students by Athabasca University was inevitable. In 1993 when the first five students convocated from the Athabasca B.Sc.N. program, an honorary degree was conferred on Helen M. Sabin, who had so capably guided the AARN through important years in its development from 1960 to 1976 as executive director of the organization. The new distance program for post-R.N. students offered by Athabasca University expanded rapidly.

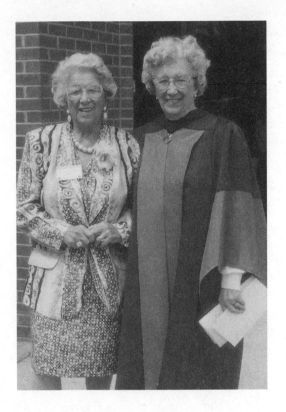

↬ *Helen M. Garfield*
Sabin (right)
following Athabasca
University
ceremony conferring
an honourary LL.D.
degree upon her; pic-
tured with her twin
sister Nettie Garfield
Pedlar. (AARN P668)

In 1995, there were 819 students enrolled from every province in Canada, nine states in the US and there were also students located in Saudi Arabia, Hong Kong and Japan.[124] A new post-baccalaureate diploma program established by Athabasca University was established in 1996 to give students the opportunity to develop advanced skills in community health nursing.

Distance education continued to be an important thrust in all universities in the province offering nursing programs. The University of Calgary made a decision to modify its post-R.N. baccalaureate program as a program which was flexible in terms of students' needs, offering a combination of distance methods, and on and off site contact with faculty members. This program has been in operation for more than a decade. Although the University of Alberta Faculty of Nursing gradually withdrew from offering its off-campus undergraduate post-R.N. program using distance methods when Athabasca University's own degree program in nursing became available, some courses in its basic collaborative program were offered via distance using interactive teaching techniques with "state of the art" interactive videoconferencing equipment acquired in 1993. With students at Red Deer College, Grande Prairie and Fort McMurray, the collaborative partnership was accompanied by resource acquisition to offer some courses in those regions at a distance. The University of Alberta also has offered graduate education in nursing at a distance. The Master of Nursing program was offered to a group of students from the Red Deer region on a pilot project basis and some courses have been offered to students in Grande Prairie. In addition, a proposal has been developed to offer the Ph.D. in Nursing program using distance delivery methods.

Baccalaureate Preparation as Entry to Practice

The Alberta Task Force on Nursing Education[125] was a committee appointed by the Alberta Government to review needs in nursing education in the province and to make recommendations to the Government. Its work became widely known across the country because of its recommendation in 1975 that the baccalaureate degree should become the basic entry qualification to the nursing profession within two decades. In its response to the Report in 1976,[126] the Alberta Association of Registered Nurses supported the goal and it was also supported by unanimous motion of the Board of Directors of the Canadian Nurses Association in February, 1982. This decision was also endorsed through a motion of support by delegates to the 1982 Biennial convention in Newfoundland. Eventually every provincial association supported the entry to practice goal. However, the profession soon found itself in conflict with the provincial government which took pains to point out that it did not support the conclusions of the Task Force it had appointed, stating that it did "not agree with making the baccalaureate degree a mandatory requirement for practice."[127] The lack of government support was an indication to the nursing profession in Alberta that it would require a concerted effort at all levels of the profession to make the goal a reality. It appeared that the Government's objection was based on the premise that offering every nurse the opportunity to take a degree program constituted an unnecessary expense for the system.

Undaunted, nurses began to make plans to consolidate all nursing education at the university level. In this, Alberta was clearly a leader in the country. Discussions between the University of Alberta Faculty of Nursing and Red Deer College to develop a basic integrated degree program began

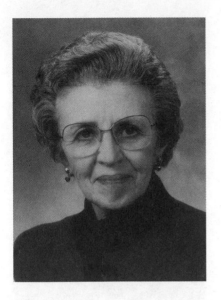

in 1985. The initiative with Red Deer College began under the leadership of Dean Jannetta MacPhail who had succeeded Dr. Amy Zelmer as Dean in 1982, and important support was given to the initiative in the planning phase. A committee was established to plan the curriculum and identify issues in the area of registration of students, fees, and collaboration between the College and the University in offering courses. After all relevant approvals had been obtained, the program got underway in the fall of 1990. It involved a unique arrangement between the two institutions and was the first in Canada between a community college and a university to offer an integrated baccalaureate degree program which was four years in length. A diploma exit of six additional months' work was available following successful completion of the second year of the program.

Dr. Marilynn Wood, who became Dean of the Faculty in 1987 upon the retirement of Dr. MacPhail, recognized the significance of the initiative for the profession from the outset and provided strong support for the collaboration with Red Deer College. She envisioned other possibilities for collaboration and extended the scope of the venture, brining in the new partners in Edmonton into the collaboration. Excellent communication and cooperation between the partner organizations were facilitated, without which the program could not have been planned and implemented. The collaborative model developed included the diploma schools of nursing at

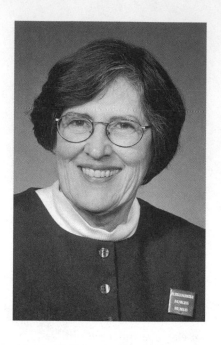

↭ *Dr. Marilynn J. Wood, Dean of the Faculty of Nursing, University of Alberta from 1987 to 1998. (Photograph courtesy of Marilynn J. Wood)*

the University of Alberta Hospitals, Grant MacEwan Community College, the Misericordia Hospital and the Royal Alexandra Hospital, and students at those sites were enrolled in the program in the fall of 1991. The extent and form of this collaborative effort between so many partners was unusual. Grande Prairie Regional College and Keyano College in Fort McMurray joined the collaboration in 1994–95, and the addition of these schools brought to seven the number of partners which had joined the collaborative endeavour with the University of Alberta. Although government approval was not strictly speaking necessary for these collaborative ventures since they did not involve the establishment of new programs, government support was sought because new funding arrangements would be necessary for the restructured programs. Given the history of opposition by the elected officials for baccalaureate entry to practice, to have gone ahead without their support could have led to confrontation and failure of the initiative.

As it was, gaining government support for the collaborative baccalaureate programs proposed by the University of Alberta and its partner diploma schools was neither easy nor simple. Even in the face of support from the AARN, AHA, nursing unions, nursing and hospital administrators, and other community organizations, government support did not come quickly. A political action committee was established by the administrative council which served as the planning and decision-making body for the collaborative ventures and a well-orchestrated campaign was carried out over a period of five months to gain the attention and support of MLAS. Approximately two hundred letters of support addressed to MLAS and cabinet ministers were delivered to the legislature each week over a period of three months and a news conference was held in mid-October, 1990 to draw public attention to the need for political support for the new collaborative B.Sc.N. programs. Finally, in late December, 1990, an announcement that government support would be forthcoming for the University of Alberta and the hospitals and colleges in the collaboration was quietly distributed to the respective parties and to the media.

In Calgary, a conjoint program developed between the Faculty of Nursing, Foothills Hospital and Mount Royal College. This proposal languished for some time awaiting government support. It differed from the University of Alberta proposal since it required new program funds. This was a time of decreasing financial support from government for higher education in general, and thus even though there was a precedent for collaboration in Northern Alberta, it took a great deal of time to work out arrangements which allowed the government to look favourably upon the proposal. Eventually, the program was approved by the Government in the fall of 1993. The unique aspect of the Calgary model was the availability of a diploma exit only following successful completion of the third year of the program. The Alberta Government announced a decision early in 1994 to close the hospital-based diploma programs in nursing in the province. However, the fact that collaborative programs had been operating for four years in Edmonton and one year in Calgary allowed for smooth curriculum transitions in a remodelled form of collaboration for university degree programs for nurses in which the universities and the colleges were the sole partners.

DEVELOPMENT OF NURSING RESEARCH

The development of nursing research in the province beginning in the 1970s was stimulated by the establishment of the first graduate program in nursing at the University of Alberta. Because a thesis was required in the program, the need for research expertise on the part of faculty was critical. Students also were required to complete rigorous preparation for research in a series of courses in statistics and research design. A strong research thrust in the Faculty was necessary to provide the guidance for students to undertake research. This recognition led to a provincial effort to develop nursing research in which the Alberta Association of Registered Nurses played a crucial role. The support of faculty in the three university schools of nursing and nursing administrators in health care agencies for the Association's efforts was strong and as a result of the representations made by the Association, the provincial government saw fit to establish the Alberta Foundation for Nursing Research in 1982. A Foundation for the exclusive support for nursing research in the province was highly unique and was a credit to the nursing leaders who saw both the need and the opportunity to develop such an organization under the auspices of the provincial government.

The window of opportunity was created by the Alberta Heritage Fund developed through oil revenues and the subsequent gift of $300,000,000 by the government of Premier Peter Lougheed to establish the Alberta Heritage Foundation for Medical Research (AHFMR). Since the AHFMR proposed to support basic biomedical research exclusively at the outset of its operations, nurses lobbied hard for support for their research. The Alberta Foundation for Nursing Research initially operated as a committee of the Department of Advanced Education and was financed by $1,000,000 from general revenues over five years, funding which was renewed in 1987. The purpose of the Foundation was to finance research projects developed by nurses in the province which had successfully met rigorous standards of peer review. This funding agency became the only research funding organization in the country to fund nursing research exclusively. The tremendous stimulation provided by this organization put both nursing research and graduate education in nursing on a firm footing in the province in a few short years. It also led to the establishment of a doctoral education in the province because of the development of faculty expertise in research. Nurses in the province were devastated at the news that funding would be withdrawn in 1994 due to cutbacks and downsizing initiated by the government of Premier Ralph Klein. Although minimal funding was forthcoming from the provincial government in 1994, the future of the agency seemed bleak. Members of the Board of Directors struggled to identify ways in which to preserve this unique funding organization for nursing research in the province and commissioned an evaluation of the Foundation.

Eventually the Board of Directors of the Foundation decided to terminate its operations, a decision which those who worked so hard to establish the organization found to difficult to accept. However, the profound impact of funding for nursing research projects awarded by the Foundation over the decade and a half of its existence will undoubtedly continue to reap positive spinoffs for years to come as researchers who gained experience and expertise through the program are able to compete successfully for funds in national and interdisciplinary competitions.

DOCTORAL EDUCATION IN NURSING AT THE UNIVERSITY OF ALBERTA

The establishment of a doctoral program in nursing at the University of Alberta on 1 January 1991 made it the first fully funded doctoral program in nursing in the country. It was a development that was long overdue, for previously nursing faculty members had had to study in other disciplines or to go to the United States in order to enter Ph.D. programs in nursing. The Faculty of Nursing had begun work on a proposal for a doctoral program in 1984 under the leadership of Dean MacPhail and Dr. Shirley Stinson who chaired the committee that prepared the initial proposal. It was approved by the University of Alberta in 1986. An announcement made by Vice-President Peter Meekison at the International Conference on Nursing Research in May, 1986 was received with enthusiasm by the 800 delegates attending the meeting. Although the Honourable James D. Horsman, Minister of Advanced Education, alluded to the likelihood of government funding of the program, it took four and a half years for this to become a reality. It required a major political campaign to convince the government of Premier Don Getty that funding of this program was a priority. A group of enterprising and politically astute graduate students including master's students, special graduate students and special case doctoral students in the Faculty were influential in lobbying for the Faculty's goal to establish the program. The thrust by the students was powerful as they were free to contact anyone they wished to press for the program and to identify why it was important to have it from a student's perspective. Dean Wood strongly supported the students' efforts and facilitated the involvement of faculty, alumnae and students in the initiative, the success of which was realized in a press release on 21 December 1990 that the program would be funded as of 1 January 1991.

Three students had been admitted to the Faculty of Nursing as special case doctoral students in nursing in 1988 as an interim step prior to the funding of the doctoral program in nursing. A fourth was admitted just after the program was funded. This meant that the first student was ready to graduate in 1993. Efforts to ensure a viable research enterprise had intensified with the development of the doctoral program and, in 1990–91 the Canadian Association of University Schools of Nursing reported that the University of Alberta held a total of $542,861 in all grants to faculty members as principal investigators.[128] By the fall of 1995, five students had graduated and there were some 27 students enrolled in the University of Alberta program. The doctoral dissertation of the first graduate of the program, Dr. Joan Bottorff, won the Region I dissertation competition of Sigma Theta Tau International. In that there were many renowned doctoral programs in Arizona, California, Oregon, and Washington in Region I, this was a remarkable accomplishment. Of the first five graduates, three were awarded substantial post-doctoral fellowships for further study by national granting agencies in which they were in competition with many other health disciplines. These were important achievements that attested to the quality of the University of Alberta program and to the competence of faculty and students.

The need for and level of interest in doctoral preparation in nursing was recognized across the province. The Faculty of Nursing at the University of Calgary had strongly supported the University of Alberta proposal and indicated its willingness to participate in the development, planning and operation of the doctoral program as this seemed appropriate and feasible. The University of Calgary Faculty of Nursing also moved to develop its resources in terms of independent offerings at the Ph.D. level and graduated its first Special Case Ph.D. student, Dr. Carol Robinson, in November 1994. The second special case Ph.D. student was well into a program of study in 1996. In 1997, the University gave approval to the development of a doctoral program in nursing.

The development of opportunities for post-doctoral education in Alberta is the next major thrust facing the profession. Post-doctoral education is relatively new in nursing, although it has been a standard requirement for those seeking research careers in many disciplines in the academic world for decades. These opportunities are essential for graduates of Ph.D. programs in nursing in order to give these new graduates an opportunity to develop research programs that they can continue as they take up academic appointments in nursing in universities. Experience across all disciplines has shown that new Ph.D. graduates require support from more experienced researchers as well as time to plan their research and submit research proposals to funding agencies. If given the opportunity to develop research proposals and conduct research on a collegial basis with established researchers, they are much more likely to be successful when they take up academic appointments. Since a great deal has been invested in these individuals in the context of Ph.D. in Nursing programs, it would seem important to offer new nursing researchers opportunities to initiate a successful research career through allowing them time for planning as well as guidance from experienced researchers.

The history of university-level nursing education in Alberta is characterized by important successes in spite of the difficult struggles which have been necessary to develop university programs of high quality for nurses. The determination of leaders in the profession to develop high standards of education and concomitantly degree programs so that all students embarking upon the study of nursing have the opportunity to complete a degree in nursing has been evident since the incorporation of the professional association in the Registered Nurses' Act passed in 1916. The goals of the profession were achieved through commitment and unity of purpose on the part of those who worked diligently for them. The process was not easy, for gender discrimination as evidenced in inadequate university support has been evident in a number of personal struggles for pioneering administrators in nursing degree programs. Despite the struggles involved in developing degree programs and securing adequate funding for undergraduate and graduate degree programs as well as for research, important successes have enabled the profession to move ahead, and indeed to become a leader in the country. Improved health for all citizens has been the fundamental aim of the nursing profession in establishing and maintaining high quality degree programs to prepare nurses for practice. A great deal has been accomplished in Alberta towards meeting this goal, and despite the fact that there is a great deal more to do, committed and knowledgeable nurses will continue to work diligently to achieve the goals of the profession in the realm of nursing education.

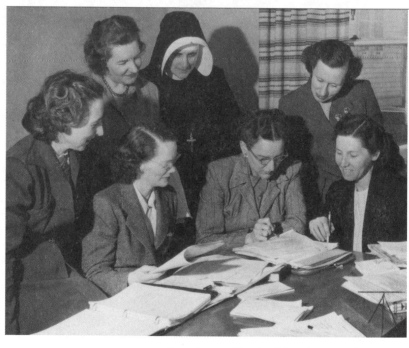

⤷ AARN *Committee on Nursing Education at work,*
*1947. (*AARN P414*)*

The Beginning
of Organized Nursing

The Alberta Association of
Registered Nurses, 1916 to 1956

The efforts of Ethel Gordon Bedford Fenwick are legendary in the annals of nursing history, for it was her foresight and drive that brought nurses around the world together to unite in an organized effort to achieve their goals. Editor of the *British Journal of Nursing*, Ethel Bedford Fenwick was a delegate to the 1893 Congress of Charities, Corrections and Philanthropy in Chicago where she met the leaders of American nursing, Isabel Hampton, Adelaide Nutting and Lavinia Dock.[1] Bedford Fenwick had been an early proponent of registration for nurses and her North American colleagues became very interested in what she told them of the struggle in Britain to achieve nursing registration. As a product of their mutual enthusiasm, a meeting of nursing representatives at the Congress was convened and an organization emerged from this historic meeting, the American Society of Superintendents of Training Schools for Nurses of the United States and Canada, later to become the National League for Nursing Education. Membership in this group consisted of qualified nurses who directed schools meeting certain standards and the first president was Isabel Hampton.[2] The goal of the organization was to raise standards of educational programs. Nurses' alumnae associations had begun to form at the large training schools in the United States after 1890, and in 1896 the Nurses' Associated Alumnae of the United States and Canada was formed with Isabel Hampton Robb as president. Membership was voluntary and composed of alumnae organizations that were eligible for membership if they were associated with hospitals having more than 100 beds and a program at least two years in length. A major purpose of the latter organization was "to secure legislation to differentiate between trained and untrained nurses."[3] This organization became the American Nurses' Association in 1911.

Bedford Fenwick returned to England with a vision of an organization of nurses that was international in scope. In 1899 she accomplished her goal and the International Council of Nurses (ICN) was founded with Britain, Germany and the United States as member organizations. Since the ICN was established as a federation of national nursing organizations, other nations could not become members of the ICN until they had first established a national nursing association. Even though there was no national nursing organization in Canada at the time of the 1899 formation of the ICN, Mary Agnes Snively, Superintendent of Nurses at Toronto General Hospital represented Canada at the 1899 meeting and was elected the first honourary treasurer of the organization.[4] Miss Snively returned to Canada and worked diligently towards the formation of a national nursing association. The Canadian Society of Superintendents of Training Schools for Nurses was formed in 1907, and in the next year the Society invited representative from all nursing organizations in Canada to meet in Ottawa to consider the formation of an organization which would truly represent nurses. At this meeting the Provisional Society of the Canadian National Association of Trained Nurses was formed with Mary Agnes Snively as president and Flora Madeline Shaw of the Montreal General Hospital as secretary-treasurer.[5] Membership in this new national organization was through affiliated societies, of which there could be several in a single province. At the ICN meeting in London in 1909, Canada became a full-fledged member of the organization. Later the CNATN streamlined its organization when the means for doing so became a reality; that is, when registration of nurses was established through legislation in each province. The organization became a federation of provincial associations in 1930 where each provincial professional association represented registered nurses in the province and was the official voice of nursing in that jurisdiction.[6]

Graduate Nurses Organize and Seek Employment

The Calgary Association of Graduate Nurses (CAGN) was formed in 1904 and was among the first to be established in the province. It was active in promoting professional interests and continuing education for nurses and as with other such organizations of nurses in the major centres, it acted as a registry for those seeking the services of private duty nurses. Correspondence between the CAGN and "the Toronto Medical Society inquiring about the possibility of a nursing journal, which would serve to keep nurses in isolated areas informed of nursing developments"[7] appears to have been influential in persuading the alumnae association of the Toronto General Hospital to initiate publication of *The Canadian Nurse* the next year under the editorial direction of Dr. Helen MacMurchy.[8] The Edmonton Association of Graduate Nurses and the CAGN had developed a united effort by 1912 to work for the passage of provincial legislation which would make registration of nurses a reality in Alberta. Nursing organizations also had been formed in other provincial centres and in 1914, the newly-formed organization called the Graduate Nurses Association of Alberta also known as the Alberta Association of Graduate Nurses gave a report to the CNATN on the progress it had made in drafting nursing legislation.[9]

With the establishment of schools of nursing, graduates of programs of training became available for work. Unfortunately earning a diploma from a school of nursing frequently carried with it the prospect of unemployment. Because hospitals were staffed primarily by students in the early years, there were relatively few opportunities for securing a staff position in a hospital upon graduation. Thus one of the early struggles relative to educational standards in which nurses became engaged following the establishment and entrenchment of the hospital-based system of nursing education was that which involved the replacement of students with graduate nurses as primary providers of nursing care.[10] Since the principal area of employment for graduate nurses for many years was private duty nursing in the homes of clients, nurses were mainly self-employed and were retained by families to give nursing care to ill family members.

Another struggle faced by the first graduates of nursing programs was the problem of the "untrained nurse." There was nothing to prevent an individual who had no training from being hired on the same basis as a graduate of a school of nursing. It could be quite difficult for the unsuspecting employer to differentiate the "trained" from the "untrained." If those without training were hired rather than those who had graduated from *bona fide* programs, there would be little incentive to complete such programs, particularly at the personal cost entailed in the long hours of work with few holidays and days off. The value of the programs offered by schools of nursing was diminished if a significant challenge in terms of the available private duty positions were to come from those who had not completed a training program:

> Nurses who were trained professionals found themselves competing for status and wages with nurses who had received little or no professional training; also, because there were no legal controls, there was no way of establishing uniformity in nursing service standards.[11]

Therefore the drive for registration became one of the early battles fought by these nurses.

THE GRADUATE NURSES ACT

The Graduate Nurses Act was passed in 1916 and with its passage nurses in Alberta had achieved their goal of establishing nursing registration. Marthe Morkin, a charter member of the Alberta Association of Graduate Nurses, the organization incorporated within the legislation, told of the onerous struggle that the nurses encountered in their campaign to secure professional legislation:

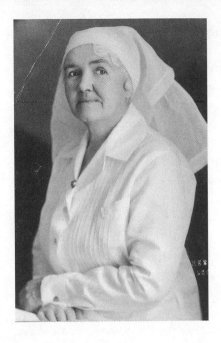

Eleanor McPhedran, one of the founding members of the AARN who served as Registrar of the Alberta Association of Graduate Nurses when it was formed in 1916, and President of the organization, 1928–1932. (AARN)

It was an uphill fight for a time. The powers that be, or were, took a dim view of women, especially nurses trying, as they felt, to unionize. The medical profession was anything but helpful. However, we had a good committee, and were persistent, and finally won out. During the 1915–16 years when I was with the department of agriculture Women's Institute, I met frequently with the nurses' group and we were all happy when we were officially launched as an organization, not a union.[12]

This was the era when women were pressing for the vote and in the same year that the Graduate Nurses Act was passed, the Alberta legislature had recorded a vote to support women's suffrage. Cashman makes note of the fact that although the road to legislative action was perceived as difficult by the small band of nurses seeking it, the support of the Minister of Health and Member of the Legislative Assembly for Athabasca, Hon. A.G. MacKay, was essential in securing passage of the Act without a dissenting vote.[13]

The first meeting of the Council of AAGN was held on 11 October 1916 in the offices of the organization's lawyer, George Ross. The meeting was chaired by Eleanor McPhedran with six other members in attendance. The organization consisted of a complement of 91 members whose names were on the register. At this historic meeting, the AAGN Council elected Victoria Winslow as its first president, allocated $200 to Eleanor McPhedran to cover expenses in maintaining the register for the year, and voted to apply to become an affiliate member of the CNATN.[14] The membership swelled to 255 at the time of the first convention of the organization in December, 1917[15] while fees were set at $10.00 to join the organization and $2.00 annually after that. Fees have often been the subject of controversy in the organization over time. However, the work of the AARN to maintain standards in practice and education led to respect both for nurses and the organization. The regulatory functions mandated by the legislation, developing and maintaining standards of education and practice and involvement in health issues of concern to nurses were essential activities for this self-regulating profession and required financial support. Although there were inevitable disputes over fees and finances, for the most part the membership of the organization recognized that designation as a self-regulating profession in legislation carried with it both privileges and responsibilities. Alberta registered nurses thus continued to support the need for a fee structure which would finance the activities of the professional association throughout the developmental stages of the organization and on into the future.

In 1917 the Minister of Education informed the Council that the Government was proposing an amendment to the Act to waive the registration examination for nurses who were in training programs in the province at the time of the passage of the Act. The Council protested that its organization was strongly opposed to such an amendment and that the Minister should be advised that "the nursing profession needs to be remedied or improved and that the Council expected to make such amendments to lay before the legislature in the next session."[16] Such was the first experience of the Council in dealing with government on a matter on which they were not in agreement. It was undoubtedly a valuable learning experience relative to the nature and extent of representations to government on contentious matters. The AAGN's statement that it would be preparing amendments for the next year did not "wash" and failed to change the government's intent to proceed with passage of its amendment. Thus, the Liberal government of the day went ahead and passed the amendment. No doubt the fact that the amendment referred only to a limited and finite number of nurses in the process of completing their educational programs at the time of the original passage of the Act made the intensity of the AAGN's opposition to the amendment fade over time. However, the impact of such a graphic example of the power of government to listen or not listen to the advice of an organization could hardly fail to have been appreciated by the members of the AAGN. In that this may have been the first sign that their quest to achieve improved standards in nursing education would not be an easy one, these nurses may well have recognized that there would be difficult issues for them and their successors to address in the years ahead.

STANDARDS OF NURSING EDUCATION

Standards of nursing education were a primary concern of the Association from the outset and the Council of the AAGN proposed amendments for changes in nursing legislation and submitted them to the Legislature. One of its first proposals was that the Association be placed under the control of the Senate of the University of Alberta. The intent in such a recommendation was undoubtedly that it was educational standards that required monitoring by the Senate.[17] The concern over inadequate educational standards in the fledgling schools of nursing around the province was related to the fact that the schools had been initiated on a service rather than an educational model in which learning and instruction had been of secondary importance. The Council also requested that the Senate of the University of Alberta appoint a nursing representative to its membership because it wanted to see the development of a standard course of study which could be implemented in all schools of nursing. The organization also discussed the possibility of a summer school offered for registered nurses under the auspices of the University of Alberta and Victoria Winslow made reference to this in her presidential address to those attending the first Convention of the AAGN in Calgary in December, 1917.[18] This reference to continuing education was perhaps modelled on that of education where summer schools were traditionally the means by which teachers upgraded their credentials. Such a program was not implemented perhaps because unlike schools, health care agencies continued to operate in the summer and nurses may have found it difficult to attend. The first registration examinations held in Calgary in 1918 included a written as well as an oral component. The examination process was carried out by the Board of Examiners also established in that year.[19] It was characteristic of the status of nursing in this era that there was general acceptance that nursing was a branch of medicine over which physicians would naturally be placed in positions of authority. Thus physicians were placed in charge of the written component of the examinations, while nurses were given responsibility for the oral or practical component.

Responsibility for monitoring standards of nursing education in schools of nursing was the subject of considerable discussion between the provincial government and the AAGN/AARN. Eleanor McPhedran advised the CNATN of the plans of the AAGN relative to the proposed nursing legislation in her 1914 report to its meeting:

> It may interest you to know that we hope to place the nursing profession on a par with other professional bodies of the province by arranging that the examinations held be under the control of the senate of the University of Alberta, and that the register be kept by the registrar of the University.[20]

Because Chapter 7 of the University Act of 1910 delegated to the University responsibility for administering examinations and appointing examiners in a number of established professions including architecture, dentistry, law, medicine and veterinary medicine, leaving the door open to the inclusion of still others,[21] it was logical that plans were made to include nursing when the legislation to regulate it was developed. It would seem unlikely that the nurses who negotiated with government about the drafting of the first nursing legislation wished to delegate responsibility to the University for establishing and monitoring the standards for nursing education in view of the statement given by Eleanor McPhedran to the CNATN on this matter: "we would like to keep the standard up to which recognized hospitals must measure, under the Nursing Association through the executive council."[22]

Despite all of these plans, the first Graduate Nurses Act did not provide either for developing or monitoring nursing education standards. It specified a common nursing examination for which responsibility was delegated to the Minister of Education, and thus was an anomaly in terms of other professional associations where the University's role was limited to the administration of examinations and the appointment of examiners. However, the AAGN began to press for the establishment of standards as it was decided at an Executive Council meeting of 12 December 1917 to request assistance from the University of Alberta Senate and the Medical Association of Alberta in developing a course of study in nursing that could be implemented in schools of nursing in order to have a uniform curriculum in schools. Other issues presented to the Senate and the physicians for their consideration included entrance requirements for applicants to schools of nursing, the need to establish a minimum number of beds for operation of a training school in conjunction with a hospital as well as the minimum number of graduate nurses that a hospital with a training school should be required to employ.[23] It may have been the case that the interference of government earlier that year relative to waiving the requirement for nursing students enroled in educational programs at the time of the passage of the legislation to write registration examinations had led to some anxiety in the AAGN January meeting. The AAGN's request for the help of the Senate of the University and the Medical Association may have been an attempt to avoid future disputes with government by aligning the AAGN with more powerful and established organizations and institutions.

There were no further developments until 1919 when legislation was passed 17 April 1919 to amend the Graduate Nurses Act of 1916.[24] This legislation gave authority to the Senate of the University of Alberta to develop examinations for registration and appoint examiners. No reference was made in the legislation to standards of nursing education and the monitoring of curricula of schools of nursing in the province. In an update on progress made in the legislation in Alberta in the *Canadian Nurse*, reference was made to the fact that the failure to designate clear authority for standards and monitoring was an oversight on the part of government. Susan Young notes that by January, 1920, a Senate committee of the Board of Examiners for nursing was engaged in developing regulations for schools of nursing in Alberta.[25] When these were finalized in May 1920, they were distributed to schools of nursing. Although the regulations were very detailed and clear, confusion continued to reign concerning the vesting of authority for standards and monitoring in nursing education. Therefore these initial regulations were stated as suggestions rather than requirements. The Graduate Nurses Act was amended once again in 1920 and through this amendment responsibility for standard setting and monitoring was given to the Senate, but only by implication:

> The Senate has the right to waive the examination and allow a person to practice if the person is from a province, state or country where provision is made for registration of nurses and in the opinion of the Senate, guarantees as high a standard of qualification as that obtained in this province . . . the Senate shall admit to practice the graduates of any hospital or training school which in its opinion gives training of as high a standard as that given by hospitals and training schools in this province.[26]

The Senate was given authority to make decisions about whether individual candidates met standards, without specifically identifying how those standards would be determined and maintained. This matter remained unclear until another amendment was passed in 1921 describing the role expected of the Senate:

> The Senate of the University of Alberta shall: 1) Satisfy itself that any person, entering upon a course of hospital training heading to registration under this act, has passed the grade eight examination of the Public School course of the province or has the equivalent educational standing; 2) Fix standards of training with regard to bed capacity, classes, lectures and other factors making for efficiency; 3) Refuse recognition to any hospital in which such standards are not consistently observed; 4) Prescribe the subjects and scope of the qualifying examination herein before referred to and appoint examiners to conduct the same.[27]

According to Young: "Now, for the first time, a specified group had the official responsibility of setting and monitoring standards in nursing education in Alberta."[28] The fact that the scope of the Senate's responsibility was considerably greater for the nursing profession than for other professions in the province made nursing a special and anomalous case. However, Alberta was not the only province to delegate responsibility for setting and monitoring standards to the University in initial nursing legislation. A similar course of action was taken in both Manitoba and Saskatchewan in their first pieces of nursing legislation. However, in both of those provinces, later amendments gave these responsibilities to the professional nursing associations. As time went on, Alberta became the only province in the country where authority for standards and monitoring in nursing education was not delegated to a nursing body.

The release of the Goldmark Report in 1923[29] drew attention to disquieting deficiencies in nursing education and had a powerful impact in Canada as well as in the United States, for similar conditions existed in the schools in both countries. The Report referred to conditions in nursing schools characterized by the "monotonous repetition of duties."[30] The recommendations of this Commission sponsored by the Rockefeller Foundation were aimed at reducing the length of nursing programs by one-fourth to avoid endless repetition of tasks by students, ensuring that there was sufficient instruction available in the schools and raising the entrance standard to nursing programs to high school graduation.[31] The AAGN had similar concerns relative to nursing education in the province, and in that achieving an entrance requirement of high school completion may not have been seen as a realistic goal for the organization to pursue at the time, it recommended continuing to support nursing programs that were three years in length.[32]

A NAME CHANGE AND NEW ALLIANCES

Because of the significance of registration to the AAGN, the Council saw fit to apply to the provincial government in 1920 to change the name of the organization to the Alberta Association of Registered Nurses. Requirements for registration included graduation from a school of nursing but were not limited to this since successful completion of registration examinations were an additional and important condition for registration.[33] In that the distinction between the "trained" and the "untrained" nurse provided the principal impetus for the development of legislation for nursing, addressing this distinction in the name of the organization seemed a reasonable and logical way to proceed. There were doubtless numerous issues facing the Alberta Association of Graduate Nurses at the time it was pressing for legislation, and those relative to the name of the organization may not have been primary at the outset. There was also uncertainty over the examinations at the time the Act was passed and it took time to establish a process for these as well as to formulate the regulations governing the process. By 1921 there were almost three hundred names on the register and the work involved in maintaining the registration records was almost beyond the ability of one individual to maintain on a voluntary basis while engaged in fulltime work in nursing. It was at this time that equipment and office furniture was purchased and a secretary engaged on a part-time basis to assist with the growing volume of work.[34]

The years following the establishment of the AAGN/AARN were tumultuous ones. As the Association came into being, World War I was in full swing and many Alberta nurses joined the war effort to support the Canadian troops overseas. During the war educational standards continued to be a primary concern of the organization and these presented some of the most trying and recurrent issues for the organization from its establishment in 1916 to the present. Other concerns arose in the period prior to the Depression over several overtures from women's organizations who wanted to join forces with the AARN in working towards common goals. The United Farm Women developed a strong lobby to work for matters pertaining to public health and pressured both the Liberal government and the United Farmers of Alberta government, which followed it in 1921, to legislate certain matters pertaining to the public health. The professional nursing association, which was barely on its feet at the time, did not see fit to develop a formal alliance with this group when an overture was made by the United Farm Women on several occasions relative to joint activity. Another group which sought some sort of formal joint association with the AAGN/AARN was the Women's Institutes of Alberta (WIA). This organization had a broadly-based membership and a great many women were active in its various branches in every corner of the province. Seeking such an alliance on the part of the WIA was reasonable as an important goal of this group was improving the health of the people. In particular, the health of women and children was of paramount concern to women's groups on the prairies because there was little to assist women during childbirth or to help them deal with health concerns relative to babies and young children. This concern was a significant one for women in the first three decades of the twentieth century.

However, there is evidence that at least two matters of interest to the AARN were sufficiently important that it was moved to act in concert with each of these women's organizations. The nursing organization added its support to that of these groups to encourage the development of a category of nursing personnel known as "trained attendants" to help ease the demand for nurses in the postwar years when such shortages were acute. Another matter involved a request made by the AARN to these organizations to encourage subscriptions to the *Canadian Nurse*. Many former nurses were members of women's groups such as the UFWA and the WIA since it was not acceptable for women to engage in paid employment after marriage, only in philanthropic work pursued on a voluntary basis.[35] The fact that these women's groups had an agenda to improve the health of people, an agenda for which they worked diligently and knowledgeably indicates that the membership was informed about these matters and the presence of former nurses among their ranks may explain this at least in part. A request that these women might support the professional nursing journal by subscribing to it would also seem to have been quite reasonable when viewed within such a membership context.

In declining to formally align itself with women's organizations, the AARN may have been making a statement on several fronts. In not wanting to join with the UFWA, it may have been signalling its unwillingness to become too closely aligned with groups that were perceived as having a political agenda. The UFWA was clearly an offshoot of a political party that was elected to government in 1921. For a professional association to join forces with an organization of this nature could be somewhat risky because of divisions within its own membership along party lines as well as potential problems with other political parties that might arise as a result of too close an association with a rival political party. However, another issue for the AARN may have been the anti-midwifery stance of nursing organizations generally in North America. To have supported this cause would have put them out of step with the thinking of other nursing organizations in Canada and the U.S. Over the years this was a pattern that continued as the AARN worked towards goals to improve public health independently of political parties and interest groups.

The relationship between nurses and women's groups has been of considerable interest over time from the standpoint of the accomplishment of goals of importance to women and of those of importance to nurses and nursing. It has also engaged attention because of assumptions made about nursing as a profession primarily composed of women. Nurses were at the forefront of women's movement from home to the workplace in the late nineteenth and early twentieth centuries as members of one of the earliest professions to beckon to women in society. In fact, nursing was second only to teaching in the order of its emergence as an acceptable avenue of work for women outside the home. Prior to the advent of these professions, women had not been permitted to work outside the home. Nightingale's campaign to find a meaningful role for herself outside marriage led to her interest in nursing and its reform so that it would become a respectable profession for lay women. These endeavours were critical in nursing's modern beginnings. Nursing was envisaged as a natural occupation for women who were believed to have certain native abilities in caring for others. Nurses as women were viewed as sharing these abilities with all women and nursing was seen as a natural activity for women. In effect, nursing was work that was taken a step further than the home, and knowledge and professional skill were downplayed in public perceptions of resources needed for nursing. The AAGN/AARN did not wholeheartedly embrace the women's suffrage movement that was in full swing at the time the campaign for nursing registration through legislation was launched, leading some to the conclusion that nurses were disinterested in the goals of the suffragists or worse rejected their initiatives. Such a view overlooks the diversity of women as a group comprising over half of the population. It also fails to account for the requirement for a fledgling organization such as the AAGN/AARN to establish its goals and work for them independently. There can be little doubt that the group as a whole was profoundly influenced by the women's movement and that it was working hard to advance the status of the profession, which at this time was composed entirely of women. In order to achieve respect for the organization, its members and its goals, it needed to pursue matters of vital importance to the organization itself in an independent, steadfast and determined manner.

The Weir Report and Standards of Nursing Education

Early in the Depression, the *Survey of Nursing Education in Canada*[36] was published. This had a great impact on every aspect of nursing in Canada. Supported jointly by the Canadian Nurses Association and the Canadian Medical Association, Dr. George Weir of the University of British Columbia undertook the survey. Its conclusions provided vindication for all of the problems about which the AARN had expressed concern over the previous decade and a half, problems which it had been attempting to have rectified in hospitals and schools of nursing. Among its major recommendations on nursing education, this comprehensive study recommended that nursing education should be integrated into the general educational system rather than continuing as a system under the control of the hospital; that the minimum number of beds for a hospital operating a school of nursing should be 75 and that the hospitals should also have a daily average census of 50 patients; that nurses should be the primary providers of instruction in schools; that better preparation should be required for nursing instructors; and that the minimum entrance standard for admission to schools of nursing should be senior matriculation.

The publication of the Weir Report provided needed support for the Association in pursuing its goals of improved standards of nursing education. It supported the AARN's repeated recommendation that schools of nursing in a number of small hospitals did not provide students with a sufficient breadth and depth of experience in clinical nursing. Other recommendations including the need for further education for nursing instructors and for raising the admission requirement to schools from grade eight to high school matriculation were also supportive to the AARN's efforts. It is a credit to the efforts of the AARN Council that the Alberta regulations for schools of nursing were changed just prior to the publication of the Weir Report and exceeded the standard proposed in the requirement that training schools have a minimum of 100 beds with a daily occupancy of 60 patients.[37] As a consequence of this change, the school of nursing in Camrose was closed due to an insufficient number of beds, and although it was recommended that St. Joseph's Hospital School of Nursing in Vegreville should be closed, the School was allowed to continue in operation on condition that the number of beds increased by 1935.[38] In her study documenting the failure of the University of Alberta to adequately monitor standards of nursing education until 1958 even though it had been delegated this responsibility, Young has asserted that "St. Mary's Hospital School of Nursing [at St. Mary's Hospital] in Camrose was the only school of nursing ever closed by the University of Alberta because of failure to meet acceptable standards."[39]

The AARN also expressed considerable concern about the initiation of a School of Nursing at the Ponoka Mental Hospital. Although Dr. C. Baragar, administrator of the hospital, applied to the University for approval to open a training school in 1932 and this was granted in 1933,[40] "The School was started prior to receiving approval from the Senate of the University of Alberta."[41] Even though this was a four-year program where the students spent two years at the Ponoka hospital and two years affiliating at three well-established schools of nursing in the province, the level of staffing and therefore of supervision for the students at the Ponoka hospital was a major issue. Young states that "The decision to approve a School of Nursing at Ponoka Mental Hospital was one in which it was clearly evident that meeting the usual standards was not considered to be a priority."[42] The staffing levels were such at Ponoka that the majority of the supervision of students was carried out by untrained attendants rather than registered nurses.

CONCERN ABOUT MEDIA PORTRAYALS OF NURSES

Nurses were concerned about the image they presented to the public and took exception to anything in the public media that maligned the image of nurses and nursing. A resolution at an October, 1934 meeting of the Edmonton Association of Graduate Nurses asked the Executive Council to ask for permission from the "Censor of Moving Pictures" to preview films that featured nursing, presumably so that nurses could ask for withdrawal of those that were deemed to be derogatory or inappropriate in terms of how nursing was depicted. A further resolution passed by the Edmonton Association perhaps went further than the authority of the group when they passed a motion that "moving pictures derogatory to the nursing pro-fession be banned in Alberta."[43] Despite the fact that the outcome of these motions is unknown, the fact that there was careful control of what the public was allowed to see at the time may have given all the professions including nursing more opportunity to have some influence on acceptable standards in the media. However, then as now, nurses were very concerned about how they were portrayed in the public media and wanted to see a reasonable and fair depiction of themselves as professionals and the profes-sional role. Nurses also wanted the public to understand their role and what they could expect from nurses. A resolution of the Council of the

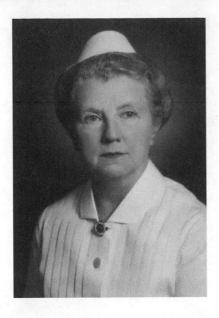

↝ *Frances (Fanny) Munroe, AARN President, 1932–1936. (Portrait by William Notman and Son, AARN)*

Executive Council of the AARN in January, 1934 called for educating the public "about the difference between Registered Nurses and others."[44]

Discussion of Health Insurance

The abject poverty experienced by people in the 1930s and their inability to secure adequate hospital, nursing and medical care led to public discussion of prepaid hospital and medical insurance. Although the first stage of a national plan was not passed for more than a decade, these matters were debated extensively over that period of time. Commercial plans developed by insurance companies began to appear almost as soon as the discussion began in the 1930s, and there were a number of public plans for prepaid care that were initiated by municipalities, hospitals and regional groups soon afterwards. The Edmonton Group Hospitalization Plan was the first known voluntary plan for prepayment of hospital care in Canada and was introduced by the four major general hospitals in 1934.[45] Plans such as the Edmonton one and the Blue Cross sponsored plans which followed required the payment of premiums by enrolees.

In 1929 the standing committee on industrial and international relations of the House of Commons recommended that "with regard to sickness

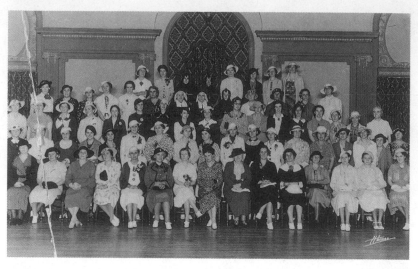

↪ AARN *Convention delegates in 1936.* (AARN P76)

insurance, the Department of Pensions and National Health be requested
to initiate a comprehensive survey of the field of public health, with special
reference to a national health programme."[46] Approval of the Report in
1933 led to action in 1935 when the Employment and Social Insurance Act
provided for collecting information and advising groups in provinces planning a health insurance program. The AARN was one such group that had
been requested by the Canadian Nurses Association to provide advice to
the Minister and President Fanny Munroe was authorized to send a night
letter to the Hon. George Hoadley on 24 April 1935 "suggesting that nursing services be included in the consideration of any plan of Health
Insurance."[47] There was also reference in the minutes of the meeting to
positive perceptions on the part of Council members about the effectiveness of the President's actions in the provincial arena in relation to health
insurance at the provincial level:

> Moved by Miss Brighty, seconded by Miss Connal, that through the
> efforts of our President Miss Munroe in promoting the interest of
> nurses in this Province, nursing services have been included in the
> recent Bill passed respecting Health Insurance in Alberta. As a Council
> may our appreciation of Miss Munroe's work be placed on record.[48]

Even though the national attempt to study health insurance issues in 1935 was sidelined by the fact that the effort was declared unconstitutional in the courts, pressure continued until another committee was constituted seven years later. Nor would the provincial Bill result in the development of a health insurance scheme, as it was never implemented.

WORKING FOR IMPROVEMENTS DURING WARTIME

Nurses were needed both at home and for the war effort, and the AARN encouraged nurses to make what contribution they could to help. In the words of President Rae Chittick: "The nursing profession has a vital part to play in developing this nationwide project."[49] The need for nurses both at home and in the service was never more acute than during this period of time and extreme shortages in the province prompted many suggested solutions to the problem. When the AARN hosted the CNA Convention in Calgary in June 1940, shortages were the topic of considerable discussion, for it was recognized that there would be pressure to lower standards of practice and education in order to prepare more nurses for the wartime emergency.[50] For its part, the AARN introduced a public relations campaign aimed at recruiting young women to nursing in 1943. Schools had increased enrolment quotas and some had experienced declines in their numbers. The intent here was to ensure that the maximum number of candidates possible was recruited to the profession. Talks were given to thousands of girls in high schools and efforts were made to secure financial assistance for those who required it. There were also news releases for radio, newspapers and films and an original script written by Kate Brighty, eighth president of the AARN, was aired on radio in major centres in the province.[51] The campaign met with limited success as schools experiencing enrolment difficulty failed to offset their enrolment declines.

It was clearly recognized that another alternative to increasing enrolments in schools of nursing was to recruit married nurses into the workforce, as there was a highly educated contingent of nurses in the community that could potentially be pressed into service. This was in fact what Dr. Angus C. McGugan, Medical Inspector of Hospitals, suggested when he addressed the AARN Annual Meeting in 1942. AARN members evidently approved of attempting to attract married nurses into the workforce to ease the shortage as they decided at this meeting to send letters to members of alumnae associations asking if they would be willing to assist with easing the shortage of nurses by returning to active duty.[52]

Recognizing that there were problems relative to working conditions for nurses and students in nursing programs, the AARN formed a committee, "The Eight-Hour Day Committee," to work for improvements.[53] At this time such a change was almost unthinkable, however important it might have been to work towards such a goal in terms of the best interests of nurses. There was also a movement to work towards better salaries for nurses as it was recognized that this could be an important factor in recruitment to the profession.[54] It was clear that there was a public perception that nursing was difficult and unrewarding in that such an active recruitment campaign reaped relatively meagre results. The AARN members who had worked so diligently in taking their campaign to the public, thought, however, that their work had not been in vain for they believed there was "due to the publicity, a greater understanding among nurses regarding their responsibility to the sick and to the community in which they served."[55]

The shortage of nurses also spawned another category of worker to assist nurses in their role. The AARN established a "Ward Aid Committee" and identified the kinds of activities that could be envisioned for those taking on this work. However, the minutes of the Annual Meeting of 1943 indicate that a survey of nurses had been carried out relative to nursing assistants or subsidiary workers, and it was clear that the majority of nurses were opposed to the creation of this category of worker.[56] However, because of the acute shortage of nurses, the idea of the nursing assistant took hold. Undoubtedly because of the economics involving lower salaries for this category of worker, hospitals hired them to ease the shortage during the war years. After the war, the role of the nursing assistant was not phased out, and training programs were later established to prepare these assistants in larger numbers. With the establishment of the first School for Nursing Aides in Calgary in 1945, the mechanism for training greater numbers of nursing assistants/aides was put in place. The nursing profession later became quite ambivalent about this worker, particularly in terms of the perceived threat to the livelihood of registered nurse through a growing share of nursing positions in hospitals being allocated to nursing assistants.

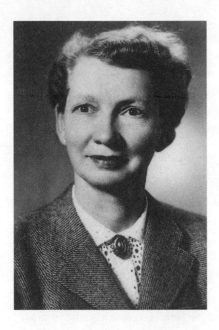

There were many aspects to standards of nursing education and the AARN attempted to work towards better standards on all fronts. Thus the recurring issue of entrance standards came up again and the grade 12 entrance standard, which nurses had wanted for a long period of time, became a reality when the Registered Nurses' Act was amended in 1941. This did not sit well with all members of the legislative assembly as the shortages of nurses became more acute as the war progressed. In 1946 the Minister of Health asked the Association to consider lowering entrance requirements to schools of nursing in the province so that more students would be admissible to schools of nursing. In that the alternative was to train more practical nurses, the AARN decided to recommend lowering the entrance standard to Grade 11 with an average of at least 50 percent. This was a difficult decision and one about which many members of the Council had misgivings, since it had taken so many years to achieve the high school matriculation standard.

On another front, plans for a ten-week course in public health nursing and one in teaching and supervision were announced at the Annual Meeting in 1943. These were to be financed by funds from the federal grant. Clinical courses were also developed with the use of these funds.

The Holy Cross Hospital in Calgary had developed a course in obstetrical nursing, but it was reported that not much interest had been shown in it. Under discussion was a course in surgical nursing to be offered in Calgary and a six-month course in psychiatric nursing in conjunction with the Ponoka Mental Hospital.[57] A number of the postgraduate courses and certificate programs offered by hospitals established during this period of time with the assistance of federal grants continued into succeeding decades. When the need for these programs was demonstrated through enrolment of students and retention of graduates in the workforce, the responsible organization offering the courses decided that it was worthwhile to continue them and to provide funding to support them. Following a meeting of the Association with Mr. Ottewell, Registrar of the University of Alberta, a recommendation was made that returning service personnel not be given concessions in university entrance requirements for nursing training programs. Since the Canadian Legion education program did not permit returning service personnel to complete high school matriculation unless only a few subjects were needed, this meant that nurses lacking high school matriculation had to acquire this before they would become eligible for the program.[58] Again the Association under the direction of President Ida Johnson did not want to compromise standards of nursing education.

In 1942, President Rae Chittick submitted a brief to the provincial government committee investigating educational opportunities at the University of Alberta, requesting consideration for the establishment of a central school for nurses in the province to be set up under the direction of the University. Ever since the publication of the Weir Report in 1932, nurses in Alberta had been pressing hard to remove nursing education from the mandate of hospitals because of the serious problems in the schools with standards. There was discussion at the twenty-fourth annual meeting in 1942 about whether raising entrance requirements for schools of nursing was contributing to reduced numbers of nursing students. However, the consensus of the group in attendance was that there were other contributing factors to low enrolment such as the various types of employment available in war industries, enrolment in Women's Auxiliary Services, difficulty in financing the three-year training period particularly in those schools in which entrance fees were charged and the lack of allowances to help students cover their expenses.[59] The next year at the annual meeting an announcement was made that financial aid was available through the Dominion-Provincial grants to girls 18 or over who were interested in nursing but unable to finance the three years of the program.[60]

The relatively low level of nursing salaries compared to both professionals and nonprofessionals continued to be an issue for nurses and the need to address it was discussed endlessly at every level in professional organizations. The CNA approval of collective bargaining by nurses with the provincial professional associations serving as bargaining agents took place in 1943 and the federal Labour Relations Act was passed the next year. Undoubtedly the general discussion at the federal level about liberalizing the legislation led the CNA to take its stand supporting collective bargaining.[61] This was an important step forward in the advancing nurses' quest to engage in meaningful and productive activity to raise the level of their salaries. The AARN Provincial Council quickly approved the formation of a Labour Relations Committee in August of 1944, but the Committee failed to materialize due to some reluctance relative to needing more information and advice about matters in this domain.[62] However, nurses still had major concerns about the level of their salaries and a resolution was passed at the AARN Convention in 1945 that salaries for Alberta nurses should be consistent with CNA salary recommendations of $1,200, $1,260 and $1,320 annually for the first, second and third years of work in addition to laundry and meals while on duty for nurses not living in the living quarters provided by hospitals for graduate nurses.[63] The Associated Hospitals of Alberta (AHA) considered this matter at its Annual Convention in 1945 and endorsed a salary of $80 per month with full maintenance and compensation for charge nurse duties. This was a considerably lower level than nurses had been asking for, and thus reflected how far apart the two groups were in their positions. Since the employer group retained ultimate control of the level at which wages and conditions were set, nurses were essentially powerless without a formal collective bargaining procedure to negotiate their compensation with their employers. Despite the fact that they had no voice in the setting of their salaries and conditions of employment, nurses were still ambivalent about collective bargaining and affiliation with trade unions and no further action was taken until a number of years had passed.

CONTINUING SHORTAGE OF NURSES
AND WORKPLACE CONCERNS

Surprisingly, the shortage of nurses was not relieved by the conclusion of hostilities and the return of those who had served overseas. The postwar economic boom began slowly, but picked up during the decade of the 50s, and since economic prosperity usually results in the availability of more health care, nursing had tended to expand during such times. The postwar period was no exception. Nursing had also gained new respect as a profession during this period of time based on its service in the war zone and nurses and nursing were highly valued both by the wounded and by the country in general. Nationally the importance of nurses to the health of the nation had been recognized and expansion of educational opportunities for nurses continue to occur over this period of time.

A Bill to allow for the licensing of Nursing Aides was assented to by the Alberta Legislative Assembly in 1947. This ended years of discussion and concern by registered nurses over the question of whether and under what conditions nursing assistants should be trained. The continuing shortage of nurses explains the government's determination to push forward with this legislation, but the financial savings for hospitals must unquestionably be considered an additional driving force.[64] In addition the minutes refer to the fact that more subsidiary workers were being employed in hospitals and more hospitals were adopting the 48-hour week. Discussion ensued also about the curriculum of the course to be given to prepare registered nursing aides and the length of the training period at 9 months with an additional period of three months' employment under supervision in an approved institution.[65]

The passage of the federal National Health Grants Act of 1948 raised further discussion about the need for nurses to staff the hospitals which would be constructed under the program. This was the first act in the series of three pieces of legislation that constituted the legislative mandate for the Canadian system of medicare. It was evident even at this stage that there was a hospital-centred focus in the system which evolved from the legislation. This resulted from financial incentives to construct hospitals and later to finance care that was provided within them. In later years, it would be recognized that this made the Canadian system relatively expensive, compared to other countries where health care was financed through public funding and where hospitals were not the central focus of the health care system.

Working conditions for nurses continued to be a matter of concern in this period and a resolution at the annual meeting of 1950 endorsed the concept of the 8-hour working day for nurses with statutory holidays and 1 1/2 days per week off duty. Another resolution passed at the meeting recommended that the Associated Hospitals of Alberta endorse a pension scheme for nurses who were employed in Alberta hospitals.[66] The shortage of nurses was raised by the matrons of small hospitals at the 1951 annual meeting where they expressed concerns that nurses in urban areas would not want to go to rural hospitals to work "where ideals are not practical because of lack of sufficient funds and equipment."[67] They further predicted that some small hospitals would be forced to close if they could not recruit sufficient numbers of registered nurses to become staff members. The minutes of the annual meeting the next year indicated that the shortage of nursing instructors was equally acute and that this compromised the work of schools of nursing. The Minister of Health announced at the meeting that a grant of $300 per graduating student would be made to schools of nursing in 1953 to provide incentives to offset the shortage of nurses. Although the AARN was still on record as supporting the idea of a central school, the Minister indicated that he did not support this concept.[68]

Nurses were seeking solutions to the lack of attention to the educational experience for nursing students. They believed that service was disguised as education and programs were unnecessarily long due to the emphasis upon service to the hospital. Thus, the Association discussed the idea of a central school for several years as a means of eliminating the problems. However in 1952 the Minister of Health, Dr. W.W. Cross, indicated that the government did not support such a concept so that there would be no public funding for it.[69] No doubt the experience in Saskatchewan with the centralized teaching program for diploma schools based in Saskatoon and Regina was a stimulus to consideration of this concept by the AARN. This was also a national issue that had engendered considerable discussion at the level of the CNA. The difficult issues that the AARN had addressed over so many years with standards in diploma schools undoubtedly led the organization to pursue this issue persistently over more than a decade.

Experimentation in Diploma Nursing Education

An interesting and important development designed to achieve similar goals in diploma education was the CNA's quest to identify whether or not a nurse could be prepared at the diploma level in a period of two years rather than three. Thus, with financing from the Canadian Red Cross Society in 1948, the CNA sponsored an experiment in nursing education in Windsor, Ontario where a demonstration school was established in association with the Metropolitan General Hospital. The school was financially independent and the question to be answered by the experiment was whether or not a nurse could be prepared in a program that was two years in length where the focus was upon instruction and quality of the learning experience. In offering such a program, the educational aspects of the program were separated from the service needs of the hospital and nursing students were not used as staff members in the hospital. A.R. Lord, who carried out the evaluation of the results of the demonstration school, stated:

> The conclusion is inescapable. When the school has complete control of students, nurses can be trained at least as satisfactorily in two years as in three, and under better conditions, but the training must be paid for in money instead of in services. Few students can afford substantial fees nor can the hospital pass on such additional costs to the "paying patient". Some new source of revenue is the only solution.[70]

Encouraged by the interest in the Demonstration School in Windsor, the CNA began in 1950 to work towards getting each provincial association to sponsor a demonstration school. Although the AARN approved of this proposal, it was not able to implement it because there was no funding for establishing and maintaining such a school on an independent basis. The Demonstration School provided nurses with some hard evidence that programs could be planned that accomplished the desired goal of preparing a nurse in less time and using more educationally sound approaches than was the case in most diploma schools of the day. This was by no means a dead issue—indeed, it was just beginning to heat up. The Association found the evaluation of the demonstration school in Windsor, Ontario very helpful in its continuing struggle to work towards the recommendation made earlier by Dr. Weir that schools of nursing should be operated within the general educational system rather than by hospitals. While Alberta was one of the last provinces to witness the shift of nursing education programs to the general educational system, it nevertheless was a gradual process that allowed for considerable discussion prior to the occurrence of major changes. The establishment of diploma nursing programs in community colleges was the first step in the process.

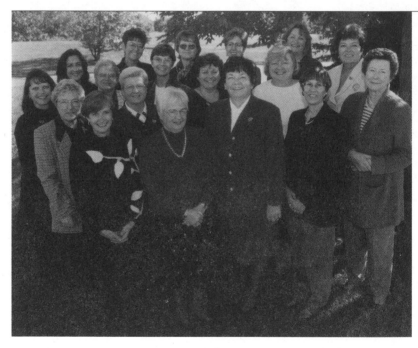

✥ *AARN Provincial Council, 1997–98. (AARN P805)*

10

Consolidation and Growth

The AARN in the Years
From 1956 to 1996

The size of the nursing workforce increased remarkably as a result of continued postwar growth and the passage of the primary pieces of federal legislation on medicare in Canada. The remarkable growth of the profession in the postwar period was reflected in the increase in the size of the AARN from 1850 active members in 1950, to 4,382 in 1960 and 11,875 by 1970. The prepayment of hospital care for all qualified residents of Canada through the provisions of the Hospital Insurance and Diagnostic Services Act of 1957, encouraged the development of hospitals

233

as the primary setting for the delivery of health care. The Medical Care Act of 1968 added prepaid medical care to the provisions already established for hospital care. The nature and extent of the stimulus given to nursing by the passage of medicare legislation has often been overlooked. However, since nursing is an essential and indeed critical component of hospital care, federal legislation establishing medicare in Canada stimulated tremendous growth in the size of the nursing workforce and the nursing profession across the country. Although community nursing remained viable and important, this was a very small sector of the total nursing enterprise.

In a society that had not yet developed a sense of limits to growth, the surging economy after the war was undoubtedly an important factor in ensuring the availability of more health care to the public resulting in a need for more nurses. However, even though more students were entering programs of nursing education than before and there was an appreciable growth of the workforce in comparison to previous years, the shortage of nurses continued. When epidemics of polio occurred in the early 1950s, nurses volunteered willingly to care for those afflicted. However, the shortage of nurses was acute and it was difficult to provide sufficient staffing in areas where care was provided to polio patients. Caring for these patients required specialized skills and nurses had to have preparation to provide this care. Therefore staffing issues were difficult. Nurses were key frontline workers and took the serious risk of exposure to the virus causing the disease. In fact, "several became permanently paralysed while others died" in Alberta.[1] Nurses volunteered to assist in the crisis in health care that the polio epidemic created, as did nursing students. During the polio epidemic of 1954, the nursing students at the Royal Alexandra Hospital volunteered to ventilate polio victims when iron lungs ceased to function during power failures[2] as they had done in the past in emergency situations in health care, and as they would continue to do in the future.

The federal government's Federal Task Force Report on the Cost of Health Services in Canada was released in 1969[3] and capped a period of substantial growth in the history of the country. The costs of health care had moved ahead rapidly over the little more than a decade since the implementation of prepaid hospital care in Canada. Awareness of the need to review and rationalize expenditures came to the fore with the realization that economic instability was just over the horizon. The AARN reviewed the report and submitted a brief to the CNA as well as to the provincial

Government.[4] The professional associations had clearly recognized how critical it was for nurses to respond to documents such as the Federal Task Force Report because of the importance of the structure of health care financing to the nursing workforce.

Another nationally-sponsored study done in the early 1970s by Dr. John Hastings, the National Study on Community Health Centres, carried with it important implications for the practice of nurses if the findings were implemented.[5] The AARN submitted a brief to Dr. Hastings and met with him during the period in which he was soliciting input from organizations about community health centres. The first recommendation of his report stands as a goal which has not yet been attained:

> The immediate and purposeful re-organization and integration of all health services into a health services system to ensure basic health service standards for all Canadians and to assure a more economic and effective use of all health care resources.[6]

Although nurses espoused the need for health care based in the community rather than in hospitals as an important direction for the future, the failure of provincial and federal governments to implement the 1972 recommendations of the Hastings Report meant that the establishment of community health centres was postponed and would not receive serious consideration by policy makers until two decades later.

STANDARDS OF PRACTICE

In its continuing concern for standards of nursing practice in the province, the AARN decided to develop a list of delegated medical responsibilities, and these were subsequently approved by Provincial Council in May of 1967.[7] The list was then forwarded to the Associated Hospitals of Alberta and the Alberta Medical Association (AMA) for approval. The need for such a list was to be found in the fact that the boundaries between nursing and medicine were somewhat grey and pressure was often placed upon nurses to perform functions that were primarily defined as medical. Even though Board-approved policies in each hospital represented the legal authority for identifying when and under what conditions nurses were permitted to perform procedures normally designated as medical acts, some policies were not clear. Agencies may have been less than clear about where responsibility rested for certain procedures. This was more often a problem in small hospitals with fewer physicians where nurses were expected to perform a greater range of activities often including medical acts. The development of a list of delegated medical responsibilities served as a guide for agencies and as a basis for discussion between nurses and the organizations in which they were employed. The updating of this list continued into the 1980s after which time it was deemed no longer necessary. For most of the period of time when it was in use, it was a collaborative project of the AARN, AHA and AMA.

New knowledge in health care accompanied by remarkable technology to assist in the diagnosis and treatment of disease, inconceivable only a few years previously, was being applied in everyday nursing practice at a brisk rate. The knowledge of practitioners was fast becoming an issue, for the ability to stay abreast of new developments and to practise safely was essential. Also assuring the competence of those who took time out from nursing for a period of years increasingly became an issue. As a self-regulating profession, there was an obligation to provide assurances to the public that those engaged in professional practice could provide safe, competent and ethical nursing care. Nursing continued to be a profession still composed primarily of women, and women's roles in society often were such that these women needed to take time out from their careers for childbearing and childrearing. Many nurses did not wish to go back to the profession after a period of years without some additional study in new developments in the field. Thus in 1958 the AARN developed standards for refresher programs for nurses so that they could be used by hospitals and educational organizations who wished to offer such programs.[8] The Association also provided support to ensure that in addition to refresher programs, short courses, workshops and lectures were available on a variety of topics which could help nurses keep up with the latest developments in their field. Guidelines for the development of continuing education programs were developed and approved in 1966 in order to assist planners in meeting the needs and interests of nurses and also to help coordinate continuing education programs offered by a variety of agencies.[9]

The possibility of sharing the work traditionally done by nurses with nursing assistants or aides had commanded the attention of the profession since the issue was first discussed during the acute nursing shortages of the war years and on through the development of a legal framework for practice for nursing aides just after the conclusion of the war. The AARN had agonized over every aspect of the practice of nursing aides following the establishment of the training program in 1946. Although certified nursing aides (CNAS) had been practising for almost a decade by the mid-fifties, there were persistent concerns about their duties and in 1959, a controversy occurred over the roles of CNAS in some hospitals in the operating room and in labour and delivery areas.[10] Clearly nurses' concerns were based at least in part upon their fear of being replaced by CNAS, even though these were prosperous times. The economy was continuing to surge, medicare was in place, and health care was booming with great expansion of hospital operations and a great increase in the number of nursing positions.

STRUCTURAL ISSUES AND LEGISLATIVE CONCERNS

By the early 1960s the AARN had 41 organizational units or chapters around the province. The chapters were units which "frequently filled volunteer needs in their communities, performed fund-raising activities, provided educational programs for nurses and the public, and held social functions for their members."[11] It appeared that the time had come to review the structure since associate members were in many cases providing the leadership and the work behind many of the volunteer activities of the chapters, and these members were not permitted to hold office in the chapters. This led to the 1965 AARN structure study carried out by a consulting firm. As a result of the study, the entire provincial and district structure of the AARN was completely reorganized into five geographic districts and the bylaws rewritten to support the new structure.[12] This represented a dramatic change, for the reorganization meant that the focus was now on the district as the organizational unit and not the chapter. There would be more attention at the district level to dealing with the business of the organization and attending to matters referred to it by Provincial Council.

At the outset of this period of time, Clara van Dusen had headed up the secretariat of the organization. However, in 1960 Helen Sabin was appointed Executive Secretary of the Association and an Assistant Secretary, Doris Price, was engaged in the same year. As the work of the organization was steadily increasing and the scope of the activities went far beyond the capabilities of two staff members to handle, an additional staff member to man-

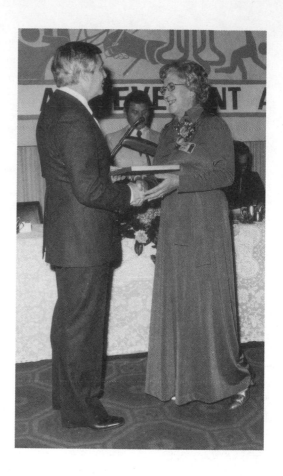

⬦ *Helen Sabin, receiving the Alberta Award of Excellence from Premier Peter Lougheed.* (AARN)

age the committees of the organization was hired two years later and a nursing counsellor was hired the following year. Thus by 1963 there were four members of staff working on a full-time basis for the Association. In 1965 as a result of the structure study and the reorganization of the Association, Muriel Garrick was appointed to the new position of Office Manager. The size of the provincial office staff of the organization continued to increase over time as the scope of its activities became even greater.

A recurring theme throughout the history of the AARN was assaults or threatened assaults on its legislation. This is not to say that there were not occasions when amendments in the legislation were not made at the request of the AARN, or other times when perfunctory amendments simply updated the Registered Nurses Act relative to changes in other legislation. An example of the former occurred when the structure study in the mid-

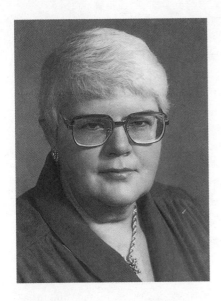

↪ *Muriel Garrick, AARN Office Manager. (AARN)*

1960s resulted in legislative changes requested by the AARN. The study was stimulated in part by the need to identify how a structure could be incorporated into the AARN. Further to its recommendations, amendments to the Registered Nurses Act in 1966 designated the AARN as a bargaining agent under the Labour Act. Thus the organization could legitimately bargain for a group of members if it was requested to do so. Although the context of the amendments to the legislation in the 1960s was relatively friendly, most decades included at least one threat or potential threat to the integrity of the nursing legislation. Assaults or threats to the legislation came primarily from outside the profession with government usually taking the initiative by announcing an intent to open the Act. In many cases, such initiatives on the part of government were encouraged by other groups with a vested interest in changing the rules governing the operation of the profession.

The first potential threat to the legislation during the time period under consideration resulted from one recommendation among several emerging from a conference on nursing held by the Minister of Health in 1961. The recommendation that immediate consideration be given to the establishment of a College of Nurses in Alberta, was investigated thoroughly by a committee headed by Ruth McClure, Director of the School of Nursing at the University of Alberta. No doubt this recommendation was stimulated by the structure created by the newly-established College of Nurses in Ontario. The Committee concluded that moving to a statutory body such as a College of Nurses responsible for regulatory functions and a professional association responsible for other professional matters was premature and might well undermine the effectiveness of the Association. The Ontario model was actually an adapted American model and the AARN committee concluded that it was not applicable in Alberta and should not be pursued. The major recommendation of the committee was that the Association should work towards mandatory registration for nurses in Alberta.

A survey of nursing education was undertaken in the early 1960s by a government appointed committee under the direction of a committee chaired by Dr. E.P. Scarlett. The Nursing Education Survey Report was released in 1963 and contained 97 recommendations concerning nursing and nursing education in Alberta.[13] Although the report generally endorsed the status quo in terms of diploma nursing education, its recommendations were wide-ranging. The recommendation to establish a Provincial Council on Nursing was of concern to the AARN because of the fact that the Scarlett Committee recommended that the regulation of nursing be carried out not by the AARN, but by a Provincial Council controlled by government. The AARN had earlier been in support of a council on nursing which it had seen as advisory, but it viewed this recommendation as quite different. Nursing would lose its status as a self-governing profession if the licensing function were to be removed from the AARN and given to a government body. If that were to happen, the profession saw it as a loss both for nurses and also the public. Because removal of licensing would have reduced the powers and scope of the AARN, the Association would also have lost its position as the voice for nurses in the province to express views on matters pertaining to nursing and health.

STANDARDS OF DIPLOMA NURSING EDUCATION

The system of nursing education continued to be scrutinized by the profession particularly in relation to the entrenchment of the service component of diploma programs and the accompanying lack of attention to the quality of the educational experience for students. The need to prepare more nurses because of continuing shortages led to continuing discussion of the standards, for external pressure to lower these was great and came from many directions. In 1958 the AARN recorded its appreciation to the University of Alberta as it had heeded their advice to appoint a qualified individual to serve as a full-time advisor to schools of nursing. The appointment of Marguerite Schumacher was applauded by the AARN because it had been requesting that the University establish such a position to help schools improve the quality of programs by assisting them to adhere to the "Regulations Governing Schools of Nursing in Alberta." Prior to this, a university nursing faculty member had been appointed on a part-time basis to carry out the monitoring role. However, this was difficult as the faculty member had to juggle the role of advisor along with teaching assignments at the University. The findings of the AARN Educational Policy Committee in 1953 had served as the catalyst for the establishment of the advisor position:

> It is true that in this Province the Regulations Governing Schools of Nursing as issued by the University, make provisions for a minimum curriculum, but these regulations are not a guarantee that all student nurses will receive a sound nursing education for at the present time no provision is made for regular and competent inspection and there is no qualified nurse advisor to Schools of Nursing. Most of the progress that has been made in the maintenance of standards is due to the fact that all students meet a common hurdle, namely the Examination for Registration.[14]

Thus, the AARN lobbied hard for the establishment of the advisor role as it viewed this as an important first step in the process of monitoring standards of nursing education.

The provincial government had earlier appointed a director of recruitment to encourage students to enter schools of nursing. During the 1950s the recruitment director was closely associated with the AARN Provincial Executive Committee, namely Frances Ferguson, President of the Association from 1950–1953. She was followed by Madeline Quirk, a member of the Executive Committee and Vice-President of the organization. While nursing schools had earlier experienced difficulty filling their quotas of students, during this period of time the enrolment of most schools was at maximum capacity. In that opportunities for women in nontraditional fields were limited following the war, nursing continued to maintain an

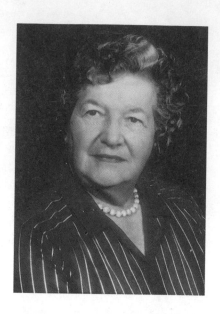

advantage as an acceptable career selection for young women. The first few men entered the profession during this period of time, but the social norms which had made nursing a sex-segregated profession meant that those men who successfully completed programs of nursing education in this era did not find it a particularly easy process.

In 1951 Dr. Mildred Montag, professor of nursing at Teacher's College, Columbia University, published her discussion of the need for nursing programs to prepare what she termed the "technical nurse" within the community college network.[15] Her work became nationally and internationally known within a short time and influenced the nursing profession around the world. Solutions had been sought for decades to inadequate educational standards in schools operated by hospitals because of the fact that the primary mission of the hospital was not education, but health care to patients. The Weir Report of 1932 had much earlier recommended that nursing education be situated within the general educational framework. Later the Royal Commission on Health Services chaired by Justice Emmett Hall recommended that additional hospital schools of nursing should not be initiated and that schools of nursing should be established within junior colleges (later termed community colleges).[16] Support was building in society generally to support the transfer of educational programs in nursing from hospitals to community colleges.

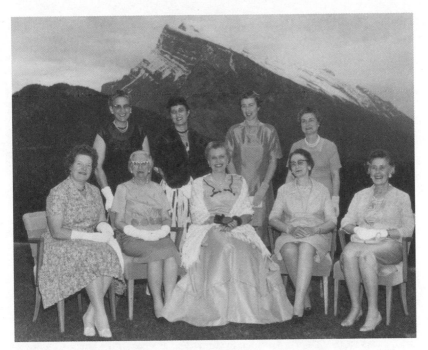

↩ *AARN presidents present and past gathered at the 1964 Convention: (front row, left to right) Frances Ferguson, Elizabeth Bietsch, Marguerite Schumacher, Ida Johnson, Margaret Street; (back row, left to right) Barbara Beattie, Claudia Tennant, Jeannie Clark, D. June Taylor. (AARN P269)*

In 1962, the AARN went on record as supporting the diploma nursing enterprise as a function of the community colleges of the province.[17] An opportunity arose for the organization to encourage this development in 1965 when the Association was asked to sponsor a study along with the Red Deer General Hospital and Red Deer College to investigate the feasibility of establishing a nursing program at Red Deer College. The resulting study confirmed the feasibility of such a program at the College.[18] The two year program at Red Deer College was approved and the AARN allocated $15,000 for a project to evaluate the program. Marguerite Schumacher, President of the AARN from 1963 to 1965, was appointed to head the new program and it got underway with the admission of its first students in September of 1968. However, the first college program established in the province was at Mount Royal College in Calgary in February of 1967 under the direction of Jean Mackie. In Edmonton, the School of Nursing at the Edmonton General Hospital was transferred to Collège St.-Jean, and that program was subsequently transferred to Grant MacEwan Community College in 1968 with Sister Thérèse Castonguay as Director. Then Lethbridge Community College established a program in the fall of 1969 under the leadership of Sister Ann Marie Cummings, President of the AARN from 1967–1969.[19] A college program was also established in this period at Medicine Hat College in 1970. It is evident that several prominent nurses who had taken major leadership roles in the AARN were involved with the development of these early college programs, thus providing evidence of the tangible support of the nursing community for the direction of events in nursing education.

An event that crystallized opposition to the movement of diploma programs from the hospitals into the colleges occurred in 1971 when a report prepared for the Alberta Colleges Commission recommended the transfer of existing hospital diploma programs to the colleges. The "Report Recommending the Transfer of All Diploma Nursing and Allied Health Programs to the Alberta College System" was prepared by Dr. R.G. Fast.[20] The recommendations of this report were so sweeping that just about every group which might have been supportive was alienated by its provisions. The report recommended that the Alberta Colleges Commission should be granted the authority to make regulations governing the education of diploma nurses. Such authority had been historically delegated to the Universities Coordinating Council through the Registered Nurses Act. This provision in the Fast Report gave the AARN cause for concern because the issue of maintaining standards in the diploma schools had been a difficult one over a long period of time. Since the professional association had the power to make such regulations in most other provinces, the AARN recommended that if authority was to be vested in a different organization, that organization should be the professional association.[21] With tremendous opposition mounting from all sectors of the nursing as well as the external community, the Report was shelved by the fledgling government of Premier Peter Lougheed.

Continuing Development of Degree Programs

The report of the national study undertaken by Dr. Helen Mussallem to determine the feasibility of and issues associated with a system of accreditation of schools of nursing in Canada recommended in 1960: "That a reexamination and study of the whole field of nursing education be undertaken."[22] This recommendation was to be realized within a very short time with the appointment of a Royal Commission by the federal government to investigate the problems and issues related to all aspects of the delivery of health services in Canada. The Royal Commission report recommended that ten more university nursing programs under administratively-autonomous schools of nursing be established in Canada as soon as possible.[23] It further recommended the elimination of nonintegrated basic programs at a time when admissions to the latter were 22 per cent higher than admissions to integrated programs. The impact of this report was impressive, for only four years later: "admission to integrated programmes constituted ninety-seven per cent of all admissions to baccalaureate programmes."[24] The recommendations of the Royal Commission provided strong support for the nursing profession in Alberta to encourage significant advances in the university nursing programs available at universities in the province. The School of Nursing at the University of Alberta under the leadership of Ruth McClure was able to revise its program from a nonintegrated five year program to a four-year integrated one just 10 years after the integrated program introduced under Helen Penhale had been terminated. In the integrated model, the arts, sciences and humanities were studied along with nursing courses throughout the four years of the program, and authority for all nursing instruction rested with the University.[25] The first class in the new integrated program at the University of Alberta enroled in the program in the fall of 1966.

Further to the Royal Commission recommendation that new university programs in nursing be established in Canada, Sister Marguerite Letourneau, a member of the Grey Nuns and a leading nursing administrator in the province was asked by the AARN to write a brief that could be submitted to the University of Calgary presenting the arguments for establishing a four-year integrated program in nursing in Calgary.[26] The brief was prepared in 1967 and presented a cogent case for the establishment of a university nursing program in south central Alberta. The University subse-

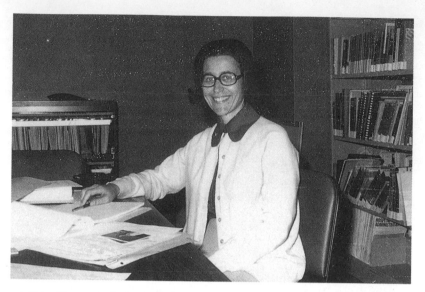

⤙ Sister Marguerite Letourneau, Superior at the Holy Cross Hospital in Calgary, later to become Superior General of the Grey Nuns order. (AARN)

quently decided to support the recommendation to establish a School of Nursing as an autonomous unit within the university administrative framework, and appointed Dr. Shirley Good as Director. The program accepted its first students the next year in the fall of 1970. Thus the 1974 convocation of the first class from the University of Calgary program meant that there were two university programs in the province preparing basic practitioners in nursing in integrated programs.

THE ENTRY TO PRACTICE POSITION

In 1974, the Minister of Advanced Education announced the Government's intention to transfer diploma schools of nursing to the general education system. Following the announcement, there were rumours that the Universities Coordinating Council would be eliminated and there was resulting concern about where the responsibility for standards for diploma programs would rest. The Alberta Task Force on Nursing Education was appointed early the next year. The mandate of the Task Force was wide-ranging and included investigating the roles to be played by nurses in the health care system; the types of nursing personnel required in the system; the educational system required to support preparation of nursing personnel; and the monitoring system required to maintain appropriate standards in nursing education. The report of the Task Force was significant in the history of nursing education in Canada in terms of its impact upon the nursing, health care and educational communities. It had a tremendous influence on policy development in terms of raising the level of initial preparation to qualify for the practice of nursing.[27] Its first recommendation was "That all nursing education be established as a component of the advanced education system."[28] However, the recommendation which commanded the most attention because of its controversial nature, was that by 1985 all those entering professional practice for the first time be qualified at the baccalaureate level. There was also a recommendation that there be only two routes to basic education for professional nursing practice: a basic program offered by a university and an articulated baccalaureate program between a university and another agency conducting a program of diploma preparation in nursing.

The controversy raised by the report produced heated discussion both within and external to the nursing profession. The AARN response to the Task Force report in 1976 was supportive, and also drew attention to the need for government support to ensure that faculty qualifications were raised and that new and well-prepared faculty were recruited.[29] Even though there was considerable diversity of opinion in the profession about the recommendations and the profession in Alberta was composed primarily of diploma graduates, the AARN was able to maintain broadly-based support within the profession for the position it had first put forward in 1976:

> The Alberta Association of Registered Nurses supports the goal of the baccalaureate degree (basic and/or post-R.N.) as the minimum educational preparation for professional nursing and further, that by the year 2000, the baccalaureate degree in nursing be the minimum requirement for entry into the nursing profession in the province of Alberta.[30]

For its part, the Government took some time to review the report of its Task Force and collected views of interested parties. Its 1977 response commented upon the desirability of baccalaureate preparation in nursing, but stopped short of approving the position that it should be required for pro-

fessional practice in nursing.[31] The lack of support for the Task Force recommendations by the Government led to ongoing discussion and disagreement between legislators and the AARN for a number of years to follow. This retreat by the Government[32] from the position on baccalaureate
entry to practice by the Task Force it had appointed, resulted in no action
on the transfer of diploma schools to Advanced Education. This matter had
to wait almost a decade until the report of the Nursing Education,
Manpower and Research Implementation Committee again recommended
the transfer, the latter finally taking place in 1983.[33]

The AARN was the first professional nursing association in the country
to take a position in support of baccalaureate preparation for entry to the
profession, a position that subsequently became known as the EP2000 position. The Association decided to take the position a step further since it had
developed a strong and committed group of councillors and others active
in the organization who felt strongly that the issue of baccalaureate preparation for entry to the profession should be widely discussed and carried to
the national level. Thus, the AARN proposed a resolution which was subsequently passed by delegates at the CNA Convention in 1980 in Vancouver to
investigate the feasibility of the baccalaureate standard for entry to professional practice. This initiated appointment of a CNA committee appointed
to study baccalaureate entry to practice. The Entry to Practice Committee
subsequently developed a "Background Paper"[34] and recommended that
baccalaureate entry be supported. The position was approved unanimously
by the Board of Directors early in 1982, and their stand was endorsed by
delegates attending the 1982 Annual Meeting in St. John's, Newfoundland.
Subsequently all professional nursing associations in Canada took a position supporting baccalaureate entry to practice.

In 1983 the AARN decided to develop a plan for the proposed implementation of the baccalaureate entry to practice position in the year 2000. A
committee was appointed to develop a document and a "Blueprint" was the
result of that effort. It was approved by Provincial Council in 1984 and it
recommended strategies to achieve the EP2000 goal focusing on students,
faculty, programs and marketing. A committee was established to develop
an action plan for implementing the recommendations of the "Blueprint,"
a plan that was approved in 1985. At this time a project director was
employed for a two-year term and an advisory committee that became the
Action Plan Advisory Committee was appointed. In 1987, a resolution

opposing the entry to practice position was approved at the annual meeting of the United Nurses of Alberta (UNA). The resolution reflected fears of UNA members about job security and mobility for diploma-prepared nurses in the future. A team of AARN/UNA members in support of the position provided information at the UNA meeting to help reduce anxiety of UNA members about these issues. This event stimulated a revision to the *Position Statement on Baccalaureate Education for Nurses* to include the statement that "Registration in accordance with other registration regulations is ensured for all diploma-prepared nurses who have graduated prior to the year 2000."[35]

In 1987, two resolutions were passed at the AARN Annual Meeting calling for widespread dissemination of the entry to practice position. In response to these resolutions, information was distributed to government ministers and leaders of a variety of groups. It was in response to these communications publicizing the AARN's position and to meetings held with cabinet ministers explaining the position that a letter was received under the signatures of two cabinet ministers, the Minister of Hospitals and Medical Care, Marvin Moore, and the Minister of Advanced Education, David Russell, indicating that the Government did not support the need for a baccalaureate degree to practise nursing. Thus it was clear that the Government's position had not changed since the publication of its response to the *Report of the Alberta Task Force on Nursing Education* in 1977. However, the entry to practice project was discontinued by the AARN in 1988 in view of the belief that the project had accomplished its goals and heightened awareness of the EP2000 position. In 1988 the Provincial Executive Committee was given responsibility for the EP2000 Action Plan and further action to support the entry to practice position.

The initiative towards collaboration between diploma and university programs in nursing was a logical step towards achieving the baccalaureate entry standard to the profession, and was an initiative that nurses in a wide variety of agencies supported enthusiastically. When the University of Alberta established its initiative to collaborate with Red Deer College and subsequently with the three hospital diploma programs and one community college diploma program in Edmonton, the AARN expressed support and a staff member participated with the partners in identifying the structure and processes to be used. The collaboration between Red Deer College and the University of Alberta got underway in 1990 and the Edmonton sites

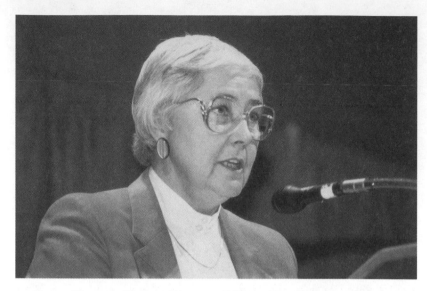

❧ *Yvonne Chapman, Director of the* AARN *Collective Bargaining Program 1970–1976, Executive Director,* AARN *1976–1990 (*AARN*)*

joined the collaboration in 1991. This was the logical next step in the transition to an all baccalaureate workforce in the nursing profession. The Government subsequently announced in 1994 that all diploma programs would be phased out and their resources cut back by 50 percent and transferred to the educational institutions. Because the structure had been put in place for a common program, disruptions in the educational process were minimized. At the University of Calgary, the proposal for a program developed through a collaborative process between all schools of nursing in Calgary, had to wait for several years for government approval for funding. Here also the AARN offered tangible support throughout the process.

Helen Sabin's retirement in 1977 as Executive Director of the AARN formally ended her outstanding leadership in the organization over a 17-year period. Under her direction, the Association grew from a small organization with relatively little power, to a much larger one that had fostered effective working relationships with Government, health care agencies and other professions. Unquestionably, she was a vital force in advancing the educational status of nurses in Alberta and her strong sense of appropriate directions for the profession saw the Association through numerous threats to the legislation. Her successor Yvonne Chapman was experienced in the

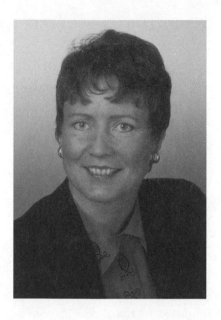

◆ Elizabeth Turnbull, appointed Executive Director of the AARN in 1994. (AARN)

workings of the Association since she had been Director of the Collective Bargaining program of the Association since 1970. She was named as Executive Director Designate in 1976 and assumed full responsibility as Executive Director on 1 March 1977. Chapman also proved to be a strong and effective leader and guided several presidents and many Council members through stormy waters. She was at the helm when the Nursing Profession Act was developed in 1984 and the leadership she provided was critical to the successful passage of the Act. The terms of Jean Smith and Bernadette Ratsoy were relatively brief, and in 1994, Elizabeth Turnbull was appointed Executive Director of the organization. As always, challenges for the executive director and the elected officers of the Association loomed on the horizon as the new government of Premier Ralph Klein took steps to establish a committee with a mandate to review the legislation governing all health professionals with a view to replacing it with omnibus legislation that for all the health professions. Hearings around the province brought to light controversy over the proposed provisions of a new legislative model and assumptions upon which it was based. As the second mandate of the Klein government began, no legislation had been passed and there were a number of unresolved issues remained including the likelihood of the passage of omnibus legislation.

Collective Bargaining Developments

In her analysis of the procedural agreement between the AARN and the AHA in 1965 at the initiation of the collective bargaining program, Chapman has noted that "an agreement was entered into by the AARN and the AHA that recognized each other as competent to bargain collectively as authorized by their respective members."[36] This would have allowed for a departure from the procedures of the Alberta Labour Act and required that "when it became necessary to go before a conciliation board, the AHA and the AARN would accept and recommend for acceptance to their respective members the conclusions of such a board."[37] The procedural agreement was replaced by one which was consistent with the steps in the Labour Act in 1972 at the instigation of the AARN because of the "potential pitfalls of being required to recommend acceptance of clauses that could be in conflict with its policies."[38]

In 1973, threat of strike action by the Staff Nurses' Association at the Royal Alexandra Hospital was narrowly averted. Chapman, the Director of the AARN's Collective Bargaining Program at the time, commented that "It was an important settlement as it clearly demonstrated the results of a positive plan of action by the nurses of the bargaining unit."[39] This was the first time since the initiation of the collective bargaining program that nurses had taken a strike vote. Nurses rejected a conciliation board award yielding only a 14 percent increase over two years and following the strike threat, the final settlement yielded 21 percent over two years. Another group of nurses in the province, the Calgary Public Health Nurses, also took a strike vote later in 1973 and voted strongly in favour of strike. The 93 nurses who went on strike were the first to do so in Alberta in a collective bargaining conflict. Their strike lasted a week and resulted in a 24.7 percent increase over a three-year period.[40]

In 1973, the Supreme Court of Canada's decision in the dispute involving the Service Employees International Union (SEIU) and the Saskatchewan Registered Nurses Association (SRNA) over the SRNA's application for certification as a bargaining agent was one that meant that professional nursing associations across the country were no longer permitted to engage in collective bargaining on behalf of members.[41] One by one, nursing unions in each province assumed the collective bargaining functions that had previously been carried out by the professional associations. In Alberta this led initially to restructuring the Collective Bargaining Program of the AARN.

The AARN moved quickly to "bring about bylaw amendments that would change the structure and establish a distinct functionally autonomous collective bargaining division."[42] Other changes were made through the bylaw amendments so that no one involved in collective bargaining could hold office in the Association. The SNAs, which had formerly been autonomous, became staff nurse divisions of the Association. Fees were divided so that those collected for collective bargaining were given directly to the Provincial Staff Nurses Committee.

The AARN attempted to address the areas of conflict identified in the legal dispute that had resulted in the Supreme Court decision in the Saskatchewan case. The restructuring of its program resulted in a collective bargaining program which operated independently from the rest of the Association. However, what amounted to an impasse developed over the fee structure between the Provincial Council and the Provincial Staff Nurses Committee in 1977, and this resulted in Council's decision to publish bylaw amendments to ensure complete separation of the collective bargaining function from the other activities of the AARN:

> Therefore be it resolved that the Provincial Council provide for the publication of Bylaw amendments that would establish the Collective Bargaining Program as independent of the AARN and further that sufficient time be given for the orderly development of an independent body to assume the collective bargaining function.[43]

This resolution was sent to all members of the Association by President Audrey Thompson on behalf of the Council to advise them of the proposal for change. A General Meeting of the Association held in Calgary on 3 May 1977 confirmed the AARN's withdrawal from collective bargaining for members. The bylaw change became effective in June of 1978 and the United Nurses of Alberta, a new organization, emerged from the controversy as the group that would take over the largest proportion of collective bargaining for nurses in the province. The SNA at the University Hospital in Edmonton continued to bargain for its nurses and its scope was eventually extended to include nurses at the Cross Cancer Institute and the Foothills Hospital in Calgary.

Standards of Practice

Standards of practice were a continuing and primary area of concern to the AARN, and a staff position for a Project Director for Standards was created within the organization in 1976. In 1977 an ad hoc committee was appointed to develop written standards of practice. This committee prepared a draft document the following year that was widely discussed within the districts during 1979 and 1980. Revisions to the document led to Provincial Council approval of the final draft of the nursing practice standards in 1981.[44] Although the practice standards were relatively general, they were based upon a number of principles believed to be fundamental in nursing practice. This was the first attempt by the AARN to develop written standards of practice, and difficult as it was to develop standards that would apply to all areas of practice and all settings, it was a historic development for the profession. Professional nursing associations in other jurisdictions took up development of such standards following the release of the AARN standards.

A plan for testing the standards in a number of practice settings was developed, and a committee was formed to guide the process. A steering committee was formed, but the effort foundered for a number of reasons, not the least of which was that members of Provincial Council believed that the focus should be broadened to that of quality assurance. The standards then moved in the direction of quality assurance and a consultant was hired to assist with the process. In 1988, the Detailed Action Plan for implementing the Long Range Plan for Quality Assurance included plans for education, nursing practice standards, consultation, networking and research. Workshops on quality assurance and other educational programs were developed on the subject and efforts were made to facilitate communication within the profession about quality assurance. The Nursing Practice Standards were completely revised as a part of this project and were approved in 1991.

Continuing Threats to the Legislation

In 1969, the now infamous Bill 119, an Act to Incorporate a Council on Nursing, was tabled in the Legislative Assembly of Alberta. This legislation would have removed the power to set standards from the professional association and as such reduced its scope considerably. Nurses around the province rallied against the proposed legislation in meetings held to discuss it. Letters and telegrams were sent to the Minister with expressions of concern by members opposing the proposed law. Concern was so great that the Government withdrew the legislation and sent it back to the drawing boards. However the legislation resurfaced in the next session as Bill 80 which was deemed by the profession to be almost more objectionable than Bill 119. The Bill proposed two standard-setting bodies, one for those eligible for registration with the AARN who would be granted a licence from the Government while the Coordinating Council on Nursing established by virtue of Bill 80 would set licensure standards for those who did not maintain registration with the AARN including those who did not qualify for registration.[45] Because its provisions would have been extremely detrimental to the independence of the AARN as a self-governing profession, nurses rallied against passage of the second version of the legislation. Once again the Bill was allowed to die on the order paper.[46]

Draft legislation for an Adult Education Act in 1975 represented an attempt on the part of Government to control "academic qualifications and standards required for entrance into professional associations."[47] While this attempted assault on the professional nursing legislation applied to all professions rather than just nursing, it was a very definite "power grab." The AARN enjoyed an advantage in this dispute over the legislation since on this occasion it was not singled out, and all professions and educational institutions faced the same issues. Therefore the response of the Council of the Professions of Alberta supported the AARN's position opposing the draft legislation,[48] and other groups and institutions also responded in the same vein until the legislation was withdrawn in 1976 because of widespread opposition to it on all sides. The concept of one act to incorporate all previous pieces of legislation in advanced education perhaps seemed advantageous to the bureaucracy of Government, but in reality it would have been difficult to recognize the diversity and uniqueness of each institution within one act. Its demise was welcome news to all of those who had opposed it.

The report of the Special Committee of the Legislative Assembly of Alberta on Professions and Occupations, also known as the Chichak Committee, was made public by the Government in 1973.[49] The mandate of the committee had been to review professional legislation in Alberta concerning regulations, licensing and the principles that distinguished between self-regulating professions and other groups that were not self-regulating. The intent had been to develop a uniform approach to legislation for the professions and occupations so that following certain principles, each professional act would be reviewed in terms of these principles guiding government policy. The report contained 25 recommendations and one referred to developing an umbrella act either for groups of professions or for all the professions and occupations. Another recommendation asserted that since a professional association's position was compromised by serving as a bargaining agent, this should not be allowed to occur. The first act to be developed after the policy was released was to serve as a "model act," and the Architect's Act was the first to be developed. There were, however, some points of departure from the policy noted in the development of this act. The AARN nevertheless took the position that systematic review of legislation for the various professions in accordance with the policy would allow it to put forward its long-term goal of mandatory registration for professional licensure.

Dispute Leads to the Nursing Profession Act

In 1981, as the bargaining agent for nurses in union locals in the majority of hospitals and in a number of other health agencies, the United Nurses of Alberta tabled a list of demands with the Alberta Hospital Association. Among these was one to remove the salary differential between registered and nonregistered (graduate) nurses. Another demand was to remove the requirement for nurses to maintain active registration with the AARN on the grounds that this should be a voluntary matter.[50] When it became known that these issues had been placed on the bargaining table and were the subject of contract negotiations, members of Provincial Council became very disturbed that the UNA had made such a proposal. Members were also shocked that registration was so seemingly fragile, depending at least in part upon a union contract. Without the salary differential and the requirement that nurses rather than employers should make the choice of whether of not to be registered, a good deal of the thrust that ensured a very high registration rate in the province (upwards of 95 percent) would be removed. Although hospital employers of nurses had traditionally been very responsible in hiring registered nurses almost exclusively, if they no longer retained the right to require nurses to be registered, it was likely that the registration rate would change quite quickly and dramatically. Because the AARN had a responsibility to the public to ensure safe, competent and ethical practice by nurses, it saw the UNA proposals as potentially very damaging to the public interest.

Special meetings of Provincial Council and the Provincial Executive were held to address the issues, and the AARN took a firm and highly public stand in opposition to the proposals put forward by the UNA. The UNA refused to change their bargaining position and eventually went on strike over all of the issues in the contract. The appointment of a Disputes Inquiry Board resolved the issue in favour of the AARN position and registration was maintained in the same form. Because nurses had gone on strike several times in the previous five years, the Government brought in the Health Services Continuation Act in 1982 that provided a mechanism for ordering nurses back to work in work stoppages and also made it illegal for nurses to go on strike. Severe penalties were incorporated in the Act for those who disregarded the law. The crisis of the moment was over for the AARN, but the issue remained because one did not know whether or not the same or similar proposals might be tabled in contract negotiations at a future date.

The Association therefore had to consider very carefully whether to take the initiative and request that the Government open the Registered Nurses Act to incorporate mandatory registration. Meetings of the Provincial Executive with cabinet ministers in the Lougheed government during the period of crisis had led to the belief that the Government would support mandatory registration in light of the fact that registration appeared rather tenuous, dependent on a union contract. The decision was taken by the Provincial Council to write to the Minister and request that the Registered Nurses' Act be opened and that mandatory registration should be the cornerstone of the new act. The decision was also made to take a proactive stance, hire a consultant and draft the legislation that could provide the basis for discussion with the Government about the details to be contained in the new act. Subsequently a legislative consultant, David Elliott was engaged to work with Yvonne Chapman, Executive Director, Janet Ross Kerr, President, and Janet Storch, Chair of the Legislation Committee to

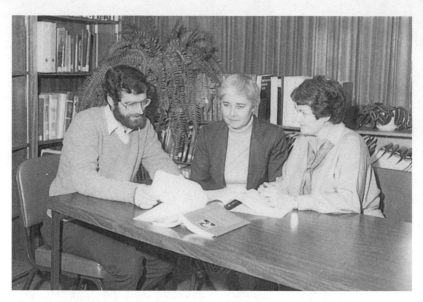

↝ *David Elliott, Janet Ross Kerr, and Yvonne Chapman working on the proposed new legislation, 1983. (AARN)*

negotiate with the Honourable David King, the minister whose portfolio included professional legislation and who carried the responsibility for taking the legislation through the Legislative Assembly.

The development of the legislation was a complex and time-consuming process, but members of Provincial Council were highly supportive and the initial draft was discussed by the negotiating team with all interested stakeholders in order to gain their support. A campaign to inform the membership about all issues in the legislation was developed and a videotape was prepared to show in the districts to serve as a focus for discussion with members. In early 1983 when the process was close to completion, the Government conveyed an impression that the legislation might need to wait for another session of the Legislative Assembly. It was clear that an intensive campaign would be needed to try to encourage early consideration of the legislation in the spring session. Buttons with "Act in Spring 1983" were distributed and worn by nurses and others, and a letter-writing campaign to the Minister and Members of the Legislative Assembly was initiated. The campaign was clearly successful and the Minister informed

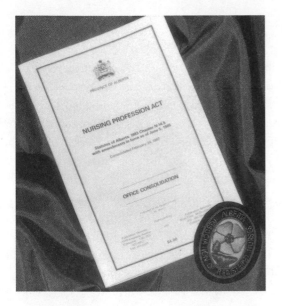

↦ *The Nursing Profession Act of 1983. (AARN)*

the President that the Government would be proceeding with the legislation to be known as The Nursing Profession Act in the spring session.

Bill 59 received first reading in late May 1983, but the Association was very disturbed by the rewording of one provision concerning setting standards of education for nursing schools. In effect the Bill removed the authority historically delegated to the Universities Coordinating Council and placed it within the powers of the Government because of the rewording of Section 54 to allow the Lieutenant Governor in Council (Cabinet) to make or amend regulations governing schools of nursing. A successful lobby of cabinet ministers by members of the Executive and negotiating team was quickly carried out in the Legislature Building, for when the bill was presented for second reading an amendment to require prior consultation with the Universities Coordinating Council had been added. Even though this was less than the Association had sought, it was better than the earlier draft and was accepted, even though such acceptance was somewhat less than enthusiastic. Royal assent was given on 6 June 1983 and following development of the regulations for the Act and negotiations between the AARN and Government, the Nursing Profession Act was proclaimed as law on 1 January 1984. Thus, mandatory registration, a long-standing goal of the Association was finally a reality.

Nursing Legislation Is Threatened Once Again

As the decade since the implementation of the Nursing Profession Act of 1984 wound to a close, yet another threat to nursing legislation appeared on the horizon. With the election of Progressive Conservative Ralph Klein as Premier in Alberta, a move to the right of the policies and programs supported by the previous Progressive Conservative administration of Don Getty took place. The shift in ideology was rapid and had far-reaching effects on all aspects of government operation. Downsizing of health care generally was extensive in Alberta and a number of major hospitals in the province were closed or reduced in size, some making the transition to community health centres. The Nursing Profession Act along with all other professional acts was targeted for review and change and the document entitled "New Directions for Legislation Change Regulating the Health Professions in Alberta"[51] prepared by the Health Workforce Rebalancing Committee was the subject of intensive study by the profession.

A special committee was appointed by the association to work on the issues and advice and consultations were sought from those with expertise in dealing with the legislative issues under consideration. Again omnibus legislation was being proposed and the Ontario model, a variant of the American approach, had surfaced once again. However, of paramount concern in the Discussion Paper,[52] was the provision to eliminate mandatory registration leaving health professionals with protection of title only. Instead, "A short list of dangerous services, which can only be provided by regulated, competent health professions will be established."[53] The AARN appeared at all of the hearings concerning the legislative proposals in several centres in the province and expressed its opposition to the proposed legislation. The Association's "Reply to the Health Workforce Rebalancing Committee" was released in October, 1994 and stated: "AARN opposed the model of legislation proposed by the Discussion Paper as ill conceived."[54] The Association further attempted to address the Rebalancing Committee's concerns in proposing this model of legislation:

> *No monopoly exists as a result of professional legislation.* To the extent that a medical monopoly exists, it is as a result of Government regulations, funding policies, and institutional structures. Correct those systems and laws and the so-called monopoly would disappear.[55]

The conclusion to this new threat to the nursing legislation is still unresolved in 1997, and legislation has not yet been introduced into the Legislature. Nevertheless, it can be seen that the current example is but another potential assault to the legislation governing nursing, of which there have been several in the past. Whether or not the resolution of the issues in this dispute will be satisfactory to the Association is not known at this time. Most nurses are hopeful that a reasonable and satisfactory solution will result that will preserve mandatory registration and the AARN's position as a self-governing profession. If this does not happen, the nurses of the province will make their views on the matter known clearly to their MLAS and to cabinet ministers of the provincial government.

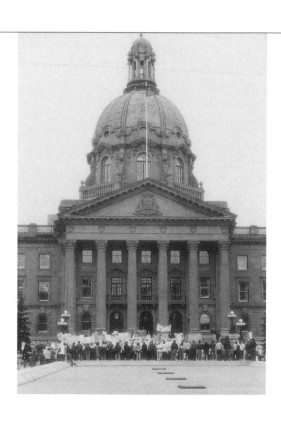

Nurses protesting government back-to-work legislation in 1977 at the Alberta Legislature. (UNA)

11

The Rise of Nursing Unions
In Alberta

At the outset of the twentieth century, the majority of graduate nurses were self-employed professionals who were engaged by families to do private duty nursing in the homes of ill family members. At this time, nurses were concerned about the credibility of the profession, recognition as respected professionals and the availability of work in the community. The major focus of their efforts in the first quarter of the twentieth century was securing legislation regulating nursing in the province so that nurses who met the standards of education and practice could be registered. Passage of the Registered Nurses Act in 1916 allowed the populace to differentiate between those who were qualified to practise nursing and those who were not. As self-employed professionals, nurses were concerned about issues that affected their work and their incomes and they were not reticent to speak out about issues of concern to them. With the founding of their professional association, they had an organization that could present their concerns and their ideas to the public, relevant groups and government.

THE ECONOMY AND THE LIVELIHOOD OF NURSES

The AARN was the host organization for the eleventh general meeting of the CNATN held in Edmonton in 1922. At this time there were two national organizations and they met together on this occasion. The Canadian Association for Nursing Education, established in 1917, was an organization that sought to further standards of nursing education. These organizations merged some two years later to form the Canadian Nurses Association.[1] At this Edmonton meeting Jean Browne, Executive Director of the Junior Red Cross, was elected President of the CNATN, and the 99 delegates heard from Marion Moodie, the first graduate of the Calgary General Hospital School of Nursing and Dr. R.G. Brett, Lieutenant-Governor of the province and founder of the Brett Sanatorium in Banff. Resolutions presented at the Convention had an economic and practical ring to them. It was hardly surprising that nurses wanted hospitals to cease hiring nurses who did not hold a diploma from a recognized school of nursing, since the distinctions between the "trained" and the "untrained" nurse had been an issue for a considerable period of time even prior to the incorporation of the AAGN/AARN. Another resolution denounced the common practice in hospitals of sending nursing students out on private duty cases and pocketing the fee. Such practices were seen as unsafe, unethical and unfair as well as posing a threat to the livelihood of the private duty nurse. They further represented to nurses an example of the pursuit of the profit motive on the part of hospitals of the time. The AARN also considered this to be exploitation of nursing students by the hospital.[2]

With the onset of the depression, the Canadian economy declined sharply, and the prairie provinces were especially hard hit. The continuing financial problems facing hospitals during the early decades of this century have been reported and analyzed. The struggle was greater in the voluntary hospital, but even among municipally owned institutions, the reluctance to

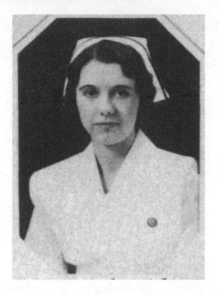

↝ *Marjorie MacDonald Chapman, graduate of the Galt Hospital School of Nursing in Lethbridge pictured with the class of 1934.* (From White Caps and Red Roses)

provide adequate funds made financing a continuing nightmare for trustees and administrators.[3] During the Depression years, a difficult situation deteriorated further until many hospitals struggled for survival because of large deficits. In the 1930s, only 40 percent to 50 percent of the patient days in public hospitals had been paid in full by 55 percent to 60 percent of the patients. Eight percent of patients paid for part of their hospital stay, and one third of those remaining were unable to pay their bill.[4] In addition, "a fairly sharp division was usually drawn between paying and non-paying patients,"[5] and extra payment for private accommodation was used to help offset deficits.

Nurses and physicians experienced financial difficulty and great hardships during this period. Since the proportion of patients unable to pay medical bills had escalated, many physicians had a difficult time financially. For instance, in Saskatchewan in "December, 1932, the provincial government was moved to provide financial assistance to physicians. Through its Relief Commission, the government made a grant of $75.00 a month to doctors in 56 rural municipalities in Relief Area 'A' and $50.00 a month in 103 rural municipalities in Relief Area 'B.'"[6] Nurses also were hard-pressed to make ends meet because graduate nursing positions in private duty nursing evaporated with the stock market crash. Calgary General Hospital graduates who were unable to get positions as special nurses, were glad to be taken on the hospital staff at a monthly salary of thirty dollars in addition to room and board. Many supervisory nurses, already on staff, had to take substantial salary reductions as the city slashed its hospital budget several times in a desperate attempt to make ends meet with the reduced taxes it was able to collect.[7]

The AARN reported that one-half to two-thirds of nurses who had worked in private duty nursing experienced unemployment. Finding themselves unable to stay afloat financially even with the minimal cost of nursing care provided by nursing students, hospitals were "discharging nurses-in-training for reasons other than those commonly accepted."[8] As Marjorie MacDonald Chapman, a 1934 graduate of the Galt Hospital School of Nursing in Lethbridge indicated:

> People were down and out financially and what assets they did have were gradually destroyed. For example, top soil drifted so much that farmers could no longer grow their crops . . . Nurses were paid a mere pittance and hard times left its mark on them personally. More than one nurse was caught shedding a few tears as she read the worried letters from home.[9]

Another graduate of the class of 1936 at the Galt School of Nursing observed that nursing students were quite lucky compared to others in a variety of walks of life:

> The depression didn't affect the student nurse very much. A young person wanting an education in nursing had an advantage over one who wanted to study law because she could trade work for room and board. But once she was out in the deflated world with her new skills she was on the same discouraging footing with the rest, trying to make a living on private duty.[10]

The Association took up the cause of the private duty nurse as the unemployment situation was critical. Prior to the Depression, nurses had worked on a daily, weekly or monthly basis. However, the AARN took up the concept of part-time work, urging members of the public to call the private duty registry for nurses who could provide service on an hourly or part-time basis. A Mutual Benefit and Loan Fund was established supported by

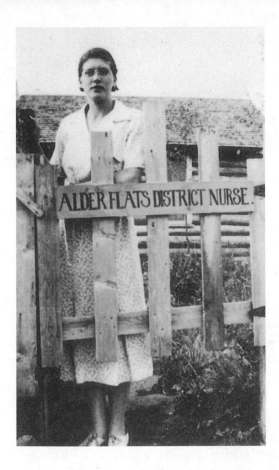

Public health nursing student at Alder Flats, 1937.
(GAA NA–3952–5)

voluntary contributions by nurses who were employed. The AARN also established a special project at Alder Flats where two nurses were engaged at salaries of $25.00 each per month to serve the community. AARN fees were lowered in 1933 in response to nurses' continuing difficulties in securing work. Although private duty nurses debated the issue of lowering their fees of $5.00 per day, they decided after much discussion of the pros and cons that the rate would remain as it was.[11] As was the case in other fields, many individuals sought to further their education during the Depression since no employment was available. Nurses were no exception and many went back to continue their education during this period of time. In order to provide encouragement and assistance to nurses to return to school to further their education, the AARN developed a scholarship program for nurses, a program which survives to the present day.

Because many patients were unable to pay their hospital bills during the Depression, hospitals struggled to remain solvent. Even so, the critical situation faced by nurses unable to find work resulted in mounting pressure on hospitals to hire graduate nursing staff. Hospitals had historically relied on students to provide the majority of the nursing service in their institutions. At the height of the Depression, unemployment of nurses led to pressure to limit the working hours of nurses to an eight-hour day, and the Eight-Hour Day Committee was established by the AARN in 1941.[12] This group focused rather broadly upon achieving more optimal working conditions for nursing staff. Although the Depression occurred barely a decade after the legal recognition of nursing in the province, it was the first period of time when nurses experienced the devastating social and economic consequences of widespread unemployment.

Hospitals gradually increased their complement of graduate nursing staff during and after the Depression, and in a relatively brief period of time, nurses moved from being almost exclusively self-employed to a situation where they were almost always employees of health care agencies. The number of nursing positions soared as a result of the post WWII expansion of hospitals stimulated by incentives for hospital construction incorporated in the 1948 National Health Grants Act. The passage of the Hospital Insurance and Diagnostic Services Act of 1957 and the Medical Care Act of 1968 by the federal government formed the cornerstone of a comprehensive national health insurance plan and created a need for even greater numbers of nurses to provide the services available under the plan. The expansionist postwar period was characterized by a surging economy and there seemed to be no limits to growth. Under these conditions, nurses were needed in ever-increasing numbers. By 1960, hospitals employed 59 percent of nurses in Alberta.[13]

THE RIGHT TO BARGAIN COLLECTIVELY

Recognition by nurses of the importance of the right to engage in collective bargaining to improve salaries and working conditions occurred over a period of several decades. The principle of collective bargaining for nurses was approved by the Canadian Nurses Association in 1944. Just as registration was an area of provincial jurisdiction, collective bargaining was also governed by provincial laws for nurses who were not federal employees. The passage of the Labour Relations Act in 1944 by the federal government gave federal employees collective bargaining rights, and was probably a factor in the CNA's decision to support collective bargaining by provincial association members of its federation. Despite approving the principle of collective bargaining, the CNA also went on record at this time as opposing strike action by groups of nurses.[14] It is unlikely that the majority of nurses in these years would have supported strikes or other forms of job action. Reflecting the CNA's position, in an address to the AARN Annual Meeting in 1946, a CNA staff member asserted that "In affiliation with trade unions, some union practices are not possible for nurses—'strike' is one word that should be unknown in the nursing profession."[15]

Collective bargaining was on the agenda of the AARN's Annual Meeting in 1944 following which an Employment Relations Committee was established to study labour relations issues and to develop recommendations concerning the socioeconomic status of nurses. Shortly thereafter, the committee recommended that the AARN urge the AHA to establish a joint committee to address salary concerns of nurses. A motion to this effect was defeated by delegates attending the AHA's 1944 Annual Meeting, but AHA officials evidently thought better of rejecting the request outright and the two groups met several months later to discuss how each organization might address changing the personnel policies for nurses.[16] For some time the AARN was content with the process of increasing nurses' salaries through nonbinding personnel policies developed annually by the AARN and discussed with the AHA, policies that employers were free to accept or reject when establishing levels of compensation for nurses. While some employers accepted the recommendations, others did not, resulting in a great deal of disparity in wages and working conditions of nurses from hospital to hospital and from urban to rural areas. The AARN reported findings from a 1953 survey that showed that nurses worked 44 hours per week in 26 hospitals and 48 hours per week in 23 others. Twenty other hospitals still employed the older split shift schedule which required nurses to be available for a much longer period of time in a day.[17] Although nurses had been unwilling to work towards certification of a bargaining unit under the provincial Labour Act following CNA's approval of collective bargaining for nurses in the 1940s, by the 1960s they began to recognize that they had failed to achieve meaningful input into the process by which salary levels and working conditions were determined. This led to the search for more effective methods of interacting with employers relative to the socioeconomic welfare of nurses in the province.

Although there was formal support for collective bargaining by the national professional association, and although the Registered Nurses Association of British Columbia became the first professional association to be certified as a bargaining agent under provincial law in 1946, nurses generally did not seem ready to take up the collective bargaining gauntlet at that time. Even though there was continual activity directed at increasing nurses' salaries, the move to establish a program of collective bargaining sanctioned by law did not begin in earnest until some two decades later. The growing assertiveness of nurses and their willingness to challenge employers over wages and working conditions appeared to parallel increased activity in the women's movement in society generally. In 1959 a resolution was passed at the AARN's annual meeting to request that government open the Registered Nurses Act to allow the Association to bargain collectively for nurses employed in health care agencies. The Executive moved forward to study techniques of collective bargaining in 1962 and prepared guidelines for the development of employee groups or staff nurses associations in 1964.

At this time, the AARN retained Ken Barrass, a labour relations consultant to provide guidance in negotiating and administering collective agreements. Hibberd commented that "Barrass played a significant role in the development of the collective bargaining program in the late 1960s, providing on-the-job training for the AARN staff as well as workshops on labour relations for the general staff nurse members."[18] The Association also established the position of Employment Relations Officer in 1964 and appointed M. Louise Tod to the position to assist groups of staff nurses to organize and to develop procedures for negotiating staff salaries and working conditions.[19] Staff nurses associations were quickly developed across the province and groups of nurses began meeting in the large urban centres to discuss strategy. There were 25 SNAs by 1965, and a year later this figure had grown to 53, with 12 of the latter groups having been certified by the Board of Industrial Relations.[20] Hibberd commented that "These developments were remarkable for the speed with which they occurred, spreading like contagion throughout the hospital industry with all the fervour of a social movement."[21] A Task Committee to Study Alternatives for Collective Bargaining chaired by Frances Moore reported to the 1965 AARN Convention on the advantages and disadvantages of engaging in collective bargaining, strike and certification as a bargaining unit.[22] The Committee recommended that the individual SNAs should be the units recognized for the purposes of collective bargaining.

AMENDMENT OF THE REGISTERED NURSES ACT[23]

The Registered Nurses Act was amended in 1966 to allow for the process of collective bargaining and the relevant clause in the amendment specified that "... the Association may: 3(2)(c) when requested to do so by a majority of a group of members, act as a bargaining agent under the Alberta Labor Act on behalf of the group of members."[24] The actual certification as a bargaining agent whether via the Labour Act or by voluntary recognition by the employer occurred in the name of the SNA since the collective agreements were made between the employer and the SNA, not between the AARN and the employer. For example, a collective agreement might be between the Royal Alexandra Hospital and the SNA of that hospital. The AARN, which served as the bargaining agent or the negotiator, attempted to come to an agreement at the provincial level with the AHA. The content of the provincial agreement was then recommended to the individual employers and SNAs and, if accepted, was incorporated in a contract at the local level. The AARN had adopted a leadership role in collective bargaining from the outset of the first discussions about it in the 1940s. In the 1960s when nurses were ready to proceed with formalizing the process, the AARN "worked to help nurses in hospitals develop staff nurses associations for bargaining"[25] and to negotiate with employers on behalf of and at the request of their SNAs.

The first SNA to become certified as a bargaining unit under the Labour Act was chaired by Beverly Palfry at the Calgary General Hospital. This organization of staff nurses had sought certification following the refusal of the Board of the Calgary General Hospital to recognize its SNA voluntarily.[26] SNAs at the Lethbridge Municipal Hospital and the Royal Alexandra Hospital achieved certification as bargaining units shortly after this. Following identification of the process to be followed, SNAs in a variety of health agencies around the province became certified in rapid succession.

At the University of Alberta Hospital, nurses who had organized the SNA attempted to become certified under the Act, but found that they could not proceed in the same way as the Calgary General Hospital and most other hospitals in the province. Under the Crown Agency Employee Relations Act, there were already provisions in place for employees to be represented by the Civil Service Association.

This was a period of turbulence as staff nurses and employers sought to master the processes of collective bargaining, and each sought to be one step ahead of the other. An example of the manoeuvering that went on is found in Bill 87, a piece of legislation which would have revoked the jurisdiction of local boards of health in the province. Public health nurses (PHNS) were very concerned about the Bill, for if passed, it would threaten their ability to be represented by groups other than the civil service union since they would become civil servants. It may have been that employers of PHNS who wished to avoid dealing with nurses directly in collective bargaining, had pressed for such legislation as they saw it as being advantageous to the employer. Representations opposing the bill were sufficiently strong that it was shelved.

Following the 1966 amendment of the Registered Nurses Act, the Employment Relations Committee of the AARN was replaced by the Provincial Staff Nurse Committee (PSNC). Membership in the latter group was restricted to those nurses who were eligible for membership in a bargaining unit since its purpose was to engage in collective bargaining. The "arms length" status of the PSNC in relation to the Provincial Council was designed to protect the independence of the bargaining process and to prevent interference by nurses holding management positions.[27] At the outset, the new structure of the Association seemed to achieve the purpose of removing bargaining from the jurisdiction of Provincial Council.

In December 1965, a Procedural Agreement was entered into by the AARN and the AHA and it specified that each organization recognized the other as competent to bargain collectively as authorized by their respective members. The steps in this agreement differed from those of the Alberta Labour Act in that if and when it became necessary to go before a Conciliation Board, the AHA and the AARN would accept and recommend acceptance of the conclusion of such a Board to their respective members. Although strike as such was not mentioned in this Procedural Agreement, the intent was clearly to avoid such an event. The potential dangers of the Procedural Agreement were readily demonstrated by the issue of the salary differential for graduates of college programs both in the negotiations for the 1969–1970 and 1971–1972 collective agrements. If the Conciliation Board had ruled in favour of the AHA, the AARN would have been obliged to recommend a clause that would have undermined the college program, a recommendation that would have been a contradiction of its position of support of the transfer of nursing programs to the educational sector.

Under the direction of Yvonne Chapman who had taken over from Louise Tod as Director of the AARN's Collective Bargaining Program in 1970, following the group bargaining and settlement of the 1971–1972 collective agreements, the PSNC reviewed the collective bargaining program and suggested to the SNAs that the Procedural Agreement be amended to simply follow the steps of collective bargaining as outlined in the Alberta Labour Act and delete the requirement of acceptance of a Conciliation Board Award by the parent bodies. The SNAs agreed with the recommendation and a termination notice was forwarded to the AHA. The AHA responded that if the Procedural Agreement was terminated that there would be a return to individual bargaining. A concerted effort by the collective bargaining arm of the AARN to have the Procedural Agreement withdrawn eventually met with success in 1972 without interference with the group-bargaining approach. Also, a new Procedural Agreement that essentially followed the steps of collective bargaining as outlined in the Alberta Labour Act was signed by the AHA and AARN in September of 1972.

THE SUPREME COURT RULING OF 1973

A decision in a Saskatchewan case which was appealed to the Supreme Court of Canada radically altered the shape and direction of labour relations in nursing in Canada in less than a decade. At issue was a dispute between the Service Employees International Union (SEIU) and the Saskatchewan Registered Nurses Association over the SRNA's application for certification as a bargaining agent. The heart of the conflict was the SEIU's charge that the potential for nurses in management positions to be elected to the governing body of the SRNA represented a conflict of interest in terms of SRNA's collective bargaining function for general staff nurses.

The Supreme Court ruled in favour of the union because the SRNA was presumed to have an inherent bias that interfered with its participation in collective bargaining. This decision ultimately required that a separate and completely independent nursing union or unions be formed to assume the collective bargaining function for general staff nurses. The transition from responsibility vested in professional associations to responsibility vested in independent nursing unions had taken place in every province in Canada by 1981. In the long run in Alberta, this historic decision meant that the amendment to the Registered Nurses Act would not be enough to maintain the collective bargaining unit within the professional association. However, at the outset an attempt was made to retain AARN control of collective bargaining with a goal of avoiding challenges to the authority of the PSNC to bargain collectively for nurses. The PSNC prepared new bylaws to ensure greater independence of its activities from the rest of the organization. These were approved by Provincial Council and provided the framework for the work of the committee until 1977.

STRIKES OR THREATENED STRIKES PRIOR TO 1977

Strike action was threatened at the Royal Alexandra Hospital by the SNA in May, 1973. Settlement of the contract came on a Thursday when the strike was to take place the following Monday. It was an important settlement as it demonstrated the results of a positive action plan by the nurses of the bargaining unit. The nurses had rejected a conciliation board award of only 14 percent over two years. Their action resulted in a review of the options by the employer group and an increase of 21 percent over two years. This was the first time that nurses had taken a strike vote in the province. The background for these events is to be found in the fact that although the salary settlement incorporated in the 1971–1972 collective agreement had been inadequate, the AARN had been obliged by the Procedural Agreement to recommend acceptance to the SNAS.

The Calgary Public Health Nurses also took a strike vote in May, 1973 and voted strongly in favour of strike action. The 93 nurses employed by the city of Calgary were the first nurses in Alberta to withdraw their services in a collective bargaining dispute. The strike lasted seven days and resulted in a three-year contract with a 24.7 percent increase over this period of time. This settlement might be considered groundbreaking for public health nurses since there is often difficulty in convincing employers of the need to remunerate nurses in this field fairly. Strike or threatened strike action by public health nurses has been more often been met with indifference by employers who believe that they can withstand such action because the needs of the consumers of these services is not as urgent as those requiring tertiary care.

THE EMERGENCE OF THE UNITED NURSES OF ALBERTA

In June, 1976, Yvonne Chapman was appointed Executive Director Designate prior to Helen Sabin's retirement. It was decided to appoint Bob Donahue, who had been Assistant Employment Relations Officer, as the Director of Collective Bargaining. Since the bylaws required that the incumbent be a nurse, Donahue was appointed Acting Director until a bylaw change could be sought. The actions of the Acting Director acting on behalf of the PSNC over the next few months presented serious dilemmas for the AARN. They first developed a long-range plan for the work of the collective bargaining program that required a substantial increase in activity and much higher levels of funding. A 150 percent increase in revenue for the PSNC was proposed to be gained through an assessment of 1/2 percent of gross basic income for each staff nurse along with payment of only 3/5 of the AARN membership fee. The latter change proved to be highly controversial and required a bylaw change in order to institute a new formula for collecting fees.

The subsequent conflict between the PSNC and the AARN Provincial Council over a number of matters pertaining to the fee assessment appeared to compromise the arm's length status of the PSNC in relation to the Provincial Council and led to the 22 April 1977 Provincial Council motion to allow the collective bargaining arm of the AARN to become an independent organization. A general meeting called for 6 May 1977 in Calgary was attended by close to 1,300 AARN members. At this meeting the facts of the dispute were reviewed by President Audrey Thompson, and those in attendance had an opportunity to ask questions. It was clear that there was support for Provincial Council's actions and Gurtey Chinell announced the PSNC's decision to form a separate organization, then

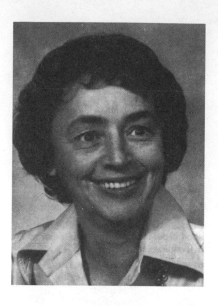

Gurtey Chinell, UNA President, 1977–1980. (UNA)

quickly moved to adjourn the meeting. Out of the separation of the two organizations, the United Nurses of Alberta under the presidency of Chinell emerged to assume authority and responsibility for labour relations on behalf of groups of nurses in a majority of health care agencies in the province. In June, 1977, the UNA packed up its bags and moved out of the AARN provincial office building into new office space located elsewhere in Edmonton. At the same time, emerging alliances between the newly-independent union and other partners in the labour union movement were an essential part of its operations as in the event of strike there was a need for assistance from other organizations both in terms of public statements of support, personnel to join picket lines and, if necessary, dollars to assist with the financial cost of a strike. Building such alliances was helpful as organizations such as the Alberta Teachers' Association, the Alberta Federation of Labour and others provided such support during nurses' strikes.[28]

CONFRONTATION AND STRIKE ACTION BY NURSES

The fledgling union had barely unpacked its effects in new quarters when it decided that the conciliation process had not yielded suitable gains for nurses. The UNA then called its first major strike in the province at seven hospitals including the Royal Alexandra Hospital, the Edmonton General Hospital, the Red Deer Hospital, the Calgary General Hospital, the Holy Cross Hospital, St. Michael's Hospital in Lethbridge and the Grande Prairie Hospital. The strike by 2,500 nurses lasted six days before nurses were ordered back to work through Order-in-Council of the provincial government. An Emergency Tribunal was appointed to achieve a settlement that would be binding for both parties to the dispute. The UNA's demand for a 36.8 percent increase was based partly on the narrowed differential between the salaries of certified nursing aides and registered nurses. The latter had occurred because of the resolution of a dispute based on a charge of discrimination under the Alberta Rights Protection Act brought by CNAs; the reason for this was that although CNAs performed the same work as nursing orderlies, their salaries were much lower.[29] UNA members were disillusioned when the arbitrator awarded a 9 percent salary increase (3 percent more than the federal wage guidelines), and bitterness remained because the settlement was viewed as a sham. The judge who arbitrated the award rejected another matter which was a part of the dispute, namely that the Rand Formula be applied to nurses so that employers would be required to deduct union dues from nurses' salary cheques and forward them directly to the union.

Following the settlement of the strike, nurses negotiated a collective agreement in 1978 that produced employer concurrence with the Rand Formula.[30] A change in management of the UNA occurred with the appointment of Simon Renouf to succeed Bob Donahue in 1979. When negotiations for the 1980 collective agreement began, nurses complained that rampant inflation had meant that following the 1977 strike, their salaries had only increased by 13.3 percent while the Consumer Price Index had risen by 18 percent.[31] Their opening position was a demand for a 33.3 percent salary increase over one year despite the provincial wage guidelines limiting the size of increases for public sector employees to 7.5–9 percent.[32] The UNA's rejection of a recommended 22 percent increase over two years by a conciliation board led to a ten-day work stoppage by 6,400 nurses in 81 hospitals.[33] According to Hibberd, the AHA concluded early in the process that strike was inevitable, because of "the massive demands, the union demonstrations of solidarity, the evidence of public support, and the restrictive provincial wage guidelines."[34] Nurses were ordered back to work by Order-in-Council of the provincial government and an Emergency

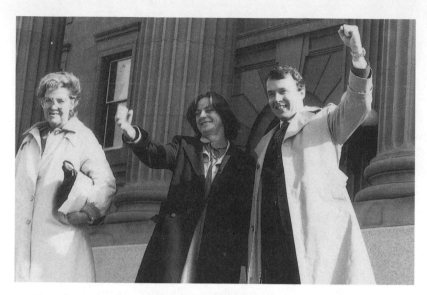

⊸ Simon Renouf, UNA Executive Director, 1979–1985 on the right with UNA President Margaret Ethier at the Alberta Legislature. (UNA)

Tribunal was appointed to hear the dispute and award a binding settlement. The award for the two-year agreement allowed for a 39.8 percent salary increase over three steps in the two-year period and many other contract enhancements. As well, professional responsibility committees were established in all hospitals. Through the committee vehicle, nurses could bring forward patient care issues of concern.

In the negotiation of the 1982 collective agreement, another impasse occurred between the UNA and the AHA. Buoyed up by the success of the previous two strikes, and in particular the 1980 strike, the UNA decided to press forward even though there was less support from both the public and from union members. The union rejected the recommendations of a Disputes Inquiry Board appointed prior to the strike and recommended a 37 percent salary increase in three stages over two years. Despite this, a number of statements made in the report were offensive to nurses and the tone of the report generally supported employers. The strike began on 16 February 1982 in 60 hospitals involving 6000 nurses and lasted 23 days. Nurses were ordered to return to their jobs by means of back to work legislation in the form of the Health Services Continuation Act and a Public

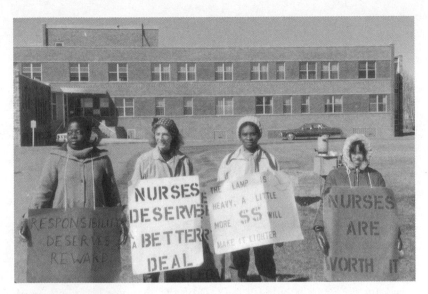

↪ *UNA strike in 1982. (UNA)*

Emergency Tribunal was appointed to deliver an arbitrated award.[35] The 16 days of public hearings convened by the Tribunal were divided between Calgary and Edmonton and produced a wage increase which at 29 percent over two years was considerably less than the Disputes Inquiry Board had recommended. Other contract enhancements were achieved but the UNA's demand to eliminate the salary differential between registered and nonregistered nurses was not upheld. Although the strike ended on 11 March, the report of the Tribunal did not come down until 16 July 1982.

Other nursing strikes occurred between 1982 and 1988 in nursing homes and health units. Generally nurses employed in health agencies other than tertiary care centres found it difficult to achieve successful outcomes through the use of the strike weapon, primarily because the services provided were not as primary or as visible as those in hospital. When one is dealing in the short term with issues of critical care often involving matters of life and death, the effect of withdrawal of nursing services is likely to be a much more dramatic than for long-term issues such as the public health concerns in the community or the care of the elderly. Therefore strike action would not have the same kind of impact upon the public and upon the work of other health professionals such as physicians. In addition, it is substantially easier for employers to make arrangements to offset strikes in settings other than tertiary care centres. It is therefore not surprising that strike outcomes achieved by the UNA in settings other than tertiary care settings have been mixed.

LEGISLATION REMOVES HOSPITAL WORKERS' RIGHT TO STRIKE

Whether or not the right to strike should be considered a fundamental right of the worker is a point that has been debated at length. Unions have maintained that the right to strike is fundamental and should never be removed, but the Supreme Court has ruled otherwise: "the guarantee of freedom of association in S. 2(d) of the Canadian Charter of Rights and Freedoms does not include (in the case of a trade union) a guarantee of the right to bargain collectively and of the right to strike."[36] Since the withdrawal of nursing services in hospitals may affect the welfare and safety of patients, strikes by nurses remain highly controversial. Judith Hibberd has noted that most nursing unions have been willing to maintain essential services during a strike, and that this has tended to defuse public anger and outrage at the consequences of strike action by nurses.[37] However, the definition of essential services is not inherently obvious and there may be considerable conflict over these even where guidelines are in place to identify how essential services should be put in place in the event of strike. Conflicting ethical positions may present dilemmas for nurses where strike action is contemplated. Whether or not to stay on the job when working conditions raise questions about patient safety must be balanced with the ethical and legal duty of a nurse to care for a patient who requires nursing care.

In response to the series of strikes by nurses and by the strident positions taken by the UNA towards government, Bill 44 was introduced in the Legislature by the Minister of Labour in April, 1983. Its major provision was the removal of the legal right to strike from all hospital workers. Compulsory arbitration rather than strike or lockout was legislated for dispute resolution. The provisions of the Bill for large fines and decertification of the union with six-month suspensions of the Rand Formula method of

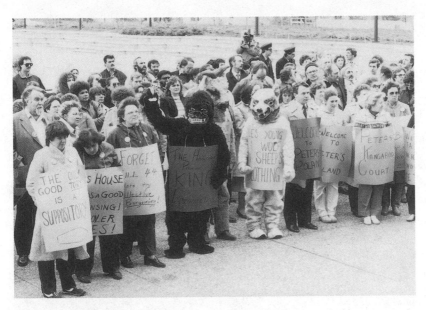

⮑ *Protesting Bill 44, 1983.* (UNA)

collection of union dues by employers for violations of the legislation were labelled Draconian by many. That the government intervened to take away nurses' right to strike has a number of possible explanations. It may have signalled a belief that the public interest had not been served by the series of nurses' strikes and also fear that there would be other strikes in the future. Another possible explanation for the introduction and passage of this legislation may have been that nurses served as a convenient scapegoat to allow the government to remove the right to strike from all hospital employees. At the time of the passage of Bill 44, many disputed the need for such severe penalties for failure to comply with the legislation. Others wondered why it was necessary to remove the right to strike when other alternatives were possible such as legislating the nature and extent of the staffing of essential services during strikes, or measures such as funding for job enhancement programs to improve the quality of nurses' worklife, ensuring that nurses have meaningful input through appointments to policy making boards of hospitals and health regions, and providing tangible support for nurses' continuing education needs.

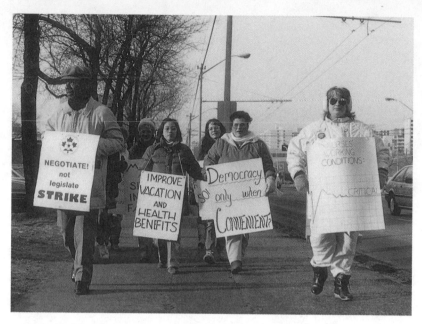

✎ *Nurses striking in 1988 in defiance of the law. (*UNA*, photograph by Andrea Waywanko, the Newsmagazine by Alberta Women)*

THE 1988 ILLEGAL STRIKE

Although it was widely believed that the passage of legislation removing nurses' right to strike would mean that there would be no further work stoppages, this was not the case. In 1988, the UNA reached an impasse with the AHA in the negotiation of a collective agreement. AHA proposals were unacceptable to the UNA because they involved rollbacks of wages and the loss of hard-fought contract provisions. When the Labour Relations Board ordered the UNA not to take a strike vote, the organization was not deterred and proceeded with the vote. Nurses voted to strike, and on 25 January 1988, 11,000 nurses in 98 hospitals left their jobs for the picket lines.[38] This was the largest strike of all since some of the Crown hospitals went out on strike along with the others. These hospitals, the Foothills, the Alberta Children's and the Glenrose Hospitals had never had the right to strike since they operated under different legislation, and in previous strikes had remained on the job. However, in this instance, none of the hospital nurses were permitted to strike, so nurses were all on the same footing and went out on an illegal strike of 19 days duration. Although criminal contempt charges were laid against the UNA and civil contempt charges against individual nurses, these did not appear to change the direction of the strike which was settled when the AHA came up with a improved contract offer. The UNA was fined $250,000 on the first charge of criminal contempt and $150,000 on the second, and individual nurses were fined up to $1,000 for civil contempt. The UNA estimated that it paid fines amounting to $426,750.[39] Although the organization appealed the criminal contempt charges to the Supreme Court of Canada, the position of the union was not upheld by the Court. The UNA did not believe that the results of the 1988 strike justified the efforts of nurses or the financial expenditures required to support it.[40] The most significant gain was seen as "forcing the employer to remove the takeaways from the table."[41]

Although illegal strikes by unions are becoming more common, that nurses have been willing to engage in them has been shocking to many. Likewise, the propensity of workers on strike including nurses to ignore court ordered injunctions has been surprising to members of the public and the health care community. The sight of nurses going out on strike and walking picket lines chanting slogans and singing solidarity songs, has been antithetical to the public stereotype of the nurse as self-effacing, kind, caring and gentle. As the women's movement gained momentum in the 1960s, nurses began to look at their own profession differently recognizing that their salaries and working conditions were differentially lower than other comparable occupational and professional groups, particularly those where men were dominant. Alberta nurses were transformed and empowered by the realization that they could confront their employers with their demands and use various strategies including strike until they had achieved them. Hibberd has reflected upon the willingness to take on an illegal strike: "Nurses were willing to disobey the law for many of the same reasons that led to their decision to abandon their no-strike policy in the 1970s. They believed that they were being unjustly treated and that they had no other recourse for bringing their case to public attention."[42]

CONTINUING LABOUR UNREST IN NURSING

Although the UNA had had its ranks decimated by the loss of nursing positions as a result of the downsizing of the acute care hospital system, and although unions of health care workers were generally believed to be on the defensive, the UNA clearly never lost sight of its goals. Protracted negotiations for the 1996 collective agreement stretched into 1997 and led to an impasse which surfaced just before the provincial election of 11 March 1997. The UNA had threatened to go out on strike a few days before the election if a favourable settlement was not forthcoming immediately. The strike vote was taken on 4 March 1997 and 85 percent voted to strike. Considerable public sympathy for nurses emerged in the conflict as a result of awareness that nurses had been the group most directly affected by the massive cuts in the health care system undertaken as part of the Klein government's restructuring of health care. The impact of the cuts had left thousands of nurses in the province unemployed and underemployed and large numbers had left the province for greener pastures, areas where their services were needed. In addition, nurses' wages had been cut by five per cent along with other public sector workers in 1994. Many asked the question: "Why must nurses be forced to threaten a strike just to secure input into working conditions, a place at the table where decisions are made, and a wage which reflects their contribution?"[43]

Following the health care cuts, the situation in Alberta hospitals was such that there was no longer the kind of flexibility that existed previously, whereby employers could sustain a strike by assigning nursing managers to give patient care. The capacity of the tertiary care hospital system had been downsized to a remarkable degree and in the process, thousands of nurses had lost their positions. No only were there markedly fewer hospital beds, but also the remaining hospital capacity was reserved for those who were critically ill and in need of treatment. There was no longer the level of registered nurse staffing at the bedside than had existed even three years earlier. The ranks of middle nursing management had largely been decimated, and Dr. Tom Noseworthy, the former president of the Royal Alexandra Hospital warned: "Expect a disaster if 12,000 nurses go on strike. . . . The walls would come tumbling down"[44] Paul Greenwood, head of the Capital Health Authority's (Edmonton) medical staff concurred, stating that "The resources are stretched to the limit. How can you possibly withdraw labor without affecting patient care?"[45] In negotiating this contract, the UNA was bargaining with regional health authorities as employers who were represented by the Provincial Health Associations of Alberta since, following restructuring the Alberta Hospital Association had been dismantled. According to UNA President Heather Smith, nurses sought not only salary increases, but also assurances that "registered nurses will be in charge of wards, plus concessions on severance pay for nurses who lose their jobs."[46] The timing of the strike vote and the threatened illegal strike just days before a provincial election undoubtedly hastened employer attempts at a settlement. The mediator's recommendation relative to the three-year agreement to run from 1 April 1996 to 31 March 1999 was an enhanced offer of a 7.1 percent with no changes in the first year, a 3.70 percent increase in the second year and a 3.40 percent increase in the third year as well as concessions on a number of patient care and other issues.[47]

THE STAFF NURSES ASSOCIATIONS OF ALBERTA

Because the United Nurses of Alberta bargains for most of the hospital nurses in the province, other unions responsible for collective bargaining for nurses are often forgotten. The largest of these has been the Staff Nurses Associations of Alberta, which represented a significant number of nurses employed in a number of health agencies including the University of Alberta Hospitals and the Cross Cancer Institute. At the time the UNA was formed in 1977, the nurses at the University of Alberta Hospital (UAH) decided to maintain their independence for purposes of collective bargaining. However, since they were employed by a Crown Corporation, the law stipulated that only the civil service union (AUPE) had the right to bargain for these nurses. In 1979 the Public Service Employee Relations Act (PSERA) was passed giving the SNA at UAH the right to bargain collectively for nurses. Shortly after this, the SNA at the UAH became certified as the bargaining agent for nurses. In 1984, the UNA sought to extend its organization to represent nurses at UAH, but UAH nurses decided to maintain their independence and voted to retain their separate union. As a result of the self-examination that had ensued from the overture from UNA to join its ranks, UAH nurses decided that they needed to expand from a complete reliance on volunteers to a more sophisticated style of operation in which they employed a labour relations consultant. This course of action required a substantially stronger financial base and was accompanied by an increase in fees. In 1986, the Staff Nurses Association of Alberta affiliated with the National Federation of Nurses Unions, a national organization supporting the interests of member unions in the provinces and territories. Also in 1986, nurses employed by the Alberta Cancer Board requested that the SNAA assume responsibility for their collective bargaining. The SNAA thus represented 2,600 registered nurses and registered psychiatric nurses. Since strikes were not allowed under the terms of the PSERA, if SNAA had recommended strike action to members, such a strike would not have been legal. The SNAA's philosophy on strike action was clearly not oriented to strike action: "SNAA respects and upholds the provisions under the Code of Ethics of the Canadian Nurses Association that any job action by nurses is directed toward securing conditions of employment that enable safe and appropriate care for clients and contribute to the professional satisfaction of nurses."[48] SNAA also referred to its experience in collective bargaining having "negotiated thirty-five Collective Agreements" and "never gone on strike."[49]

The attitudes of nurses in a union not on strike during a strike by a large nursing union were studied by Judith Hibberd and Judy Norris.[50] Members of the SNAA have been in this kind of situation a number of times when the UNA has been on strike. They pointed out that "there is much evidence to suggest that nurses believe strikes are damaging both to nursing's public image and to their own self-esteem as professionals."[51] The ambivalence of those who were not on strike about strike action and their concern for the high level of acuity of the patients for whom they were caring was evident in this study. The conclusion confirmed that "to strike places nurses in the dilemma of having to choose between loyalty to patients in providing uninterrupted services, and loyalty to peers in collectively pursuing improvements in working conditions and socio-economic status."[52] Such choices are never easy, and nurses have found them particularly difficult.

RELATIONSHIPS BETWEEN
PROFESSIONAL ASSOCIATIONS AND UNIONS

The separation of professional associations from unions as a result of the Supreme Court decision of 1973 ensured that there would be a separate organization in each jurisdiction in Canada to carry out the collective bargaining function. In Alberta, the period of time after the establishment of the UNA as an independent and autonomous organization in 1977 was characterized by acrimony. This was due to a complex interplay of factors, and the hostile relationships between the AARN and the UNA did not dissipate quickly. During Margaret Ethier's term as president of the UNA from 1980 to 1988, relationships were particularly difficult but the AARN did not sit back and accept the UNA's demand that the salary differential between registered and nonregistered nurses be eliminated in the negotiation of the 1982 contract. It went to the public with its concern and for its part, the UNA initiated a lawsuit against the AARN charging that the AARN had implied that it was not concerned about the quality of nursing care when it informed the public of the change that would occur if the salary differential were incorporated in the collective agreement. Although the UNA demand was not upheld in the report of the Tribunal, the AARN's concern over it led directly to the drive to incorporate mandatory registration for nurses in the province, a goal that was achieved when the Nursing Profession Act was proclaimed on 1 January 1984. Relationships gradually improved following election of Heather Smith to the presidency of the UNA in 1988. The UNA eventually withdrew its lawsuit against the AARN after a number of years had passed and it was all but forgotten. Relationships which each of the nursing unions had maintained with the AARN differed, with those between the SNAA and the AARN being more cordial than those between the AARN and the UNA. This may have been related to differing organizational orientations or simple varying approaches of executive and staff members. Times change though and eventually members of the SNAA decided to amalgamate with the UNA. Beginning in October, 1997, the UNA represented all organized registered nurses in Alberta.

The history of collective bargaining in Alberta reflects a remarkable transition in the awareness of nurses of the need for justice in the terms and conditions of work and in their willingness to stand behind their demands in the labour relations arena. The development of expertise in collective bargaining began when labour relations was the responsibility of the professional association and continued when independent nursing unions were formed. Beginning in the late 1970s, nurses began to use more confrontational tactics with employers leading to a number of high profile nursing strikes. When legislation passed in 1983 prohibited strikes by all

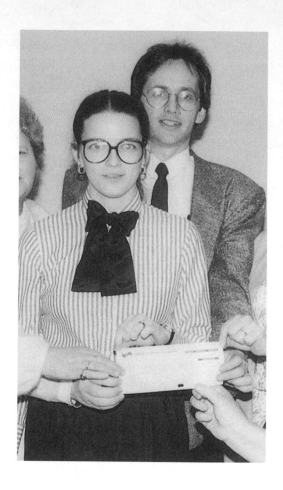

↬ *Heather Smith, UNA President, with $250,000 cheque to pay the fine assessed by Court. (UNA)*

hospital workers, nurses were incensed and were unwilling to relinquish what they saw as their right to bargain collectively complete with the power that the right to strike carried with it. Therefore the last major nursing strike in the province was an illegal one in which nurses in 98 hospitals went out on an illegal strike with minimal regard for the personal and organizational reprisals that could and did result. They demonstrated their willingness to take these risks once again in 1997 when they took a strike vote and prepared to go out on another illegal strike during the provincial election campaign. The settlement of the strike just prior to election day demonstrated the collective clout that nurses continued to wield despite the restructuring and downsizing of Alberta hospitals which had had such a devastating effect upon nurses' salaries and working conditions as well as the number of nursing positions in health care agencies. The signals were loud and clear that nurses were not prepared to yield ever again to the forces of oppression: "The history of organized nursing has been the history of a profession seeking to assert itself, to define and control its own body of knowledge and practice, to win recognition, respect and just reward for its contributions."[53]

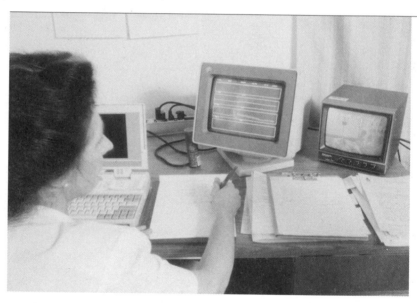

↩ *Ph.D. candidate in nursing Ginette Rodger studying tapes of nursing interventions. (Faculty of Nursing, University of Alberta)*

12

Issues, Commitments, and Directions as the Nursing Profession Approaches the 21st Century

Extraordinary shifts in the nature of public policy discussions about health care and concomitant questioning of fundamental values about health in Canadian society have occurred in the last decade of the twentieth century. As provincial and federal governments have questioned the level of health expenditures and downsized expenditures for health and social services, stormy public debate has ensued. At 9.9 percent of Gross Domestic Product in 1991,[1] national expenditures for health care became an obvious target for cuts and downsizing of health programs. Nurses comprise the largest group of health professionals, the large majority of whom (75 percent) are employees of acute and long-term care hospitals in a system supported virtually in its entirety by provincial and federal taxation.[2] As governments have moved forward with health system restructuring, this may signal in some sense a recognition of limits to growth in a post-industrial society. Deep cuts to the health system in Alberta between 1993 to 1996 resulted in lower health expenditures in Alberta than in any other province.[3] A concomitant questioning of values driven by questions about the financing of the system, has left nurses as primary targets of deep cuts in acute care budgets.[4]

The program of restructuring predicated upon a new system of regionalization and markedly lower budget allocations for health care took place on a very rapid timetable. Although the new regional health authorities were mandated with the responsibility for funding health care delivery in each region, they were allocated reduced funds with which to do this by the provincial ministry of health. The timetable for downsizing has been a contentious issue as the major cuts were orchestrated for the first two years of the Klein government's first mandate beginning in 1993. In the second half of the mandate, the cuts were less severe. If one were to look at developing a reasonable plan for rationalizing and restructuring the system with concomitant downsizing of certain areas, it is likely that a more gradual process would be selected in order to allow for time for public discussion and to reduce hardship among professionals displaced in the process and among consumers of health care, particularly vulnerable groups such as the elderly and the disabled.

The cuts have meant that nurses as the largest group of health professionals employed in the system have been on the leading edge of large-scale layoffs in tertiary care hospitals. Growing unemployment amongst nurses has not been seen in Canada since the Depression in the 1930s when widespread unemployment among registered nurses occurred for the first time when families who engaged nurses privately on a fee for service to care for their ill members in their homes could no longer afford their services. In some ways it seems as if history is repeating itself, as nurses whose positions have disappeared have set up private practices and are offering their nursing services to individuals and families in their homes and through in-person and telephone consultations in relation to their health. Nurses have had to be resourceful because, for the most part they have been offered little in the way of compensation for the loss of their positions and they have had to be creative in finding new avenues for using their knowledge and skills.

Nurses have been on record as supporting health care reform for decades. It has been obvious that the health system as it has developed in Canada under a system of national health insurance has been relatively costly. While many other countries have established national health systems that are publicly funded, the Canadian system employs a private overlay on a public system. Excess capacity in certain sectors including acute care, remuneration for certain categories of health professionals on a costly fee for service basis and over-development of some services with little attention to whether or not these were needed have characterized the system. In addition, financial incentives to the provinces to develop systems based upon hospital and physician-centred care have added considerably to overall health expenditures. Because of these incentives, the total cost of the system has been higher than would have been the case if certain other policy directions had been taken.

The political will to reform the system has not been there until recently, and whether true reform will occur or just window-dressing remains to be seen. Since political will is driven by the ability to garner votes from the electorate, the shape of reform may be such that a publicly-funded health system may be less attractive to the politicians than one with more privately funded services than previously. Politicians have historically found it much easier to support the high cost elements of the system such as physicians' services since these individuals constitute a powerful pressure group in society. Politicians ultimately responsible for health policy have always found it difficult to address the aspects of the system which most need reform in order to ensure that the publicly funded system of health care remains viable. Among these are included the need to shift the acute care focus of the system to a focus which is based in community health centres; streamlining the method of payment for health to exclude fee-for-service and include remunerating health professionals on a salary or contract basis; identifying how many professionals are needed in the system and limiting the number practising in the system to the number required; limiting the facilities where the work of the health system is carried on to those which are required and closing those not needed. Rationalization of the system could lead to the establishment of community health centres where a range of services provided by health professionals could be offered. This could potentially facilitate collaboration and coordination of care and reduce costs through efficiencies achieved through common use of facilities and interdisciplinary teamwork. The need to address these matters in order to preserve a publicly funded and effective health system is critical.

Health care reform as envisioned by nurses, would see the primary focus of health care moving to the community in primary health centres from its traditional base in tertiary care hospitals. In the Alberta context it is really too early to tell whether funding which has been taken out of the acute care system will find its way to support care in the community. The movement of health care policy development and decision making relative to health care delivery to the new health authorities in a regionally-based system required major transitions in a relatively short period of time. The closing of acute hospital beds was accompanied by a promise to shift care to the community with the development of community health centres. However, it is still early in the process to identify just how these concepts will be translated into action. The shift to a regional system of health care has been advantageous as it has moved responsibility for the operation of health systems to the regions from the large Alberta Health bureaucracy. It may require an overall agency such as Alberta Health though to become the arbiter of standards, as the regions develop in remarkably disparate ways. Regionalization has also done much to end competition between tertiary care institutions and consequent duplication of services and programs offered within these. There were two exceptions in Alberta relative to the powers granted to the regions to develop health care. These exceptions were physicians' services and mental health. The mental health decision was a temporary one as mental health was slated to move into the regional system within a specified period of time. At that time the funds for mental health will also be given to the regions to manage. That funding for physicians' services has not been part of the budgets of regional health authorities has been problematic, since this is one of the most costly items in the health care system. True reform of the system requires hard decisions about care and the best ways of providing it to people by qualified professionals. If the hands of the regional health authorities are tied by not having jurisdiction over all services required for care such as medical care, those services will continue to be fragmented and expensive. To restructure a health system in such a dramatic way without including physicians' services in that restructuring would seem to indicate that the government lacks the political will to make the changes that are so badly needed in the financing of medical care.

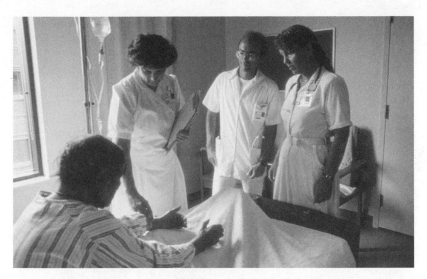

↪ *University of Alberta Faculty of Nursing students in clinical area with instructor. (Faculty of Nursing, University of Alberta)*

To date, nurses have not been engaged in substantial numbers for the delivery of primary health care, but it entirely possible that this will occur in the future with the development of community health centres. It is likely that changes in the way in which nursing is practised will continue as society becomes more aware of the benefits of health promotion and the need to develop healthier life-styles to prevent disease. Alternatives to hospitalization for tertiary and long-term or continuing care, in the form of home care and ambulatory care, appear attractive at both the personal and societal levels. It must be recognized, however, that all levels of hospitalization will continue to be required to meet the needs of people. In the rhetoric about downsizing the tertiary care hospital and moving services to the community, it must be recognized that high quality tertiary care services are critical to a well-functioning system. Nurses have been preparing for their new roles in community and long-term care settings and have the knowledge and the communication and interactional skills to assist consumers in meeting health goals. The system of nursing education has responded to the need for nurses to be prepared for primary health care roles and post-baccalaureate and master's degree programs have been modified to serve these needs. Nurses are well-poised and positioned to

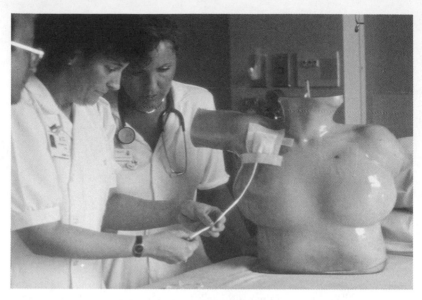

↪ *Nursing instructor helping student learn subclavian line care. (Faculty of Nursing, University of Alberta)*

serve society in a health system which is centred in the community and based on the primary health care model in which consumer education and control over personal health decision-making are prominent.

The history and traditions of nursing education in Alberta are long and impressive. A system of diploma nursing education first became available in Alberta over 100 years ago and it has been 78 years since the first courses in public health nursing were offered by the University of Alberta in 1919. Currently the system of diploma nursing education has been phased into collaborative or conjoint baccalaureate programs offered by the community colleges acting with the University of Alberta or the University of Calgary. Increased availability of baccalaureate programs in nursing will provide a stronger basis for the practice of nursing. The University of Alberta was a pioneer in distance delivered degree programs as the first university in the country to offer an entire degree program at a distance more than a decade ago. While teleconferencing was the initial distance method which was employed, the transition was made to video-enhanced teleconferencing and finally to videoconferencing and computer conferencing. Athabasca University developed a distance degree program for post-R.N. graduates offered to nurses in other provinces and countries as well as in Alberta. It has emerged as a leader in Canada as a postsecondary institution offering distance programs. The University of Calgary developed its post-R.N. program entirely on a distance education basis. The development of a context-based learning program in the University of Alberta's undergraduate program implemented in the fall of 1997 was another innovative development in degree programs in nursing education in Alberta.

Graduate programs at the master's level have been available in the universities in both Calgary and Edmonton since the initiation of master's degree programs at the University of Alberta in 1975 and at the University of Calgary in 1981. Experimentation in offering graduate education at the master's level has been undertaking by the University of Alberta employing distance delivery, principally videoconferencing to groups of students in Red Deer and Grande Prairie on a pilot project basis. Alberta had the distinction of mounting the first doctoral program in nursing in the country beginning on 1 January 1991 at the University of Alberta. The initiation of doctoral education has been an important milestone for the profession, since preparing nurses to contribute to the discovery of nursing knowledge through theory and research will lead to improved care. Planning for "flexible Ph.D." offerings on a distance basis is underway. Undergraduate and graduate programs offered by the universities in the province are considered to be among the best in Canada, and Alberta university nursing faculty have been at the forefront nationally in graduate education and research.

Nursing has made great progress in improving its standards and it would appear that the long and difficult campaign of the AARN to raise standards in the schools of the nursing in the province were not in vain, for today Alberta is a leader in nursing education in the country. It was apparent by the 1960s and 1970s that as in the rest of the country the system of diploma nursing education in Alberta was undergoing a profound transformation as it moved to the general educational system. Widespread debate about the quality of instruction had been heard in the profession in Alberta from the earliest part of the century. The professional association worked very hard to ensure awareness of the deficiencies and the need for reform. The publication of the Weir Report[5] in 1932 corroborated the AARN's criticisms and paved the way for further changes in the system of nursing education. While some of the reforms advocated in the Weir Report had been implemented in Alberta prior to its publication, it would take decades for others to reach fruition both in Alberta and elsewhere. Some recommendations have just seen full implementation in the mid-1990s in the province, undoubtedly an indication that in making some of his recommendations, Dr. Weir was on target and considerably ahead of his time.

In reviewing the history of nursing education in the province, it is apparent that there has been a progression in thinking over time about schools of nursing and about the system of nursing education. Nevertheless, certain principles have continued to characterize the approaches that the profession and those engaged in the educational system have taken to the improvement of standards and monitoring the quality of education in programs. The importance of engaging well-qualified instructors, selecting appropriate content, retaining a strong clinical focus, and maintaining appropriate admission standards have been elements which have been concerns over time. The concern for standards of education and practice has been a fundamental one in view of the responsibility for providing safe and competent care to clients. However, dynamic leadership will be required to provide direction to new generations of skilled practitioners and to ensure that their talents are used to the fullest extent for the benefit of the public.

With the development of the discipline and the expansion of the knowledge base, the appropriateness of the environment in which learning takes place is at issue. Improvement in the status of women combined with the fact that nursing remains as one of the last sex-segregated professions has led to attention to the potential for differential treatment and stereotyping of nurses' roles. Systematic undervaluing of the contributions of the profession continues and is evident in the published histories of many health care institutions in which nurses contributions have been downplayed, when in fact nurses have almost always contributed significantly to the implementation and management of care. Nevertheless, nurses have developed strong organizations to put forward the perspective of the profession on health policy issues and these organizations have demonstrated their effectiveness in the public policy debate. Given that nurses believe deeply in the importance of their contribution to public health, it is unlikely that they will ever again take a back seat in health policy debates. Although it is difficult to say what the next 100 years hold for Alberta nurses and their profession, it is likely that they will continue to perform a highly valued service in the health care system and that they will be respected for their knowledge, skill and contributions to the health of people.

Notes

INTRODUCTION

1. Susan Jackel, "Women in Canadian Universities: A historical overview," unpublished keynote address to the Conference and Annual Meeting, Western Region, Canadian Association of University Schools of Nursing, University of Alberta, Edmonton, AB, 17 February 1985.
2. Angus McGugan, *The First Fifty Years: A History of the University of Alberta Hospital 1914–1964* (Edmonton, AB: The University of Alberta Hospital, 1964); J. Ross Vant and Tony Cashman, *More Than a Hospital: University of Alberta Hospitals 1906–1986* (Edmonton, AB: The University Hospitals Board, 1986).

3. Susan M. Reverby, *Ordered to Care: The Dilemma of American Nursing, 1850–1945* (New York: Cambridge University Press, 1987), p. xi.

4. Kathryn McPherson, *Bedside Matters: The Transformation of Canadian Nursing, 1900–1990* (Toronto, ON: Oxford University Press, 1996), p. 8.

5. S.J. Roberts, Oppressed group behavior: Implications for nursing. *Advanced in Nursing Science 5* (4).

6. Abraham Flexner, "Is Social Work a Profession?" in *Proceedings of the National Conference of Charities and Corrections* (Chicago: Heldermann Printing Co., 1915), pp. 578–581.

7. Amatai Etzioni, ed., *The Semi-Professions and Their Organization: Teachers, Nurses, Social Workers.* (New York: Free Press, 1969).

8. Heber C. Jamieson, *Early Medicine in Alberta: The First Seventy-Five Years* (Edmonton, AB: The Canadian Medical Association, Alberta Division, 1947).

9. Esther Lucile Brown, *Nursing for the Future* (New York: Russell Sage Foundation, 1948).

1   THE ORIGINS OF NURSING

1. Irene M. Spry, *The Palliser Expedition: An Account of John Palliser's British North American Expedition, 1857–1860* (Toronto: Macmillan, 1963).

2. James MacGregor, *A History of Alberta* (Edmonton: Hurtig Publishers, 1972), p. 80.

3. Robin W. Winks, *Canada and the United States: The Civil War Years* (Baltimore: Johns Hopkins University Press, 1971).

4. Ibid., p. 42.

5. Archives des Soeurs Grises de Montréal (ASGM), "Journal de Voyage" de Soeur Alphonse, *Lettres de St-Albert 1858–1877*, Copie de l'ancien cahier numéro un, ASGM. An identical copy of this document was also found in the Archives des Soeurs Grises de Montréal, Province de St-Albert, Edmonton (ASGME) Document 23, Lac Sainte-Anne Historique.

6. MacGregor, p. 73.

7. ASGM, "Journal de Voyage" de Soeur Alphonse," *Lettres de St-Albert 1858–1877*, Copie de l'ancien cahier numéro un, ASGM.

8. Sister Emery stated: "It is likely that the location of the mission will change. Here, agriculture is quite difficult; the wheat doesn't ripen and one can only cultivate barley and potatoes." Translated from the original French: "Il est tout probable que la mission va changer de place. . . . Ici c'est tout à fait désagréable pour la culture, le blé ne murit pas, il n'y a que l'orge et les patates que l'on puisse récolter." ASGME, Soeur Emery, Lettre à Mère Deschamps, 13 avril 1860, *Lettres de St-Albert, 1858–1877*.

9. Marcel Giraud, *Le Métis canadien* (Winnipeg: Les Editions du Blé d'Or, 1984), pp. 1080–86.

10. ASGME, Lettre de Soeur Emery à Mère Slocombe, St-Albert, 11 décembre 1864, *Lettres de St-Albert, 1858–1877*.

11. MacGregor, p. 62.

12. Translated from the original French: "La maladie fait de terribles ravages, et nous avons déjà quatre de nos enfants de mort; un cinquième touche à sa fin. Il n'y a rien de si pitoyable, c'est une vrai corruption! Toutes les fois que nous l'approchons, il faut se bander le nez bien fort. Les personnes du dehors meurent très vite parce que les soins leur manquent." ASGME, Lettre de Soeur Emery à Mère Slocombe, 27 novembre 1870, St-Albert, pp. 231–39.

13. ASGME, Lettre de Soeur Charlebois à Mère Slocombe, St-Albert, 20 décembre 1871, *Lettres de St-Albert 1859–1877*.

14. Lorraine Bizon, *"Grey Nuns": Pioneer missionary contributions in Alberta*. ASGM (1978), pp. 3–12.

15. ASGME, Lettre de Soeur Ward, 4 septembre 1878, *Circulaire mensuelle*. *Hôpital-Général* (Montréal: octobre, 1878), no. 9, pp. 315–16.

16. John Gibbon and Mary Mathewson, *Three Centuries of Canadian Nursing* (Toronto: The MacMillan Co., 1947).

17. Ibid., p. 1.

18. Canadian Nurses Association, *The Leaf and the Lamp* (Ottawa: The Association, 1968).

19. Meredith Hill, "The women workers of the diocese of Athabasca; 1930–1970," *Journal of the Canadian Church Historical Society* 28 (1986): 64.

20. Ibid.

21. Tony Cashman, *Heritage of Service: The History of Nursing in Alberta* (Edmonton: Alberta Association of Registered Nurses, 1966), p. 19.

22. *Edmonton Bulletin*, 7 August 1886.

23. Cashman, *Heritage of Service*, p. 19.

24. Olive I. Ziegler, "Outpost hospitals—a fine achievement," *The Canadian Hospital* 18, no. 2 (1941): 17.

25. Cashman, *Heritage of Service*, pp. 42–107.

26. Ibid., p. 71.

27. Gibbon and Mathewson, pp. 484–89.

28. Ibid.

29. Ibid.

30. Ibid.

31. Ibid.

32. Ibid.

33. Ibid.

34. Ibid.

35. *Grande Prairie Herald*, 23 October 1914.

36. Cashman, *Heritage of Service*, pp. 42–107.
37. Lacombe medical history, undated [circa 1964–1965], AARN Archives.
38. D. Schurerman, "History of Nursing in Rimbey," undated [circa 1964–1965], AARN Archives.
39. Cashman, *Heritage of Service*, pp. 42–107.
40. Letter from Thelma A. McIntyre, Vulcan, undated [circa 1964–1965], AARN Archives.
41. Letter from Mrs. Willis Teskey, Rocky Mountain House, 11 April 1964, AARN Archives.
42. Letter from E. Mayan to Tony Cashman, Bluesky, AB, 29 June 1965, AARN Archives.
43. Gibbon and Mathewson, p. 269.
44. Ibid., pp. 250–76.
45. Ibid., p. 269.
46. Freda Viste, *No Doctor in the house, In Hanna North, A Rural History 1908–1978* (Hanna: Hanna North Book Club, 1978), pp. 42–43.
47. Ibid., p. 43.
48. Ibid.

2 NURSES AND THE ESTABLISHMENT OF EARLY HOSPITALS

1. Charles E. Rosenberg, *The Care of Strangers* (New York: Basic Books, 1987), pp. 1–11.
2. Ibid.
3. J.G. Nelson, *The Last Refuge* (Montreal: Harvest House Ltd., 1973), p. 109.
4. C.M. MacInnes, *In the Shadow of the Rockies* (London: Rivington, 1930), p. 64.
5. Doug Owram, *Promise of Eden: The Canadian Expansionist Movement and the Idea of the West 1856–1900* (Toronto: University of Toronto Press, 1980).
6. *RCMP Quarterly* 24, no. 1 (July, 1958).
7. Fort McLeod Chapter, Alberta Association of Registered Nurses (unsigned), Letter to Tony Cashman written 28 April 1965, Archives of the Alberta Association of Registered Nurses, Edmonton, Alberta.
8. Joy Duncan, *Red Serge Wives* (Edmonton: Lone Pine Publishing, 1985).
9. D. Scollard, *Hospital—A Portrait of Calgary General* (Calgary: Calgary General Hospital, 1981), p. 12.
10. Ibid., p. 13.
11. Barbara Kwasny, *Nuns and Nightingales: A History of the Holy Cross School of Nursing—1907–1979* (Calgary: Alumnae Association of the Holy Cross School of Nursing, 1982), p. 13.
12. Ibid., p. 14.

13. Ibid., p. 16.
14. J.G. Calder, *Excerpt from annual report for 1892: Medicine Hat General Hospital*, Medicine Hat Archives, M-14A. M83.15.11, p. 1.
15. Leah Poelman, *White Caps and Red Roses: History of the Galt School of Nursing, Lethbridge, Alberta, 1910–1979* (Lethbridge: Galt School of Nursing Alumnae Society of Alberta, 1979), p. 11.
16. J.B. Peters, *Excerpt from annual report of 1894: Medicine Hat General Hospital*, Medicine Hat Archives, M-14A. M83.15.11.
17. These words of Mrs. Higinbotham were quoted in the *Lethbridge Herald*. Although the content seems plausible it was impossible to verify authenticity. The quote was found in an article entitled: "Extension to the Galt hospital," 20 June 1931, p. 3, Galt Museum and Archives, Lethbridge.
18. Susan Jackel, *A flannel shirt and liberty: British emigrant gentlewomen in the Canadian West, 1880–1914* (Vancouver: UBC Press, 1982), p. 123–25.
19. Ibid., p. 147.
20. Ted Byfield, ed., *Alberta in the 20th Century: The Great West before 1900* (Edmonton: United Western Communications Ltd., 1991), pp. 166–67.
21. Ted Byfield, ed., *Alberta in the 20th Century: The Birth of the Province 1900–1910* (Edmonton: United Western Communications Ltd., 1992), p. 115.
22. Discussions of this episode in Edmonton hospital history may be found in Janet Ross Kerr and Pauline Paul, "Nurses and hospitals in Edmonton at the turn of the century," *Proceedings of the Qualitative Health Research Conference* (Edmonton: University of Alberta, 22 February 1991); Janet Ross Kerr, Pauline Paul and Alice MacKinnon, *The Origins of Nursing in Alberta: 1859–1909* [Final Research Report to the Alberta Foundation for Nursing Research] (Edmonton: Faculty of Nursing, University of Alberta, 1992); and Pauline Paul and Janet Ross Kerr, "A philosophy of care: The Grey Nuns of Montreal," in Bob Hesketh and Frances Swyripa, eds., *Edmonton, The Life of a City* (Edmonton: NeWest Publishers, 1995), pp. 126–34.
23. Grey Nuns' Archives, Edmonton Hôpital Historique, Document 58, 1899.
24. Grey Nuns' Archives, Edmonton Hôpital Historique, Document 9, 1894.
25. Ibid.
26. Ibid.
27. Grey Nuns' Archives, Edmonton Hôpital Historique, Document 11, 1894.
28. Grey Nuns' Archives, Edmonton Hôpital Historique, Document 15, 1894.
29. Grey Nuns' Archives, Edmonton Hôpital Historique, Document 18, 1894.
30. Grey Nuns' Archives, Edmonton Hôpital Historique, Document 23, 1895.
31. Grey Nuns' Archives, Edmonton Hôpital Historique, Document 25A, 1907.
32. Grey Nuns' Archives, Edmonton Hôpital Historique, Document 58, 1899.
33. Ibid.
34. Edmonton Hospital Board minutes, 1899–1939. Public Hospital Minutes 1BT.E24h. City of Edmonton Archives.

35. Ibid.

36. Christina Dorward and Olive Tookey, *Below the Flight Path* (Edmonton: Alumnae Association of the Royal Alexandra Hospital School of Nursing, 1968), p. 1.

37. "Citizens Favour Hospital By-Law," *Edmonton Bulletin*, 20 June 1910, City of Edmonton Archives.

38. John Gilpin, *The Misericordia Hospital: 85 years of service in Edmonton* (Edmonton: Misericordia Hospital, 1986), p. 3.

39. Ibid., p. 19.

40. Ibid., p. 13.

41. Ibid., p. 15.

42. Ibid., p. 31.

43. Ibid., p. 32.

44. Ibid., p. 33.

45. "A Quarantine Hospital," *Edmonton Bulletin*, 18 February 1901. City of Edmonton Archives.

46. Ibid.

47. Maureen Riddell, *Toward a Healthier City: A History of the Edmonton Local Board of Health and Health Department 1871–1979* (Edmonton: Local Board of Health, 1980), p. 25.

48. Riddell, p. 26.

49. J. Ross Vant and Tony Cashman, *More than a Hospital: University of Alberta Hospitals 1906–1986* (Edmonton: University of Alberta Hospitals Board, 1986), p. 5.

50. Ibid., p. 6.

51. Ibid., p. 35.

52. Ibid., p. 35.

53. Ibid., p. 36.

54. Rosenberg, p. 5.

3 DILIGENCE, DEDICATION AND DISTINGUISHED SERVICE: *NURSES IN THE MODERN HOSPITAL ERA*

1. Jannetta MacPhail, "Men in nursing," in Janet Ross Kerr and Jannetta MacPhail, eds., *Canadian Nursing: Issues and Perspectives* (Toronto: Mosby-Year Book, 1996).

2. Janet Ross Kerr, "Emergence of nursing unions as a social force in Canada," in Janet Ross Kerr and Jannetta MacPhail, eds., *Canadian Nursing: Issues and Perspectives* (Toronto: Mosby-Year Book, 1996).

3. George M Weir, *Survey of Nursing Education in Canada* (Toronto: University of Toronto Press, 1932).

4. Sister Marie Bonin, "Trends in Integrated Basic Degree Nursing Programs in Canada: 1942–1972," Ph.D. dissertation, University of Ottawa, 1976, pp. xii–xiii.

5. Alberta Association of Registered Nurses, Minutes of 17th Annual Convention, Edmonton, AB, 23 March 1932, p. 298.

6. Mabel Holt, "Staffing with graduate nurses," *The Canadian Nurse* 32 (January 1936): 10.

7. Cashman, *Heritage of Service*, p. 93.

8. G. Harvey Agnew, *Canadian Hospitals 1920–1970: A Dramatic Half Century* (Toronto: University of Toronto Press, 1974), p. 150.

9. Ibid.

10. Deborah Gorham, "'No longer an invisible minority': Women physicians and medical practice in late twentieth-century North America," in Dianne Dodd and Deborah Gorham, eds., *Caring and Curing: Historical Perspectives on Women and Healing in Canada* (Ottawa: University of Ottawa Press, 1994), p. 183.

11. Ibid.

12. Kathryn McPherson, "Science and technique: Nurses' work in a Canadian hospital, 1920–1939, " in Dianne Dodd and Deborah Gorham, eds., *Caring and Curing: Historical Perspectives on Women and Healing in Canada* (Ottawa: University of Ottawa Press, 1994), p. 71.

13. Ibid., p. 78.

14. Ibid., p. 82.

15. Ibid., pp. 80–81.

16. Ibid., p. 79.

17. Ibid., p. 80.

18. Ibid., p. 82.

19. A. Worcester, "Is nursing really a profession?" *American Journal of Nursing* 2 (Aug. 1902): 908–17.

20. Janet C. Kerr, "Provincial variation in nursing functions," in Shirley R. Good and Janet C. Kerr, eds., *Contemporary Issues in Canadian Law for Nurses* (Toronto: Holt, Rinehart and Winston Inc., 1973), pp. 83–93.

21. M. Johnson and H. Martin, "A sociological analysis of the nurse's role," *American Journal of Nursing* 58, no. 3 (1958), p. 3.

22. American Nurses Association, *Educational Preparation for Nurse Practitioners and Assistants to Nurses: A Position Paper* (New York: American Nurses Association, 1965).

23. H. Thurston, "Education for episodic and distributive care," *Nursing Outlook* 20, no. 8 (1972): 519–23.

24. Martha Rogers, "To be or not to be," *Nursing Outlook* 20, no. 1 (1972): 42–46.

25. Murray Ross, "The evolution of hospital care in Alberta," *Dimensions in Health Service* 57, no. 4, p. A4, 1980.

26. Vant and Cashman, p. 188.

27. Ibid.

28. George M. Weir, *Survey of Nursing Education in Canada* (Toronto:University of Toronto Press, 1932).

29. Cashman, *Heritage of Service*, pp. 281–84.

30. Ibid., p. 283.

31. Poelman, p. 114.

32. Ibid.

33. Alberta Association of Registered Nurses, Minutes of the Annual Meeting, 8 and 9 April 1946, AARN Archives.

34. Rae Chittick, "Let us take pride in our craft," *The Canadian Nurse* 44, no. 9 (1948), pp. 705–6.

35. Ibid., p. 706.

36. Alberta Association of Registered Nurses, Minutes of Annual Convention, 21 May 1952, Edmonton, AB, AARN Archives.

37. Kathryn McPherson, *Bedside Matters: The Transformation of Canadian Nursing, 1900–1990* (Toronto: Oxford University Press, 1996), p. 206.

38. Alberta Association of Registered Nurses, Minutes of Annual Meeting of 1939, April 1939, AARN Archives.

39. Ruth Roach Pierson, *They're Still Women After All: The Second World War and Canadian Womanhood* (Toronto: McClelland and Steward, 1986), p. 53.

40. Alberta Association of Registered Nurses, Minutes of Annual Meeting, 13, 14 and 15 April 1950, Edmonton, AB, AARN Archives.

41. Sheila Abercrombie, *Alberta Hospital Edmonton 1923 to 1983, An Outline of History to Commemorate the 60th Anniversary* (Edmonton: Alberta Hospital, 1983), pp. 23, 38.

42. W.R.N. Blair, *Mental Health in Alberta*, A Report on the Alberta Mental Health Study (Edmonton: Queen's Printer, 1969).

43. Alberta Association of Registered Nurses, Minutes of Annual Meeting of 1918, AARN Archives.

44. Alberta Association of Registered Nurses, Minutes of Annual Meeting, 11 and 12 October 1939, AARN Archives.

45. Abercrombie, p. 43.

46. Ibid.

47. Edmonton Association for Retarded Children, unpublished manuscript, 24 June 1965, AARN Archives, p. 1.

48. Staff Nurses Association of Alberta, "Patient care in region 10: Registered nurses' professional concerns and solutions," November 6, 1996, citing figures from Alberta Health. As cited by Kevin Taft, *Shredding the Public Interest: Ralph Klein and 25 Years of One-party Government* (Edmonton, Alberta: University of Albeta Press and the Parkland Institute, 1997), p. 29.

49. Taft, p. 31.

1. J.J. Heagerty, "The development of public helath in Canada," in C. Meilicke, and J.L. Storch, eds., *Perspectives on Canadian Health and Social Services Policy: History and Emerging Trends* (Ann Arbor, MI: Health Administration Press, 1980), p. 142.

2. G. Miller, ed., *Letters of Edward Jenner and Other Documents Concerning the Early History of Vaccination* (Baltimore: Johns Hopkins University Press, 1983).

3. C.A. Dawson and E.R. Younge, *Pioneering in the Prairie Provinces: The Social side of the Settlement Process* (Toronto: Macmillan, 1940), p. 244.

4. Adelaide Schartner, *Health Units of Alberta* (Edmonton: Coop Press, 1982), p. 8.

5. Heagerty, p. 142.

6. Ibid., p. 10.

7. Riddell, p. 6–7.

8. Schartner, p. 7.

9. Riddell, pp. 7–8.

10. Heber Jamieson, *Early Medicine in Alberta: The First Seventy-five Years* (Edmonton: Canadian Medical Association, Alberta Division, 1947), pp. 73–74.

11. Adelaide Schartner, *Health Units of Alberta* (Edmonton: Coop Press, 1982), p. 22.

12. Ibid., p. 24.

13. Ibid., p. 33.

14. Ibid., p. 24; Riddell, p. 7.

15. Schartner, p. 25.

16. Riddell, p. 23.

17. That the native peoples appreciated the skills of the nursing orders was evident because they sought their ministrations. Nevertheless one should qualify such discussions with acknowledgement of the knowledge that native peoples had developed herbal remedies for health problems and the effects of their own spiritual approaches to healing.

18. Margaret M. Allemang, "Development of community health nursing in Canada," in Miriam J. Stewart, ed., *Community Nursing: Promoting Canadians' Health* (Toronto: W.B. Saunders, 1995), p. 3.

19. Ibid.

20. Beverly Boutilier, "Helpers or heroines? The National Council of Women, Nursing, and 'Woman's Work' in late Victorian Canada," in Dianne Dodd and Deborah Gorham, eds., *Caring and Curing: Historical Perspectives on Women and Healing in Canada* (Ottawa: University of Ottawa Press, 1994), p. 17.

21. Ibid., pp. 19–21.
22. Ibid., pp. 41–42.
23. Collins, p. 4.
24. Collins, p. 9.
25. *Edmonton Journal*, 6 February 1919.
26. Cashman, *Heritage of Service*, p. 191.
27. Jamieson, pp. 73–74.
28. Irene Stewart, *These Were Our Yesterdays: A History of District Nursing in Alberta* (Calgary: Friesen Printers, 1979), p. 7.
29. Jamieson, pp. 73–74.
30. "Alberta health department sent out 200 nurses," *Edmonton Bulletin*, 18 January 1919, Provincial Archives of Alberta, Acc. No. 75–454.
31. "Public health work by nurses," *Edmonton Bulletin*, 23 January 1919, Provincial Archives of Alberta, Acc. No. 75–454.
32. Schartner, p. 44.
33. Ibid.
34. Ibid., p. 45.
35. Stewart, p. 11.
36. Marion Lavell, Transcript of an interview for the Glenbow Museum by Jerry Dunsmore, 16 March 1973, Glenbow Museum Archives.
37. Stewart, p. 11.
38. Mary Watt, Transcript of interview done for the Glenbow Museum by Jerry Dunsmore, 13 March 1973, Glenbow Museum Archives.
39. Ibid.
40. Schartner, p. 43.
41. Ibid.
42. Paul V. Collins, "The Public Health Policies of the United Farmers of Alberta Government, 1921–1935," unpublished Master of Arts thesis, Faculty of Graduate Studies, The University of Western Ontario, London, ON, 1969, p. 4.
43. Canadian Red Cross Society, *The Canadian Red Cross Society: The Role of One Voluntary Organization in Canada's Health Services—A Brief to the Royal Commission on Health Services* (Toronto: Canadian Red Cross Society, 1962), p. 98.
44. Canadian Red Cross Society, p. 116.
45. Ibid., pp. 98–99; Gibbon and Mathewson, p. 342.
46. Gibbon and Mathewson, p. 276.
47. Ibid.
48. Meryn Stuart, "Shifting professional boundaries: Gender conflict in public health, 1920–1925," in D. Dodd and D. Graham, eds., *Caring and Curing: Historical Perspectives on Women and Healing in Canada* (Ottawa: University of Ottawa Press, 1994), p. 53.
49. Stuart, pp. 49–70.

1. The Public Health Nurses Act 1919, Chapter 7, Section 49.
2. Stewart, p. 13.
3. Malcolm R. Bow and F.T. Cook, "The History of the Department of Public Health of Alberta," *Canadian Journal of Public Health* 26, no. 8 (1935): 390.
4. Ibid.
5. Mabel Jacques, *District Nursing* (1911), p. 4.
6. Government of Alberta. Department of Public Health. "Annual Report, 1929–1935."
7. Suzanne Buckley, "Ladies or midwives? Efforts to reduce infant and maternal mortality," in Linda Kealey, ed., *A Not Unreasonable Claim: Women and Reform in Canada 1880s–1920s* (Toronto: The Women's Educational Press, 1979), pp. 131–49.
8. Lavinia L. Dock, "The history of public health nursing," in Mazyck L. Ravenel, ed., *A Half Century of Public Health: Jubilee Historical Volume of the American Public Health Association* (Lynn, MA: American Public Health Association, 1921), p. 439.
9. Government of Alberta. Department of Public Health. "Annual Report", 1930–1935.
10. Dominion Bureau of Statistics, Government of Canada, *Vital Statistics 1921, First Annual Report* (Ottawa: F.A. Acland, 1921), p. xv.
11. Ibid., p. xiii.
12. *Hanna Herald*, 11 April 1919.
13. Collins, p. 9.
14. D.G. Lent, *Alberta Red Cross in Peace and War, 1917–1947* (Alberta, 1947), p. 61.
15. Ibid., p. 10.
16. Gibbon and Mathewson, p. 276.
17. John Gibbon, *The Victorian Order of Nurses for Canada* (Montreal: Southam Press, 1947), p. 51.
18. Sheila Penney, *A Century of Caring 1887–1997: The History of the Victorian Order of Nurses for Canada* (Ottawa: VON Canada, 1991), p. 50.
19. Alberta Association of Graduate Nurses, Minutes of meeting of 22 May 1917, AARN Archives.
20. Canadian National Association of Trained Nurses, Minutes of the Annual Meeting 1917, AARN Archives.
21. Alberta Association of Graduate Nurses, Minutes of meeting of 7 May 1918, AARN Archives.
22. Ibid.
23. Alberta Association of Graduate Nurses, Minutes of meeting of 1 July 1918, AARN Archives.
24. Ibid.

25. Alberta Association of Registered Nurses, Minutes of meeting of 14 May 1920, AARN Archives.

26. Alberta Association of Registered Nurses, Minutes of Annual Convention of 16 October 1923, AARN Archives.

27. Alberta Association of Registered Nurses, Minutes of meeting of 26 May 1925, AARN Archives.

28. Penney, p. 50.

29. Marion Cran, "A woman in Canada," in Susan Jackel, ed., *A Flannel Shirt and Liberty: British Emigrant Gentlewomen in the Canadian West, 1880–1914* (Vancouver: University of British Columbia Press, 1982), pp. 126–49.

30. Ibid., p. 144.

31. Ibid., p. 146.

32. Ibid.

33. Penney, p. 52.

34. Ibid.

35. Ibid., p. 50.

36. Ibid., p. 52.

37. Ibid.

38. Malcolm R. Bow, "The history of the Department of Public Health of Alberta," *Canadian Journal of Public Health* 26, no. 8 (1935): 385.

39. Stewart, p. 19.

40. Ibid., p. 29.

41. Ibid.

42. Ibid., p. 65.

43. Ibid., p. 64.

44. Ibid.

45. Ibid., pp. 80–81.

46. Ibid., p. 37.

47. Philippa Chapman, from interview by Margaret Maw, 11 October 1967, Department of Public Health Archives, Provincial Archives of Alberta, p. 2.

48. Ibid., p. 4.

49. Ibid., p. 7.

50. Laura Attrux, As cited in report of interview with Susan Fierbach, July 1987. AARN Archives, p. 4.

51. Ibid., p. 5.

52. Ibid., p. 3.

53. Ibid., p. 5.

54. Ibid., p. 3.

1. Monica Baly, *As Miss Nightingale Said . . .* (London: Scutari Press, 1991), p. 33.

2. Baly, p. 30.

3. Canadian Nurses Association, *The Leaf and the Lamp*, p. 63.

4. Ibid.

5. Gibbon and Mathewson.

6. Ibid., pp. 290–91.

7. Ibid., pp. 290.

8. Ibid., p. 296.

9. Ibid., p. 297.

10. Nicholson, p. 98.

11. Ibid., p. 99.

12. Cashman, *Heritage of Service*, p. 109.

13. Cashman, *Heritage of Service*, pp. 108–9.

14. G.W.L. Nicholson, *Canada's Nursing Sisters* (Toronto: A.M. Hakkert Ltd.), p. 52.

15. Jennifer Sherwood and Eve Henderson, "Our history—A proud heritage: The Alberta Association of Registered Nurses, 1916–1991," AARN *Newsletter* 46, no. 8 (1990), p. 34.

16. Nicholson, pp. 103–6.

17. Sherwood and Henderson, "Our history . . . 1916–1991," p. 34.

18. Nicholson, p. 106.

19. Ibid.

20. Ibid.

21. Ibid., p. 109.

22. Gibbon and Mathewson.

23. Ibid., p. 465.

24. Ibid., p. 467.

25. Ibid., p. 462.

26. Canadian Nurses Association, *The Leaf and the Lamp*, p. 65.

27. Cashman, *Heritage of Service*, p. 229.

28. Ibid., p. 229.

29. Ibid., p. 230.

30. Ibid.

31. Ibid., p. 231.

32. Nursing Sisters' Association of Canada, *Commemorative Issue and National Directory* (Ottawa: Author, 1994), p. 24.

33. Ibid., p. 25.

34. Ibid., p. 31.

35. Transcript of interview with Nettie Garfield Pedlar, 9 February 1982, Glenbow Alberta Archives.

36. Ruth Roach Pierson, *They're Still Women After All: The Second World War and Canadian Womanhood* (Toronto: McClelland and Stewart, 1986), p. 125.

1. Esther Lucile Brown, *Nursing for the Future* (New York: Russell Sage Foundation, 1948), p. 164.
2. Susan L. Young, "Standards in Diploma Nursing Education: The Involvement of The University of Alberta, 1920–1970," unpublished Master of Nursing thesis, University of Alberta, Edmonton, AB, 1994, p. 12.
3. Ibid.
4. Canadian Nurses Association, *Report on the Canadian Nurses Association School Improvement Program* (Ottawa: Canadian Nurses Association, 1965).
5. George Weir, *Survey of Nursing Education in Canada* (Toronto: University of Toronto Press, 1932); Helen K. Mussallem, *Spotlight on Nursing Education: The Report of a Pilot Project for the Evaluation of Schools of Nursing in Canada* (Ottawa: Canadian Nurses Association, 1960)
6. Muriel Elizabeth Chapman, "Nursing Education and the Movement for Higher Education for Women: A Study of Interrleationship, 1870–1900," Doctor of Education Thesis, Teachers College, Columbia University, New York, NY, 1969, p. 528.
7. Young, p. 12.
8. Minutes of the Committee on Nursing Education, 29 June 1953, University of Alberta Archives.
9. J.G. Calder, Excerpt from annual report for 1892 Medicine Hat General Hospital, Medicine Hat Archives, M-14A. M83.15.11, p. 1.
10. Poelman, p. 11.
11. Histoire de l'école [history of the school], Edmonton General Hospital, ASGME.
12. Betty Wilson, *To Teach This Art, The History of the Schools of Nursing at the University of Alberta 1924–1974* (Edmonton: Hallamshire Publishers, 1977), pp. 9–10.
13. Poelman, p. 13.
14. Christina Dorward and Olive Tookey, *Below the Flight Path* (Edmonton: The Alumnae Association, 1968), p. 15; Barbara Kwasny, *Nuns and Nightingales, A History of the Holy Cross School of Nursing 1907–1979* (Calgary: The Alumnae Association, 1982), p. 29.
15. Florence A. Love, *The Lamp Is Golden, Lamont and its Nurses 1912–1962* (Edmonton: Alumnae Association, 1962), p. 31.
16. Kwasny, p. 61
17. D. Scollard, *Hospital—A portrait of the Calgary General* (Winnipeg: Hignell Printing Ltd., 1981), p. 17.
18. Weir, p. 329.
19. Scollard, p. 33.

20. *Première réunion des soeurs missionnaires dans nos hôpitaux de l'ouest, compte rendu des réunions de juillet 1917*, School of Nursing File, EGH, ASGME.

21. Dorward and Tookey, pp. 25–34.

22. Ibid., p. 21.

23. John Gilpin, *The Misericordia Hospital, 85 Years of Service in Edmonton* (Edmonton: Misericordia Hospital, 1986), p. 77.

24. Poelman, p. 48.

25. Cashman, *Heritage of Service*, p. 58.

26. Kwasny, pp. 30–31.

27. Dorward and Tookey, p. 25.

28. Love, p. 29; Pauline Paul, "A History of the Edmonton General Hospital: 1895–1970, 'Be faithful to the duties of your calling'," unpublished Ph.D. dissertation, The University of Alberta, Edmonton, AB, 1994, p. 76.

29. Ibid., p. 41.

30. Summary of the school of Nurse's Enrolment 1908–1971, EGH, ASGME.

31. Alvine Cyr Gahagan, *Yes Father, Pioneer nursing in Alberta* (Manchester, NH: Hammer Publications Inc., 1979), p. 67.

32. Scollard, p. 36.

33. Dorward and Tookey, p. 31.

34. Dorward and Tookey, p. 32.

35. Considering this difficulty and the fact that most of the schools for which information was available existed for only short periods of time, it is possible that a few schools which might have existed are not acknowledged in this chapter. Nonetheless it is unlikely that if other schools existed that they would have been much different from those for which information was available.

36. Young.

37. Cashman, *Heritage of Service*, p. 34.

38. Ibid., p. 65.

39. Ibid., p. 165.

40. Ibid., p. 167.

41. Kwasny, p. 95.

42. Poelman, p. 268.

43. EGHS, EGH, ASGME, 1959.

44. Scollard, *Hospital—A Portrait of Calgary General*, p. 45.

45. Ibid., p. 47.

46. Young, p. 131.

47. Wilson, *To Teach This Art*, p. 119.

48. Alberta Department of Health, *Report of the Nursing Education Survey Committee, Province of Alberta, 1961–1963* (Edmonton: Queen's Printer, 1963), pp. 50–51.

49. Ibid., p. 195.

50. Ibid., p. 191.

51. Cashman, *Heritage of Service*, p. 318.

52. Janet Ross Kerr, "The Origins of Nursing Education in Canada: An overview of the Emergence and Growth of Diploma Programs: 1874–1974," in Janet Ross Kerr and Jannetta MacPhail, eds., *Canadian Nursing: Issues and Perspectives*, 3rd edition (Toronto: Mosby-Year Book, 19961), p. 302.

53. Marguerite Létourneau, "Trends in Basic Diploma Nursing Programs Within Provincial Systems of Education in Canada, 1964–1974," Ph.D. dissertation, University of Ottawa, Ottawa, ON, 1975, p. 240.

54. Minutes of the joint meeting on two-year nursing program, Edmonton General and Misericordia Hospitals, 6 April 1967, School of Nursing File, Edmonton General Hospital, ASGME.

55. G.L. Pickering, Keynote address to graduating nurses, 19 August 1973, School of Nursing File, EGH, ASGME.

56. Alberta Advanced Education and Manpower, *The Final Report of the Nursing Manpower and Education and Research Implementation Committee* (Edmonton: Alberta Advanced Education and Manpower, 1983), p. 4.

57. Kwasny, p. 38.

58. The Alberta Task Force on Nursing Education, *The Report of the Alberta Task Force on Nursing Education* (Edmonton: Alberta Advanced Education and Manpower, 1975).

59. Janet Ross Kerr, "Entry to practice: Striving for the Baccalaureate Standard," in Janet Ross Kerr and Jannetta MacPhail, eds., *Canadian Nursing: Issues and Perspectives*, 3rd edition (Toronto:, Mosby-Year Book, 1996), pp. 328–29.

$\mathcal{8}$ THE EMERGENCE AND GROWTH
OF UNIVERSITY NURSING EDUCATION

1. Alice Baumgart and Rondalyn Kirkwood, "Social reform versus education reform: University nursing education in Canada, 1919–1960," *Journal of Advanced Nursing* 15, no. 5 (1990): 510.

2. Gibbon and Mathewson, p. 342.

3. Canadian Red Cross Society, "The Role of One Voluntary Organization in Canada's Health Services: A Brief to the Royal Commission on Health Services" (Toronto: Canadian Red Cross Society, 1962), p. 96.

4. Ibid.

5. Canadian Red Cross Society, pp 98–99; Gibbon and Mathewson, p. 342; Betty Wilson, *To Teach this Art* (Edmonton: Hallamshire Publishers, 1977), p 14.

6. Cashman, *Heritage of Service*, p. 116.

7. Wilson, p. 14.

8. Department of Public Health, *Annual Report, 1918*, Provincial Archives of Alberta.

9. Stewart, p. 10.

10. Revised Statutes of Alberta, *The Public Health Nurses Act*, Assented to 17 April 1919, Operative 17 May 1919, Section 38, p. 793.

11. Ibid.

12. Stewart, p. 7.

13. Cashman, *Heritage of Service*, p. 193.

14. Ibid., p. 192

15. Ibid., p. 163.

16. University of Alberta, Financial Statements for 1930–31 and 1940–41.

17. While the Financial Statements of the University of British Columbia for the years 1930–31 and 1940–41 showed a decline in revenues, this decline was 8 percent ($932,640 to $855,494) over the 10-year period, rather than the 18 percent which occurred at the University of Alberta.

18. Wilson, p. 55.

19. Canadian Nurses Association, *A Supplement to a Proposed Curriculum for Schools of Nursing in Canada* (Montreal: Canadian Nurses Association, 1940).

20. E. Kathleen Russell, "The Teaching of Public Health Nursing in the University of Toronto" in *Methods and Problems of Medical Education* (The Rockefeller Foundation, 1932).

21. Helen M. Carpenter, "The University of Toronto School of Nursing: An Agent of Change," in Mary Q Innis, ed., *Nursing Education in a Changing Society* (Toronto: University of Toronto Press), p. 90.

22. Wilson, p. 55.

23. Ibid.

24. Ibid., p. 23.

25. Ibid., pp. 27–28.

26. Cashman, *Heritage of Service*, p. 157.

27. "Appointments at University Are Announced," *Edmonton Bulletin* reprint, Helen Penhale file, Archives of the University of Alberta, Acc. no. 1120–2 (hereafter cited as AUA), 9 March 1946.

28. George M. Weir, *Survey of Nursing Education in Canada* (Toronto: University of Toronto Press, 1932).

29. Cashman, *Heritage of Service*, p. 187.

30. Janet C. Ross Kerr, "Financing University Nursing Education in Canada: 1919–1976," unpublished Ph.D. dissertation, University of Michigan, Ann Arbor, Michigan, 1978, pp. 110–33.

31. Ibid., p. 90.

32. Ibid., pp. 110, 113.

33. Ibid., p. 258.

34. Ibid., p. 259.

35. Royal Commission on Health Services, *Report,* Vol. 1 (Ottawa: Queen's Printer, 1964).

36. A more detailed version of the Penhale research was published in the *Canadian Journal of Nursing Research* by Janet Ross-Kerr and Pauline Paul, entitled "Visions realised and dreams dashed: Helen Penhale and the first basic integrated program in nursing in the West at the University of Alberta, 1952–1956," *Canadian Journal of Nursing Research* 27, no. 3: 39-63.

37. Royal Commission on Health Services, *Report.*

38. Minutes of the regular meeting of September 14, 1945, University Hospital Board Meeting Minutes, Archives of the University of Alberta Hospital, Book No. 4 (June, 1940-February, 1948), pp. 188–89 (hereafter cited as UHBMM/AUAH).

39. Ibid.

40. Ibid.

41. Ibid.

42. Ibid.

43. Minutes of the regular meeting of November 23, 1945, UHBMM/AUAH, Book No. 4 (June, 1940-February, 1948), p. 199.

44. Minutes of the regular meeting of September 13, 1946, UHBMM/AUAH, Book No. 4 (June, 1940-February, 1948), p. 234.

45. Ibid.

46. Minutes of the regular meeting of January 10, 1947, UHBMM/AUAH, Book No. 4 (June, 1940-February, 1948), p. 247.

47. Ibid.

48. Ibid.

49. Ibid.

50. Ibid.

51. Minutes of the regular meeting of January 24, 1947, UHBMM/AUAH, Book No. 4 (June, 1940-February, 1948), p. 248.

52. Ibid.

53. Ibid.

54. Ibid.

55. Ibid.

56. Minutes of the regular meeting of February 14th, 1947, UHBMM/AUAH, No. 4 (June, 1940-February, 1948), p. 250.

57. Minutes of the regular meeting of December 12, 1947, UHBMM/AUAH, Book No. 4 (June 1940-February, 1948), p. 290.

58. Helen Penhale, "The spirit of achievement," *The Canadian Nurse* 50, no. 4 (April 1954): 258.

59. Minutes of the Council Meeting of May 9, 1952, Council of the Faculty of Medicine Minutes, AUA Acc. no. 68–1–1052, box 93, p. 9.

60. Wilson, p. 95 (from an interview with Miss Penhale in the mid 1970s).

61. Ibid.
62. Minutes of the Executive Committee of 3 March 1948, Board of Governors, AUA Acc. No. 71–164–10–12, p. 13.
63. Ross Kerr, "Financing University Nursing Education," pp. 110–33.
64. Ibid., pp. 96–137.
65. Minutes of the regular meeting of May 13, 1949, UHBMM/AUAH, Book No. 5 (March, 1948-April, 1953), p. 63.
66. Ibid.
67. Ibid.
68. Minutes of the regular meeting of June 10, 1949, UHBMM/AUAH, Book No. 5 (March, 1948-April, 1953), p. 67.
69. Ibid.
70. Ibid.
71. Minutes of the regular meeting of June 27, 1949, UHBMM/AUAH, Book No. 5 (March, 1948-April, 1953), p. 71.
72. Ibid.
73. Ibid.
74. Ibid.
75. Letter from President Newton to Miss Helen Penhale, 20 June 1950, School of Nursing-General, AUA Acc. no. 68–1–1070, box 95.
76. Minutes of the regular meeting of February 23, 1951, UHBMM/AUAH, Book No. 5 (March, 1948-April, 1953), p. 153.
77. Ibid.
78. Minutes of the regular meeting of November 23, 1951, UHBMM/AUAH, Book No. 4 (March, 1948-April, 1953), p. 190.
79. Ibid.
80. Dr. Andrew Stewart had succeeded Dr. Robert Newton as President of the University of Alberta in 1950; see Walter H. Johns, *A History of the University of Alberta, 1908–1969* (Edmonton: University of Alberta Press, 1981), p. 489.
81. Minutes of the regular meeting of March 28, 1952, UHBMM/AUAH, Book No. 5 (March, 1948-April, 1953), p. 213.
82. Dr. John Scott succeeded Dr. J.J. Ower as Dean of the Faculty of Medicine in 1948; see Elise A. Corbet, *A History of Medical Education and Research at the University of Alberta* (Edmonton: University of Alberta Press, 1990), p. 198.
83. Ibid.
84. Minutes of the regular meeting of the Council of the School of Nursing, 28 January 1953, School of Nursing, AUA Acc. no. 68–1–1069, box 94.
85. Ibid.
86. Ibid.
87. Minutes of the special meeting of November 9, 1953, UHBMM/AUAH, Book No. 6 (May, 1953-January, 1958), p. 25.
88. Ibid.

89. Ibid.

90. Ibid.

91. Minutes of the Executive Committee Meeting, 24 November 1953, Board of Governors and Executive Committee Minutes, AUA (January, 1953-October, 1954), p. 146.

92. Ibid.

93. Ibid.

94. Minutes of the regular meeting of December 18, 1953, UHBMM/AUAH, Book No. 6 (May, 1953-January, 1958), p. 33.

95. Ibid.

96. Ibid.

97. Minutes of the Executive Committee Meeting, 23 March 1956, Board of Governors and Executive Committee Minutes, AUA, Acc. no. 71–164–13–15 (November 22, 1954-February 1, 1957).

98. Angus McGugan, *The first fifty years. A history of the University of Alberta Hospital—1914–1964* (Edmonton: University of Alberta Hospital, 1964), p. 37.

99. Ibid., p. 38.

100. Wilson, p. 171.

101. Wilson, p. 171.

102. Ibid.

103. Nursing School-General, AUA Acc. no. 64–1–1430, box 142, p. 182.

104. Wilson, p. 99.

105. Cashman, p. 530.

106. Rondalyn Kirkwood, "Blending vigorous leadership and womanly virtues: Edith Kathleen Russell at the University of Toronto, 1920–52," *Canadian Bulletin of Medical History* 11, no. 2 (1994): 189.

107. Rondalyn A. Kirkwood, "Discipline discrimination and gender discrimination: The case of nursing in Canadian universities, 1920–1950." *Atlantis* 16, no. 2 (1991): 52; Mary L. Kinnear, "Disappointment in discourse: Women university professors at the University of Manitoba before 1970," *Historical Studies in Education* 4, no. 2 (1992): 269.

108. Rondalyn Kirkwood and Jeanette Bouchard, *"Take counsel with one another" A Beginning History of the Canadian Association of University Schools of Nursing 1942–1992* (Kingston: Canadian Association of University Schools of Nursing, 1992) p. 13.

109. Ibid., pp. 36–38.

110. Young, p. 222.

111. Ross Kerr, "Financing University Nursing Education in Canada," pp. 60–77.

112. Royal Commission on Health Services, *Report* (Ottawa: Royal Commission on Health Services, 1964).

113. Wilson, p. 137.

114. Ibid., p. 135.

115. Johns, p. 445.

116. ASGME, EGH, School of Nursing File, Minutes of Joint meeting, 17 December 1967.

117. Paul, "A History of the Edmonton General Hospital," pp. 336–54.

118. Royal Commission on Health Services, p. 68.

119. Ibid.

120. Sister Marguerite Letourneau, *A Brief to the University of Calgary* (Edmonton: Alberta Association of Registered Nurses, 1967), p. 51.

121. The writer held a position as Assistant Professor and Administrative Assistant to Dr. Good at the time this leadership crisis occurred and was involved in a protest to the Board of Governors of the way in which these matters had been handled by the President.

122. Nora Greenley was the special case student referred to and the writer was appointed as her supervisor. This means of initiating graduate education in the Faculty prior to the formal approval of a master's degree program allowed faculty members to gain experience in teaching graduate students sooner than would otherwise have been the case.

123. These events are recounted on the basis of experience as the writer was involved in the negotiations with the Faculty of Graduate Studies and the Department of Advanced Education and manpower in relation to the new program. She was then appointed as Associate Dean with responsibility for the master's degree program when it became a reality.

124. Joy Fraser, personal communication, 18 December 1995

125. Alberta Task Force, *Report.*

126. Alberta Association of Registered Nurses, *The Response of the Alberta Association of Registered Nurses to the Government of Alberta's Position Paper on Nursing Education* (Edmonton: Alberta Association of Registered Nurses, 1976).

127. Government of Alberta, *Position paper on nursing education: Principles and issues* (Edmonton: Government of Alberta, 1977), p. 6.

128. Janet Ross Kerr, "The financing of nursing research in Canada," in Janet Ross Kerr and Jannetta MacPhail, eds., *Canadian Nursing: Issues and Perspectives*, 3rd ed. (Toronto: Mosby-Year Book, 1996), p. 143.

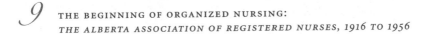

9 THE BEGINNING OF ORGANIZED NURSING:
THE ALBERTA ASSOCIATION OF REGISTERED NURSES, 1916 TO 1956

1. The early leadership in American nursing included Canadian nurses who went to the United States for their profession education and remain there. Isabel Hampton Robb became the first Principal of the School of Nursing of Johns Hopkins Hospital her efforts resulted in the first course for graduate nurses at a North American university at Columbia University. Mary Adelaide Nutting from Quebec became the first full-time Director of the

Department of Nursing and Health at Teacher's College, Columbia University and the first nurse in the world to hold a professorship.

2. Canadian Nurses Association, *The Leaf and the Lamp*, pp. 34–35.
3. Ibid., p. 35.
4. Ibid., p. 36.
5. Ibid.
6. Ibid., pp. 38–39.
7. Ibid., p. 56.
8. Ibid., p. 83.
9. Ibid., p. 56.
10. Ross Kerr, "Financing University Nursing Education in Canada," pp. 41–42.
11. Canadian Nurses Association, *The Leaf and the Lamp*, p. 38.
12. Cashman, *Heritage of Service*, p. 113.
13. Ibid., p. 114.
14. Sherwood and Henderson, "Our history . . . 1916–1991," p. 19.
15. Cashman, *Heritage of Service*, p. 116
16. Sherwood and Henderson, "Our history . . . 1916–1991," p. 19.
17. Sherwood and Henderson, "Our history . . . 1916–1991," p. 19.
18. Cashman, *Heritage of Service*, pp. 116–17.
19. Sherwood and Henderson, "Our history . . . 1916–1991," p. 19.
20. Eleanor McPhedran, Report of the Graduate Nurses Association of Alberta, *Canadian Nurse* X, no. 10, pp. 634–35.
21. Government of Alberta, *Statutes of Alberta*, Chapter 18 (Edmonton, AB, 1910).
22. McPhedran, p. 634–35.
23. Alberta Association of Graduate Nurses, Minutes of the Executive Council Meeting, 12 December 1917, AARN Archives, p. 40.
24. Government of Alberta, *Statutes of Alberta*, Chapter 47 (Edmonton, 1919).
25. Young, p. 29.
26. Government of Alberta, *Statutes of Alberta* (Edmonton, 1920).
27. Government of Alberta, *Statutes of Alberta*, Chapter 18 (Edmonton, 1910).
28. Young, p. 32.
29. Josephine Goldmark, *Nursing and Nursing Education in the United States* (New York: The MacMillan Co., 1923).
30. Ibid., p. 460.
31. Goldmark Report.
32. Young, p. 32.
33. Cashman, *Heritage of Service*, p. 177
34. Ibid.
35. Sherwood and Henderson, "Our history . . . 1916–1991," p. 34.
36. George M. Weir, *Survey of Nursing Education in Canada* (Toronto: University of Toronto Press, 1932).
37. Minutes of Provincial Council, 24 April 1931, Alberta Association of Registered Nurses (AARN Archives), p. 272.

38. Minutes of Provincial Council, October, 1933, Alberta Association of Registered Nurses (AARN Archives), p. 334.

39. Young, p. 61.

40. Minutes of the Committee on Small Hospitals, 25 November 1932, University of Alberta (University of Alberta Archives).

41. Sherwood and Henderson, "Our history—A proud heritage, the 1930s . . . dirty and depressing," *AARN Newsletter* 46, no. 9 (1990), p. 31.

42. Young, p. 63.

43. Jennifer Sherwood and Eve Henderson, "Our history . . . 1930s," p. 31.

44. Ibid.

45. Agnew, p. 65.

46. Agnew, p. 165.

47. Alberta Association of Registered Nurses, Minutes of Provincial Council, 14 May 1935 (AARN Archives).

48. Ibid.

49. Alberta Association of Registered Nurses, *AARN Annual Report*, 1040, p. 3.

50. Cashman, p. 235.

51. Jennifer Sherwood and Eve Henderson, "Our history—A proud heritage—The war years and beyond—1940–1949," *AARN Newsletter* 46, no. 10 (1990), p. 22.

52. Alberta Association of Registered Nurses, Minutes of Provincial Council (Edmonton: AARN, 1942) (AARN Archives).

53. Cashman, *Heritage of Service*, p. 235.

54. Sherwood and Henderson, "Our history . . . 1940–1949," p. 23.

55. Sherwood and Henderson, "Our history . . . 1940–1949," p. 22.

56. Alberta Association of Registered Nurses, Minutes of Annual Meeting (Edmonton: AARN, 1943) (AARN Archives).

57. Alberta Association of Registered Nurses, Minutes of Annual Meeting (Edmonton: AARN, 1943) (AARN Archives).

58. Alberta Association of Registered Nurses, Minutes of Annual Meeting (Edmonton: AARN, 1945) (AARN Archives).

59. Alberta Association of Registered Nurses, Minutes of Provincial Council (Edmonton: The Association, 1942) (AARN Archives).

60. Alberta Association of Registered Nurses, Minutes of Annual Meeting (Edmonton: AARN, 1943) (AARN Archives).

61. Alberta Association of Registered Nurses, Minutes of Annual Meeting (Edmonton: AARN, 1944) (AARN Archives).

62. Sherwood and Henderson, "Our history . . . 1940–1949," p. 23.

63. Sherwood and Henderson, "Our history . . . 1940–1949," p. 23.

64. Alberta Association of Registered Nurses, Minutes of Annual Meeting (Edmonton: AARN, 1948) (AARN Archives).

65. Ibid.

66. Alberta Association of Registered Nurses, Minutes of Annual Meeting (Edmonton: AARN, 1950) (AARN Archives).

67. Alberta Association of Registered Nurses, *Minutes of Annual Meeting* (Edmonton: AARN, 1951) (AARN Archives).

68. Alberta Association of Registered Nurses, *Minutes of Annual Meeting* (Edmonton: AARN, 1952) (AARN Archives).

69. Alberta Association of Registered Nurses, *Minutes of Annual Meeting* (Edmonton: AARN, 1952) (AARN Archives).

70. A.R. Lord, *Report of the Evaluation of the Metropolitan School of Nursing, Windsor, Ontario* (Ottawa: Canadian Nurses Association, 1952), p. 54.

10 CONSOLIDATION AND GROWTH: THE AARN IN THE YEARS FROM 1956 TO 1996

1. Jennifer Sherwood and Eve Henderson, "Our history—A proud heritage, the 1950s," *AARN Newsletter* 46, no. 11 (1990): 11.

2. Russell F. Taylor, *A Memorial for Russell Frederick Taylor, Polio '53* (Edmonton: The University of Alberta Press, 1990).

3. Government of Canada, *Federal Task Force Report on the Cost of Health Services in Canada* (Ottawa: Government of Canada, 1969).

4. Yvonne Chapman, "Our history—A proud heritage, 1970–1974," *AARN Newsletter* 47, no. 6 (1991): 14.

5. John E.F. Hastings, *The Community Health Centre in Canada: Report of the Community Health Centre Project to the Conference of Health Ministers* (Ottawa: Conference of Health Ministers of Canada, 1972).

6. Ibid., p. 47.

7. Jennifer Sherwood and Eve Henderson, "Our history—A proud heritage, 1965–69," *AARN Newsletter* 47, no. 2 (1991), p. 17.

8. Alberta Association of Registered Nurses, *Minutes of Provincial Council* (Edmonton, AB, AARN, 1958) (AARN Archives).

9. Alberta Association of Registered Nurses, *Minutes of Provincial Council* (Edmonton, AB, AARN, 1966).

10. Alberta Association of Registered Nurses, *Minutes of the Annual Meeting* (Edmonton, AB, AARN, 1959) (AARN Archives).

11. Sherwood and Henderson, "Our history—A proud heritage,1960–64," *AARN Newsletter* 47, no. 1 (1991), p. 11.

12. Alberta Association of Registered Nurses, *Minutes of Provincial Council* (Edmonton, AB, AARN, October, 1965).

13. Government of Alberta, *Nursing Education Survey Report* (Edmonton: Author, 1963).

14. Alberta Association of Registered Nurses, *Minutes of the Provincial Council* (Edmonton, AB, AARN, 18 May 1952) (AARN Archives).

15. Mildred L. Montag, *The education of nursing technicians* (New York: G.P. Putnam's Sons, 1951).

16. Royal Commission on Health Services, Report, vol. 1 (Ottawa: Queen's Printer, 1964).
17. Alberta Association of Registered Nurses, Minutes of Provincial Council (Edmonton, AB, AARN, 1962) (AARN Archives).
18. Alberta Association of Registered Nurses, Minutes of Annual Meeting (Edmonton, AB, AARN, 1965) (AARN Archives).
19. Sherwood and Henderson, "Our history . . . 1965–69," p. 15.
20. R.G. Fast, "A Report Recommending the Transfer of All Diploma Nursing and Allied Health Programs to the Alberta College System" (Edmonton: Alberta Colleges Commission, 1971).
21. Chapman, "Our history . . . 1970–1974," p. 13.
22. Mussallem, Spotlight on Nursing Education, p. vii.
23. Royal Commission on Health Services, p. 68.
24. M. Kathleen King, "The development of university nursing education," in M. Q. Innes, Nursing Education in a Changing Society (Toronto: University of Toronto Press, 1970), pp. 78–79.
25. An integrated program had been initiated some 14 years previously at the University of Alberta under the direction of Helen Penhale, but it survived only two years. It was offered only for the classes enroling in 1952 and 1953 and was terminated because of opposition to it coming principally from the hospital and medical communities.
26. Sister Marguerite Letourneau, "A Brief to the University of Calgary" (Edmonton: AARN, 1967).
27. Alberta Task Force, Report.
28. Alberta Task Force, Report, p. 113.
29. Alberta Association of Registered Nurses, The Response of the Alberta Association of Registered Nurses to the Government of Alberta's Position Paper on Nursing Education (Edmonton: Alberta Association of Registered Nurses, 1976).
30. Alberta Association of Registered Nurses, "Position Sttement on Baccalaureate Education for Nurses (Edmonton: AARN, 1979), p. 1.
31. Government of Alberta, Position Paper on Nursing Education: Principles and Issues (Edmonton: Government of Alberta, 1977).
32. Alberta Task Force, Report.
33. Department of Advanced Education and Manpower, The Final Report of the Nursing Manpower and Education and Research Implementation Committee (Edmonton: Department of Advanced Education and Manpower, 1983), p. 4.
34. Canadian Nurses Association, Entry to the Practice of Nursing: A Background Paper (Ottawa: Canadian Nurses Association, 1982).
35. Alberta Association of Registered Nurses, Position Statement on Baccalaureate Education for Nurses (Edmonton: AARN, 1988).
36. Chapman, "Our history . . . 1970–1974," p. 14.
37. Ibid.

38. Ibid.

39. Ibid., p. 15.

40. Ibid.

41. Ross Kerr, "Emergence of nursing unions," p. 269.

42. Chapman, "Our history . . . 1970–1974," p. 15.

43. Alberta Association of Registered Nurses, Minutes of Provincial Council (Edmonton, AB, AARN, 22 April 1977).

44. Alberta Association of Registered Nurses, Minutes of Provincial Council Meeting (Edmonton, AB, AARN, February, 1981).

45. Chapman, "Our history . . . 1970–1974."

46. Ibid.

47. Yvonne Chapman, "Our history—A proud heritage, 1975–1979," AARN Newsletter 47, no. 7 (1991): 15–17.

48. Chapman, "Our history . . . 1975–1979," p. 16.

49. Government of Alberta, *Policy Governing Future Legislation for the Professions and Occupations* (Edmonton: Government of Alberta, 1973).

50. These concerns were brought to me as president of the AARN two weeks after I had assumed the presidency. This was the beginning of a crisis for the Association which did not end until the new Nursing Profession Act was passed in June, 1983 and proclaimed in January, 1984.

51. Health Workforce Rebalancing Committee, "New Directions for Legislation Changes Regulating the Health Professions in Alberta" (Edmonton: Government of Alberta, 1993).

52. Health Workforce Rebalancing Committee, *New Directions for Legislation Regulating the Health Professions in Alberta* (Edmonton: Government of Alberta, 19 August, 1994).

53. Ibid., p. 27.

54. Ibid., p. i.

55. Ibid., p. 42.

11 THE RISE OF NURSING UNIONS IN ALBERTA

1. Cashman, *Heritage of Service*, p. 178.

2. Ibid.

3. G. Harvey Agnew, *Canadian Hospitals, 1920 to 1970: A Dramatic Half Century* (Toronto: University of Toronto Press, 1974), p. 149.

4. Ibid., p. 151.

5. Ibid., p. 153.

6. *Canadian Medical Association Journal*, 1953, p. 671.

7. Agnew, p. 150.

8. Sherwood and Henderson, "Our history . . . 1930s," p. 10.

9. Marjorie MacDonald Chapman, "Nursing in the depression years," in Leah Poelman, *White Caps and Red Roses: History of the Galt School of Nursing, Lethbridge, Alberta, 1910–1979* (Lethbridge: Galt School of Nursing Alumnae Society of Alberta), p. 78.

10. Alma Wagner Donaldson, as cited in Cashman, p. 209.

11. Sherwood and Henderson, "Our history . . . The 1930s," p. 10.

12. AARN Provincial Council Minutes, June 1941, AARN Archives.

13. Trudy Richardson, *United Nurses of Alberta: History* (Edmonton: United Nurses of Alberta, 1993), p. 3.

14. Helen K. Mussallem, "Nurses and political action," in Betsy LeSor and M. Ruth Elliott, eds., *Issues in Canadian Nursing* (Scarborough: Prentice-Hall, 1977), pp. 154–81.

15. AARN Annual Meeting Minutes, April, 1946, AARN Archives.

16. AARN Provincial Council Minutes, July, 1945, AARN Archives.

17. AARN Annual Meeting Minutes, May, 1953, AARN Archives.

18. Judith M. Hibberd, "Labour Disputes of Alberta Nurses: 1977–1982," unpublished PhD dissertation, The University of Alberta, Edmonton, AB, 1987, p. 117.

19. Alberta Association of Registered Nurses, Minutes of Annual Meeting (Edmonton, AB, AARN, 1964) (AARN Archives).

20. Hibberd, p. 110.

21. Ibid., p. 111.

22. Sherwood and Henderson, "Our history . . . 1965–69," pp. 21–22.

23. The author is grateful to Yvonne Chapman for reading this section and the succeeding section of this chapter and for suggesting revision to accurately portray the events that took place.

24. Revised Statutes of Alberta, 1966, The Labour Act, 3 (2) (c).

25. Ross Kerr, "Emergence of nursing unions," p. 273.

26. Richardson, p. 3.

27. Ibid.

28. Hibberd, p. 173.

29. Hibberd, pp 2,170.

30. Richardson, p. 7.

31. Hibberd, pp. 147–48.

32. See Chronology of the 1980 strike by Hibberd, pp. 327–31.

33. Hibberd, p. 2.

34. Ibid., p. 267.

35. Ibid., pp. 2–3.

36. Re: Public Service Employee relations Act, Labour Relations Act and Police officers Collective Bargaining Act (1987), 38 D.L.R. (4th), p. 161.

37. Judith M. Hibberd, "Strikes by nurses: the nature of strikes," Part 1, *Canadian Nurse* 88, no. 2 (1992), p. 25.

38. Judith M. Hibberd, "Strikes by nurses—incidence, issues and trends," Part 2, *Canadian Nurse* 88, no. 3 (1992), p. 28.

39. Ibid.

40. Richardson, p. 13.

41. Ibid.

42. Ibid., p. 28.

43. Liane Faulder, "Nurses have proven their worth—and then some," *The Edmonton Journal,* 4 March 1997, B1.

44. Ed Struzik and Paul March, "Readying for chaos—Exhausted nurses set to fight for better standards," *The Edmmonton Journal,* 4 March 1997, p. B1

45. Rick Pedersen, "Nurse strike 'would be devastating' —Hospitals stressed, says MD," *The Edmonton Journal,* 25 February 1997, p. A1.

46. Rick Pedersen and Andy Ogle, "Nurses vote 85% for illegal strike," *The Edmonton Journal,* 5 March 1997, p. A1.

47. Provincial Health Authorities of Alberta, Memorandum regarding mediator's recommendation to effect a settlement multi-health authority (facility)/UNA negotiations to chief executive officers of regional health authorities, Provincial Mental Health Advisory Board and voluntary organizations, Appendix 1, Total Compensation Summary, p. 2, 5 March 1997.

48. SNAA Information Package, "Bargaining," March, 1997.

49. Ibid.

50. Judith M. Hibberd and Judy Norris, "Strike by nurses: Perceptions of colleagues coping with the fallout," *Canadian Journal of Nursing Research* 23, no. 4 (1991): 51.

51. Ibid.

52. Ibid., p. 52.

53. Anne Zimmerman, "Collective bargaining in the hospital: The nurse's right, the professional association's responsibility," in Joanne McCloskey and Helen Grace, eds., *Current issues in nursing* (Boston: Blackwell Scientific Publications), p. 603.

12 ISSUES, COMMITMENTS, AND DIRECTIONS AS
THE NURSING PROFESSION APPROACHES THE 21ST CENTURY

1. Health Canada, *Preliminary estimates of health expenditures in Canada: Provincial-Territorial Summary Report, 1987–1991* (Ottawa: Health Information Division, Policy and Consultation Branch, Health Canada, 1994).

2. Canadian Centre for Health Information, *Registered Nurses Management Data* (Ottawa: Statistics Canada, 1992), pp. 18, 20.

3. Taft, p. 29.

4. Ibid., p. 29. According to Taft, "From 1992 to 1995, the total province-wide loss of employed registered nurses was estimated at almost 8,275, or a staggering 43% of all employed nurses in Alberta."

5. George M. Weir, *Survey of Nursing Education in Canada* (Toronto: University of Toronto Press, 1932).

Bibliography

ARCHIVES

Alberta Association of Registered Nurses Archives, Edmonton, Alberta.
Alberta Association of Registered Nurses, AARN *Annual Report,* 1040.
Edmonton Association for Retarded Children, unpublished manuscript, 24 June 1965, AARN Archives.
Fort McLeod Chapter, Alberta Association of Registered Nurses (unsigned), Letter to Tony Cashman, written 28 April 1965, AARN Archives.
Lacombe medical history, undated [circa 1964–1965], AARN Archives.
Letter from Thelma A. McIntyre, Vulcan, undated [circa 1964–1965], AARN Archives.
Letter from Mrs. Willis Teskey, Rocky Mountain House, 11 April 1964, AARN Archives.

Letter from E. Mayan to Tony Cashman, Bluesky, AB, 29 June 1965, AARN Archives.
Minutes of meeting, Edmonton: AARN, 22 May 1917, AARN Archives.
Minutes of the Executive Council Meeting, Edmonton: Alberta Association of
Graduate Nurses, 12 December 1917, AARN Archives.
Minutes of the Annual Meeting, Edmonton: Canadian National Association of
Trained Nurses, 1917, AARN Archives.
Minutes of meeting, Edmonton: Alberta Association of Graduate Nurses, 7 May
1918, AARN Archives.
Minutes of meeting, Edmonton: Alberta Association of Graduate Nurses, 1 July,
1918, AARN Archives.
Minutes of Annual Meeting, Edmonton: AARN, 1918, AARN Archives.
Minutes of Annual Meeting, Edmonton: AARN, 14 May 1920, AARN Archives.
Minutes of Annual Convention, Edmonton: AARN, 16 October 1923, AARN Archives.
Minutes of meeting, Edmonton: AARN, 26 May 1925, AARN Archives
Minutes of Provincial Council, Edmonton: AARN, 24 April 1931, AARN Archives.
Minutes of 17th Annual Convention, Edmonton: AARN, 23 March 1932, AARN
Archives.
Minutes of Provincial Council, Edmonton: AARN, October, 1933, AARN Archives.
Minutes of Provincial Council, Edmonton: AARN, 14 May 1935, AARN Archives.
Minutes of the Annual Meeting, Edmonton: AARN, April, 1939, AARN Archives.
Minutes of Annual Meeting, Edmonton: AARN, 11 and 12 October, 1939, AARN
Archives.
Minutes of Provincial Council, Edmonton: AARN, June 1941, AARN Archives.
Minutes of Provincial Council, Edmonton: AARN, 1942, AARN Archives
Minutes of Annual Meeting, Edmonton: AARN, 1943, AARN Archives.
Minutes of Annual Meeting, Edmonton: AARN, 1944, AARN Archives.
Minutes of Annual Meeting, Edmonton: AARN, 1945, AARN Archives.
Minutes of Provincial Council, Edmonton: AARN, July, 1945, AARN Archives.
Minutes of the Annual Meeting, Edmonton: AARN, 8 and 9, 23 April, 1946, AARN
Archives.
Minutes of Annual Meeting, Edmonton: AARN, 1948, AARN Archives.
Minutes of Annual Meeting, Edmonton: AARN, 13, 14 and 15 April 1950, AARN
Archives.
Minutes of Annual Meeting, Edmonton: AARN, 1950, AARN Archives.
Minutes of Annual Meeting, Edmonton: AARN, 1951, AARN Archives.
Minutes of Annual Convention, Edmonton: AARN, 21 May 1952, AARN Archives.
Minutes of Provincial Council, Edmonton: AARN, 18 May 1952, AARN Archives.
Minutes of Annual Meeting, Edmonton: AARN, 1952, AARN Archives.
Minutes of Annual Meeting, Edmonton: AARN, May, 1953, AARN Archives.
Minutes of Provincial Council, Edmonton: AARN, 1958, AARN Archives.
Minutes of Annual Meeting, Edmonton: AARN, 1959, AARN Archives.
Minutes of Provincial Council, Edmonton: AARN, 1962, AARN Archives.
Minutes of Annual Meeting, Edmonton: AARN, 1964, AARN Archives.

Minutes of Annual Meeting, Edmonton: AARN, 1965, AARN Archives.
Minutes of Provincial Council, Edmonton: AARN, October, 1965, AARN Archives.
Minutes of Provincial Council, Edmonton: AARN, 1966, AARN Archives.
Minutes of Provincial Council, Edmonton: AARN, 22 April 1977, AARN Archives.
Minutes of Provincial Council Meeting, Edmonton:AARN, February, 1981, AARN
    Archives.
Report of Interview with Susan Fierbach, July 1987, AARN Archives.
Schurerman, D. "History of Nursing in Rimbey," undated [circa 1964–1965], AARN
    Archives.

City of Edmonton Archives, Edmonton, Alberta

"A Quarantine Hospital," *Edmonton Bulletin*, 18 February 1901, City of Edmonton
    Archives.
"Citizens Favour Hospital By-Law," *Edmonton Bulletin*, 20 June 1910, City of
    Edmonton Archives.
Edmonton Hospital Board minutes, 1899–1939. Public Hospital Minutes 1BT.E24h.
    City of Edmonton Archives.

Galt Museum and Archives, Lethbridge, Alberta

"Extension to the Galt hospital" *Lethbridge Herald*. 20 June 1931, p. 3, Galt Museum
    and Archives.

Glenbow Museum Archives, Calgary, Alberta

Lavell, Marion. Transcript of an interview for the Glenbow Museum by Jerry
    Dunsmore, 16 March 1973, Glenbow Museum Archives.
Pedlar Garfield, Nettie. Transcript of an interview, 9 February 1982, Glenbow
    Museum Archives.
Watt, Mary. Transcript of interview done for the Glenbow Museum by Jerry
    Dunsmore, 13 March 1973, Glenbow Museum Archives.

Grey Nuns Archives (Archives des soeurs grises de Montréal, Edmonton),
Edmonton, Alberta

Archives des Soeurs Grises de Montréal (ASGM), "Journal de Voyage" de Soeur
    Alphonse, *Lettres de St-Albert 1858–1877,* Copie de l'ancien cahier numéro
    un, ASGM; copy in the Archives des Soeurs Grises de Montréal, Province de
    St-Albert, Edmonton (ASGME) Document 23, Lac Sainte-Anne Historique.
ASGME, EGH, School of Nursing File, Minutes of Joint meeting, 17 December 1967.
Bizon, Lorraine. *"Grey Nuns": Pioneer missionary contributions in Alberta.* ASGM
    (1978), pp. 3–12.
Edmonton General Hospital. (1967). Minutes of the joint meeting on two-year
    nursing program, Edmonton General and Misericordia Hospitals, 6 April
    1967, School of Nursing File, ASGME.
Histoire de l'école [history of the school], Edmonton General Hospital, ASGME.

Pickering, G.L. (1973). Keynote address to graduating nurses, 19 August 1973, School of Nursing File, EGH, ASGME.

Première réunion des soeurs missionnaires dans nos hôpitaux de l'ouest, compte rendu des réunions de juillet 1917, School of Nursing File, EGH, ASGME.

Summary of the school of Nurse's Enrolment 1908–1971, EGH, ASGME.

Medicine Hat Archives, Medicine Hat, Alberta

Calder, J.G. *Excerpt from annual report for 1892: Medicine Hat General Hospital*, Medicine Hat Archives, M-14A. M83.15.11.

Peters, J.B. *Excerpt from annual report of 1894: Medicine Hat General Hospital*, Medicine Hat Archives, M-14A. M83.15.11.

Provincial Archives of Alberta

"Alberta health department sent out 200 nurses," *Edmonton Bulletin*, 18 January 1919, Provincial Archives of Alberta, 75–454.

Chapman, Philippa, from interview by Margaret Maw, 11 October 1967, Department of Public Health Archives, Provincial Archives of Alberta.

Department of Public Health, *Annual Report, 1918*, Provincial Archives of Alberta.

"Public health work by nurses," *Edmonton Bulletin*, 23 January 1919, Provincial Archives of Alberta, 75–454.

University of Alberta Hospitals Archives, Edmonton, Alberta

Minutes of University Hospital Board meetings, 1946–1956.

Minutes of University Hospital Board Meeting Minutes, Archives of the University of Alberta Hospital, Book No. 4: June, 1940 -February, 1948.

Minutes of the regular meeting of 23 November 1945, UHBMM/AUAH, Book No. 4: June, 1940 -February, 1948, p. 199.

Minutes of the regular meeting of 13 September 1946, UHBMM/AUAH, Book No. 4: June, 1940 -February, 1948, p. 234.

Minutes of the regular meeting of 10 January 1947, UHBMM/AUAH, Book No. 4: June, 1940 -February, 1948, p. 247.

Minutes of the regular meeting of 24 January 1947, UHBMM/AUAH, Book No. 4: June, 1940 -February, 1948, p. 248.

Minutes of the regular meeting of 14 February 1947, UHBMM/AUAH, No. 4: June, 1940 -February, 1948, p. 250.

Minutes of the regular meeting of 12 December 1947, UHBMM/AUAH, Book No. 4: June 1940 -February, 1948, p. 290.

Minutes of the regular meeting of 13 May 13 1949, UHBMM/AUAH, Book No. 5: March, 1948 -April, 1953, p. 63.

Minutes of the regular meeting of 10 June 1949, UHBMM/AUAH, Book No. 5: March, 1948 -April, 1953, p. 67.

Minutes of the regular meeting of 23 November 1951, UHBMM/AUAH, Book No. 4 March, 1948 -April, 1953, p. 190.

Minutes of the regular meeting of 27 June 1949, UHBMM/AUAH, Book No. 5: March, 1948-April, 1953, p. 71.

Minutes of the regular meeting of 23 February 1951, UHBMM/AUAH, Book No. 5: March, 1948-April, 1953, p. 153.

Minutes of the regular meeting of 28 March 1952, UHBMM/AUAH, Book No. 5: March, 1948-April, 1953, p. 213.

Minutes of the special meeting of 9 November 1953, UHBMM/AUAH, Book No. 6: May, 1953-January, 1958, p. 25.

Minutes of the regular meeting of 18 December 1953, UHBMM/AUAH, Book No. 6: May, 1953-January, 1958, p. 33.

University of Alberta Archives, Edmonton, Alberta

Minutes of the Committee on Small Hospitals, 25 November 1932, University of Alberta, University of Alberta Archives.

"Appointments at University Are Announced," *Edmonton Bulletin*, 9 March 1946. Edmonton Bulletin reprint, Helen Penhale file, Archives of the University of Alberta, Acc. no. 1120–2.

Letter from President Newton to Miss Helen Penhale, 20 June 1950, School of Nursing-General, AUA Acc. no. 68–1–1070, box 95.

Minutes of the Council Meeting of 9 May 1952, Council of the Faculty of Medicine Minutes, AUA Acc. no. 68–1–1052, box 93, p. 9.

Minutes of the Committee on Nursing Education, 29 June 1953, University of Alberta Archives.

Minutes of the regular meeting of the Council of the School of Nursing, 28 January 1953, School of Nursing, AUA Acc. no. 68–1–1069, box 94.

Minutes of the Executive Committee of 3 March 1948, Board of Governors, AUA Acc. No. 71–164–10–12, p. 13.

Minutes of the Executive Committee Meeting, 24 November 1953, Board of Governors and Executive Committee Minutes, AUA: January, 1953-October, 1954, p. 146.

Minutes of the Executive Committee Meeting, 23 March 1956, Board of Governors and Executive Committee Minutes, AUA, Acc. no. 71–164–13–15: November 22, 1954-February 1, 1957).

Nursing School, General, AUA Acc. no. 64–1–1430, box 142, p. 182.

Abercrombie, Sheila. (1983). *Alberta Hospital Edmonton 1923 to 1983, An Outline of History to Commemorate the 60th Anniversary.* Edmonton: Alberta Hospital.

Agnew, G. Harvey. (1974). *Canadian Hospitals, 1920 to 1970: A Dramatic Half Century.* Toronto: University of Toronto Press.

Alberta Advanced Education and Manpower. *(1983). The Final Report of the Nursing Manpower and Education and Research Implementation Committee.* Edmonton: Alberta Advanced Education and Manpower.

Alberta Association of Registered Nurses. (1976). *The Response of the Alberta Association of Registered Nurses to the Government of Alberta's Position Paper on Nursing Education.* Edmonton: AARN.

———. (1979). *"Position Statement on Baccalaureate Education for Nurses.* Edmonton: AARN.

———. (1988). *Position Statement on Baccalaureate Education for Nurses.* Edmonton: AARN.

Alberta Department of Health. (1963). *Report of the Nursing Education Survey Committee, Province of Alberta, 1961–1963.* Edmonton: Queen's Printer.

The Alberta Task Force on Nursing Education. (1975). *The Report of the Alberta Task Force on Nursing Education.* Edmonton: Alberta Advanced Education and Manpower.

Allemang, Margaret M. (1995). "Development of community health nursing in Canada," in Miriam J. Stewart, ed., *Community Nursing: Promoting Canadians' Health.* Toronto: W.B. Saunders.

American Nurses Association. (1965). *Educational Preparation for Nurse Practitioners and Assistants to Nurses: A Position Paper.* New York: American Nurses Association.

Baly, Monica. (1991). *As Miss Nightingale Said . . .* London: Scutari Press.

Blair, W.R.N. (1969). *Mental Health in Alberta,* A Report on the Alberta Mental Health Study. Edmonton: Queen's Printer.

Bonin, Sister Marie. (1976). "Trends in Integrated Basic Degree Nursing Programs in Canada: 1942–1972," Ph.D. dissertation, University of Ottawa.

Brown, Esther Lucile. (1948). *Nursing for the Future.* New York: Russell Sage Foundation.

Boutilier, Beverly. (1994). "Helpers or heroines? The National Council of Women, Nursing, and 'Woman's Work' in late Victorian Canada," in Dianne Dodd and Deborah Gorham, eds., *Caring and Curing: Historical Perspectives on Women and Healing in Canada.* Ottawa: University of Ottawa Press.

Buckley, Suzanne. (1979). "Ladies or midwives? Efforts to reduce infant and maternal mortality," in Linda Kealey, ed., *A Not Unreasonable Claim: Women and Reform in Canada 1880s–1920s.* Toronto: The Women's Educational Press.

Byfield, Ted, ed. (1992). *Alberta in the 20th Century: The Birth of the Province 1900–1910.* Edmonton: United Western Communications Ltd.

————. (1991). *Alberta in the 20th Century: The Great West before 1900.* Edmonton: United Western Communications Ltd.

Canadian Centre for Health Information. (1992). *Registered Nurses Management Data.* Ottawa: Statistics Canada.

Canadian Nurses Association. (1982). Entry to the Practice of Nursing: A Background Paper. Ottawa: Canadian Nurses Association.

————. (1968). *The Leaf and the Lamp.* Ottawa: The Association.

————. (1965). *Report on the Canadian Nurses Association School Improvement Program.* Ottawa: The Association.

————. (1940). *A Supplement to a Proposed Curriculum for Schools of Nursing in Canada.* Montreal: The Association.

Canadian Red Cross Society. (1962). *The Canadian Red Cross Society: The Role of One Voluntary Organization in Canada's Health Services—A Brief to the Royal Commission on Health Services.* Toronto: Canadian Red Cross Society.

Carpenter, Helen M. (1970). "The University of Toronto School of Nursing: An Agent of Change," in Mary Q Innis, ed., *Nursing Education in a Changing Society.* Toronto: University of Toronto Press, p. 90.

Chapman, Muriel Elizabeth. (1969). "Nursing Education and the Movement for Higher Education for Women: A Study of Interrleationship, 1870–1900," Doctor of Education Thesis, Teachers College, Columbia University, New York, NY.

Cashman, Tony. (1966). *Heritage of Service: The History of Nursing in Alberta.* Edmonton: Alberta Association of Registered Nurses.

Collins, Paul V. (1969). "The Public Health Policies of the United Farmers of Alberta Government, 1921–1935," unpublished Master of Arts thesis, Faculty of Graduate Studies, The University of Western Ontario, London, ON.

Corbet, Elise A. (1990). *A History of Medical Education and Research at the University of Alberta.* Edmonton: University of Alberta Press.

Cran, Marion. (1982). "A woman in Canada," in Susan Jackel, ed., *A Flannel Shirt and Liberty: British Emigrant Gentlewomen in the Canadian West, 1880–1914.* Vancouver: University of British Columbia Press.

Dawson, C.A. and Younge, E.R. (1940). *Pioneering in the Prairie Provinces: The Social side of the Settlement Process.* Toronto: Macmillan.

Dock, Lavinia L. (1921). "The history of public health nursing," in Mazyck L. Ravenel, ed., *A Half Century of Public Health: Jubilee Historical Volume of the American Public Health Association.* Lynn, MA: American Public Health Association.

Dominion Bureau of Statistics, Government of Canada. (1921). *Vital Statistics 1921, First Annual Report.* Ottawa: F.A. Acland.

Dorward, Christina and Tookey, Olive. (1968). *Below the Flight Path.* Edmonton: Alumnae Association of the Royal Alexandra Hospital School of Nursing.

Duncan, Joy. (1985). *Red Serge Wives.* Edmonton: Lone Pine Publishing.

Fast, R.G. (1971). "A Report Recommending the Transfer of All Diploma Nursing and Allied Health Programs to the Alberta College System". Edmonton: Alberta Colleges Commission.

Gahagan, Alvine Cyr. (1979). *Yes Father, Pioneer nursing in Alberta.* Manchester, NH: Hammer Publications Inc.

Gibbon, John. (1947). *The Victorian Order of Nurses for Canada.* Montreal: Southam Press.

Gibbon, John and Mathewson, Mary. (1947). *Three Centuries of Canadian Nursing.* Toronto: The MacMillan Co.

Gilpin, John. (1986). *The Misericordia Hospital: 85 years of service in Edmonton.* Edmonton: Misericordia Hospital.

Goldmark, Josephine. (1923). *Nursing and Nursing Education in the United States.* New York: The MacMillan Co.

Gorham, Deborah. (1994). 'No longer an invisible minority': Women physicians and medical practice in late twentieth-century North America, in Dianne Dodd and Deborah Gorham, eds. *Caring and Curing: Historical Perspectives on Women and Healing in Canada.* Ottawa: University of Ottawa Press.

Giraud, Marcel. (1984). *Le Métis Canadien.* Winnipeg: Les Editions du Blé d'Or.

Government of Alberta. (1977). Position Paper on Nursing Education: Principles and Issues. Edmonton: Author.

———. (1976). Position paper on nursing education: Principles and issues. Edmonton: Author.

———. (1973). Policy Governing Future Legislation for the Professions and Occupations. Edmonton: Author.

———. (1963). Nursing Education Survey Report. Edmonton: Author.

———. (1919). *Statutes of Alberta,* Chapter 47. Edmonton, Author.

———. (1910). *Statutes of Alberta,* Chapter 18. Edmonton, Author.

———. Department of Public Health. "Annual Report", 1930–1935, Author.

———. Department of Public Health. "Annual Report", 1929–1935, Author.

Government of Canada. (1969). *Federal Task Force Report on the Cost of Health Services in Canada.* Ottawa: Author.

Hastings, John E.F. (1972). *The Community Health Centre in Canada: Report of the Community Health Centre Project to the Conference of Health Ministers.* Ottawa: Conference of Health Ministers of Canada.

Health Canada. (1994). *Preliminary estimates of health expenditures in Canada: Provincial-Territorial Summary Report, 1987–1991.* Ottawa: Health Information Division, Policy and Consultation Branch, Health Canada.

Heagerty, J.J. (1980). "The development of public health in Canada," in C. Meilicke, and J.L. Storch, eds., *Perspectives on Canadian Health and Social Services Policy: History and Emerging Trends.* Ann Arbor, MI: Health Administration Press.

Health Workforce Rebalancing Committee. (1994). *New Directions for Legislation Regulating the Health Professions in Alberta.* Edmonton: Government of Alberta.

Health Workforce Rebalancing Committee. (1993). *New Directions for Legislation Changes Regulating the Health Professions in Alberta.* Edmonton: Government of Alberta.

Hibberd, Judith M. (1987). "Labour Disputes of Alberta Nurses: 1977–1982," unpublished Ph.D. dissertation, The University of Alberta, Edmonton, AB.

Jackel, Susan. (1982). *A flannel shirt and liberty: British emigrant gentlewomen in the Canadian West, 1880–1914.* Vancouver: UBC Press.

Jamieson, Heber. (1947). *Early Medicine in Alberta: The First Seventy-five Years.* Edmonton: Canadian Medical Association, Alberta Division.

Jacques, Mabel. (1911). *District Nursing.*

Johns, Walter H. (1981). *A History of the University of Alberta, 1908–1969.* Edmonton: University of Alberta Press.

Kerr, Janet C. (1973). Provincial variation in nursing functions," In Shirley R. Good and Janet C. Kerr, eds., *Contemporary Issues in Canadian Law for Nurses.* Toronto: Holt, Rinehart and Winston Inc.

King, M. Kathleen. (1970). "The development of university nursing education," in M.Q. Innes, *Nursing Education in a Changing Society.* Toronto: University of Toronto Press, pp. 78–79.

Kirkwood, Rondalyn and Bouchard, Jeanette. (1992). *"Take counsel with one another" A Beginning History of the Canadian Association of University Schools of Nursing 1942–1992.* Kingston: Canadian Association of University Schools of Nursing.

Kwasny, Barbara. (1982). *Nuns and Nightingales: A History of the Holy Cross School of Nursing—1907–1979.* Calgary: Alumnae Association of the Holy Cross School of Nursing.

Lent, D.G. (1947). *Alberta Red Cross in Peace and War, 1917–1947.* Alberta.

Létourneau, Marguerite. (1975). "Trends in Basic Diploma Nursing Programs Within Provincial Systems of Education in Canada, 1964–1974," Ph.D. dissertation, University of Ottawa, Ottawa, ON.

Letourneau, Sister Marguerite. (1967). *A Brief to the University of Calgary.* Edmonton: Alberta Association of Registered Nurses.

Lord, A.R. (1952). *Report of the Evaluation of the Metropolitan School of Nursing, Windsor, Ontario.* Ottawa: Canadian Nurses Association.

Love, Florence A. (1962). *The Lamp Is Golden, Lamont and its Nurses 1912–1962.* Edmonton: Alumnae Association.

MacGregor, James. (1972). *A History of Alberta.* Edmonton: Hurtig Publishers.

MacInnes, C.M. (1930). *In the Shadow of the Rockies.* London: Rivington.

McGugan, Angus. (1964). *The first fifty years. A history of the University of Alberta Hospital—1914–1964.* Edmonton: University of Alberta Hospital.

MacDonald Chapman, Marjorie. (1979). "Nursing in the depression years," in Leah Poelman, *White Caps and Red Roses: History of the Galt School of Nursing, Lethbridge, Alberta, 1910–1979.* Lethbridge: Galt School of Nursing Alumnae Society of Alberta.

MacPhail, Jannetta. (1996). "Men in nursing," in Janet Ross Kerr and Jannetta MacPhail, eds., *Canadian Nursing: Issues and Perspectives.* Toronto: Mosby-Year Book.

McPhedran, Eleanor. (1914). Report of the Graduate Nurses Association of Alberta, *Canadian Nurse X*, no. 10, pp. 634–35.

McPherson, Kathryn. (1996). *Bedside Matters: The Transformation of Canadian Nursing, 1900–1990.* Toronto: Oxford University Press.

———. (1994). Science and technique: Nurses' work in a Canadian hospital, 1920–1939. In Dianne Dodd and Deborah Gorham, eds., *Caring and Curing: Historical Perspectives on Women and Healing in Canada.* Ottawa: University of Ottawa Press.

Miller, G., ed. (1983). *Letters of Edward Jenner and Other Documents Concerning the Early History of Vaccination.* Baltimore: Johns Hopkins University Press.

Montag, Mildred L. (1951). *The education of nursing technicians.* New York: G.P. Putnam's Sons.

Mussallem, Helen K. (1960). *Spotlight on Nursing Education: The Report of a Pilot Project for the Evaluation of Schools of Nursing in Canada.* Ottawa: Canadian Nurses Association.

———. (1977). "Nurses and political action," in Betsy LeSor and M. Ruth Elliott, eds., *Issues in Canadian Nursing.* Scarborough: Prentice-Hall.

Nelson, J.G. (1973). *The Last Refuge.* Montreal: Harvest House Ltd.

Nicholson, G.W.L. (1975). *Canada's Nursing Sisters.* Toronto: Samuel Stevens, Hakkert Ltd.

Nursing Sisters' Association of Canada. (1994). *Commemorative Issue and National Directory.* Ottawa: Author.

Owram, Doug. (1980). *Promise of Eden: The Canadian Expansionist Movement and the Idea of the West 1856–1900.* Toronto: University of Toronto Press.

Paul, Pauline. (1994). "A History of the Edmonton General Hospital: 1895–1970, 'Be faithful to the duties of your calling,'" unpublished Ph.D. dissertation, The University of Alberta, Edmonton.

Paul, Pauline and Ross Kerr, Janet. (1995). "A philosophy of care: The Grey Nuns of Montreal," in Bob Hesketh and Frances Swyripa, eds., *Edmonton, The Life of a City.* Edmonton: NeWest Publishers.

Penney, Sheila. (1991). *A Century of Caring 1887–1997: The History of the Victorian Order of Nurses for Canada.* Ottawa: VON Canada.

Poelman, Leah. (1979). *White Caps and Red Roses: History of the Galt School of Nursing, Lethbridge, Alberta, 1910–1979.* Lethbridge: Galt School of Nursing Alumnae Society of Alberta.

Provincial Health Authorities of Alberta. (1997). Memorandum regarding mediator's recommendation to effect a settlement multi-health authority (facility)/UNA negotiations to chief executive officers of regional health authorities, Provincial Mental Health Advisory Board and voluntary organizations, Appendix 1, Total Compensation Summary, p. 2, 5 March 1997, Edmonton: author.

The Public Health Nurses Act 1919, Chapter 7, Section 49.

Public Service Employee relations Act, Labour Relations Act and Police officers Collective Bargaining Act (1987), 38 D.L.R. (4th).

Revised Statutes of Alberta, *The Public Health Nurses Act,* Assented to 17 April 1919, Operative 17 May 1919, Section 38.

Revised Statutes of Alberta, 1966, The Labour Act, 3 (2) (c).

Richardson, Trudy. (1993). *United Nurses of Alberta: History.* Edmonton: United Nurses of Alberta.

Riddell, Maureen. (1980). *Toward a Healthier City: A History of the Edmonton Local Board of Health and Health Department 1871–1979.* Edmonton: Local Board of Health.

Roach Pierson, Ruth. (1986). *They're Still Women After All: The Second World War and Canadian Womanhood.* Toronto: McClelland and Steward.

Rosenberg, Charles E. (1987). *The Care of Strangers.* New York: Basic Books.

Ross Kerr, Janet. (1996). "The financing of nursing research in Canada," in Janet Ross Kerr and Jannetta MacPhail, eds., *Canadian Nursing: Issues and Perspectives,* 3rd ed. Toronto: Mosby-Year Book.

———. (1996). "Emergence of nursing unions as a social force in Canada," in Janet Ross Kerr and Jannetta MacPhail, eds., *Canadian Nursing: Issues and Perspectives.* Toronto: Mosby-Year Book.

———. (1996). "The Origins of Nursing Education in Canada: An overview of the Emergence and Growth of Diploma Programs: 1874–1974," in Janet Ross Kerr and Jannetta MacPhail, eds., *Canadian Nursing: Issues and Perspectives,* 3rd edition. Toronto: Mosby-Year Book

———. (1996). "Entry to practice: Striving for the Baccalaureate Standard," in Janet Ross Kerr and Jannetta MacPhail, eds., *Canadian Nursing: Issues and Perspectives,* 3rd edition. Toronto: Mosby-Year Book.

———. (1978). "Financing University Nursing Education in Canada: 1919–1976," unpublished Ph.D. dissertation, University of Michigan, Ann Arbor, Michigan.

Ross Kerr, Janet, Paul, Pauline and MacKinnon, Alice. (1992). *The Origins of Nursing in Alberta: 1859–1909.* Final Research Report to the Alberta Foundation for Nursing Research. Edmonton: Faculty of Nursing, University of Alberta.

Royal Commission on Health Services (1964). Report, Vol. 1. Ottawa: Queen's Printer.

Russell, E. Kathleen. (1932). "The Teaching of Public Health Nursing in the University of Toronto" in *Methods and Problems of Medical Education.* The Rockefeller Foundation.

Schartner, Adelaide. (1982). *Health Units of Alberta.* Edmonton: Coop Press.

Scollard, D. (1981). *Hospital—A Portrait of Calgary General.* Calgary: Calgary General Hospital.

Staff Nurses Association of Alberta Information Package, "Bargaining," March, 1997. Edmonton: Author.

Spry, Irene M. (1963). *The Palliser Expedition: An Account of John Palliser's British North American Expedition, 1857–1860.* Toronto: Macmillan.

Stewart, Irene. (1979). *These Were Our Yesterdays: A History of District Nursing in Alberta.* Calgary: Friesen Printers.

Stuart, Meryn. (1994). "Shifting professional boundaries: Gender conflict in public health, 1920–1925," in D. Dodd and D. Graham, eds., *Caring and Curing: Historical Perspectives on Women and Healing in Canada.* Ottawa: University of Ottawa Press.

Taft, Kevin. (1997). *Shredding the Public Interest: Ralph Klein and 25 Years of One-party Government.* Edmonton, Alberta: University of Alberta Press and the Parkland Institute.

Taylor, Russell F. (1990). *A Memorial for Russell Frederick Taylor, Polio '53.* Edmonton: The University of Alberta Press.

Vant, J. Ross and Cashman, Tony. (1986). *More than a Hospital: University of Alberta Hospitals 1906–1986.* Edmonton: University of Alberta Hospitals Board.

Viste, Freda. (1978). *No Doctor in the house, In Hanna North, A Rural History 1908–1978.* Hanna: Hanna North Book Club.

Weir, George M. (1932). *Survey of Nursing Education in Canada.* Toronto: University of Toronto Press.

Wilson, Betty. (1977). *To Teach This Art, The History of the Schools of Nursing at the University of Alberta 1924–1974.* Edmonton: Hallamshire Publishers.

Winks, Robin W. (1971). *Canada and the United States: The Civil War Years.* Baltimore: Johns Hopkins University Press.

Young, Susan L. (1994). "Standards in Diploma Nursing Education: The Involvement of The University of Alberta, 1920–1970," unpublished Master of Nursing thesis, University of Alberta, Edmonton, AB.

Zimmerman, Anne. (1981). "Collective bargaining in the hospital: The nurse's right, the professional association's responsibility," in Joanne McCloskey and Helen Grace, eds., *Current issues in nursing.* Boston: Blackwell Scientific Publications.

ARTICLES

Baumgart, Alice and Kirkwood, Rondalyn. (1990). "Social reform versus education reform: University nursing education in Canada, 1919–1960," *Journal of Advanced Nursing* 15, no. 5: 510.

Bow, Malcolm, R. (1935). "The history of the Department of Public Health of Alberta," *Canadian Journal of Public Health* 26, no. 8: 385.

Bow, Malcolm, R and Cook, F.T. (1935). "The History of the Department of Public Health of Alberta," *Canadian Journal of Public Health* 26, no. 8: 390.

Chapman, Yvonne. (1991). "Our history—A proud heritage, 1975–1979," *AARN Newsletter* 47, no. 7: 15–17.

————. (1991). "Our history—A proud heritage, 1970–1974," *AARN Newsletter* 47, no. 6: 14.

Chittick, Rae. (1948). "Let us take pride in our craft," *The Canadian Nurse* 44, no. 9: 705–6.

Edmonton Bulletin, 7 August 1886.

Edmonton Journal, 6 February 1919.

Faulder, Liane. (1997). "Nurses have proven their worth—and then some," *The Edmonton Journal,* 4 March 1997, B1.

Godkin, Dianne, M. and Bottorff, Joan. (1991). "Doctorate in nursing: Idea to reality," *Canadian Nurse* 87, no. 111: 31–34.

Grande Prairie Herald, 23 October 1914.

Hanna Herald, 11 April 1919.

Hibberd, Judith M.(1992). "Strikes by nurses: the nature of strikes," Part 1, *Canadian Nurse* 88, no. 2: 25.

————. (1992). "Strikes by nurses—incidence, issues and trends," Part 2, *Canadian Nurse* 88, no. 3: 28.

Hibberd, Judith M and Judy Norris. (1991). "Strike by nurses: Perceptions of colleagues coping with the fallout," *Canadian Journal of Nursing Research* 23, no. 4 : 51.

Hill, Meredith. "The women workers of the diocese of Athabasca; 1930–1970," *Journal of the Canadian Church Historical Society* 28 (1986): 64.

Holt, Mabel. (1936). "Staffing with graduate nurses," *The Canadian Nurse* 32 (January).

Kinnear, Mary L. (1992). "Disappointment in discourse: Women university professors at the University of Manitoba before 1970," *Historical Studies in Education* 4, no. 2: 269.

Kirkwood, Rondalyn. (1994). "Blending vigorous leadership and womanly virtues: Edith Kathleen Russell at the University of Toronto, 1920–52," *Canadian Bulletin of Medical History* 11, no. 2: 189.

————. (1991). "Discipline discrimination and gender discrimination: The case of nursing in Canadian universities, 1920–1950." *Atlantis* 16, no. 2: 52.

Johnson, M. and Martin, H. (1958). "A sociological analysis of the nurse's role," *American Journal of Nursing* 58, no. 3.

Pedersen, Rick. (1997). "Nurse strike 'would be devastating' —Hospitals stressed, says MD," *The Edmonton Journal,* 25 February 1997, p. A1.

Pedersen, Rick and Ogle, Andy. (1997). "Nurses vote 85% for illegal strike," *The Edmonton Journal,* 5 March 1997, p. A1.

Penhale, Helen. (1954). "The spirit of achievement," *The Canadian Nurse* 50, no. 4: 258.

RCMP Quarterly 24, no. 1 (July, 1958).

Rogers, Martha. (1972). "To be or not to be," *Nursing Outlook* 20, no. 1: 42–46.

Ross, Murray. (1980). "The evolution of hospital care in Alberta," *Dimensions in Health Service* 57, no. 4, p. A4.

Ross Kerr, Janet and Paul, Pauline. (1991). "Nurses and hospitals in Edmonton at the turn of the century," *Proceedings of the Qualitative Health Research Conference*. Edmonton: University of Alberta.

Sherwood Jennifer and Henderson, Eve. (1990). "Our history—A proud heritage, 1965–69," *AARN Newsletter* 47, no. 2: 17.

———. (1990). "Our history—A proud heritage, the 1950s," *AARN Newsletter* 46, no. 11: 11.

———. (1990). "Our history—A proud heritage, the 1930s…dirty and depressing," *AARN Newsletter* 46, no. 9: 31.

———. (1990). "Our history—A proud heritage: The Alberta Association of Registered Nurses, 1916–1991," *AARN Newsletter* 46, no. 8: 34.

———. (1990). "Our history—A proud heritage, 1960–64," *AARN Newsletter* 47, no. 1: 11.

Struzik, Ed and March, Paul. (1997). "Readying for chaos—Exhausted nurses set to fight for better standards," *The Edmmonton Journal*, 4 March 1997, p. B1.

Thurston, H. (1972). "Education for episodic and distributive care," *Nursing Outlook* 20, no. 8: 519–23.

University of Alberta, Financial Statements for 1930–31 and 1940–41.

Worcester, A. (1902). "Is nursing really a profession?" *American Journal of Nursing* 2, 908–17.

Ziegler, Olive I. (1941). "Outpost hospitals—a fine achievement," *The Canadian Hospital* 18, no. 2: 17.

Index

* *Photographs are indicated in bold italics.*